"Communicating in Spanish for Medical Personnel"

Julia Jordán Tabery
Marion R. Webb
Beatriz Vásquez Mueller

Communicating in Spanish for Medical Personnel

Communicating in Spanish for Medical Personnel

Julia Jordán Tabery
Bilingual Education Specialist,
Head Start Leadership Development Program
Texas Southern University, and
Special Lecturer,
Texas Woman's University, Houston

Marion R. Webb
Assistant Professor in Spanish,
Houston Baptist University, Houston

Beatriz Vásquez Mueller
Formerly Charge Nurse,
St. Joseph Hospital, and
Volunteer Nursing Consultant,
American Red Cross, Houston

Little, Brown and Company   Boston

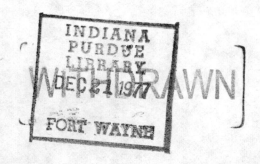

To our nurses -- and all nurses

Preface

Medical personnel increasingly recognize the need for learning to communicate with Spanish-speaking patients. The fundamental concept of this text is that the medically oriented student can learn, in a limited time, the specialized vocabulary and structures needed to communicate with patients at a basic level. Structures included in the text are those most useful to basic communication between health care provider and patient rather than those considered essential to a general study of Spanish. The text is unique in that it presents a broad range of medical vocabulary integrated into simple structures for ready functioning in a specialized area of the language.

To serve the diverse needs of medical personnel, the text is designed to be used at any level of language study, for credit or noncredit courses, for in-service workshops, and for self-study. If the student already has a background in Spanish, he can review and improve his conversational skills while at the same time mastering an area of vocabulary new to him. For the student who has no familiarity with the language, the book serves as a conversational introduction to a specialized area of Spanish, and it gives him the opportunity to acquire vocabulary that he can use immediately. Even advanced classes and bilingual students can profit from conversation practice with the technical vocabulary, much of which will be new to them.

This is a language text rather than a medical one. It attempts to give the student facility in communicating his own knowledge to the patient and in understanding the patient's needs; it does not teach medical information per se. The lessons are arranged according to practical or medical topics to make this a useful reference book in the hospital, but the Spanish structures to be learned dictate the order of material within each lesson.

The core of each lesson is given in both Spanish and English. The Spanish conversation practice and other materials to be studied by the English-speaking student appear on the right-hand page of the text. On the left-hand page, applicable parts of the lesson are given in English. Thus tedious reference to vocabularies or previous lessons is avoided — an asset to the mature, career-oriented student. Because the student does not become hopelessly lost if he has insufficient study time or misses a lesson or two, the high dropout rate common in noncredit language programs is avoided. The material is particularly appropriate for in-service training and for the student who may study no more than one session or one semester of Spanish. In addition, since the core of each lesson is bilingual, the text may even serve to teach some basic English structures and specialized vocabulary to Spanish-speaking medical personnel.

We are grateful to the many persons who have helped us in the preparation of this text. Deserving of special mention are our colleagues, Dorothy Caram and Josephine W. Rodgers; our co-workers, Judy Penney and Mary Lou Moore; our editors, Sarah Boardman and Nancy Megley; the typist who prepared the camera copy for the printer, Elisabeth Humez; and especially our nursing students at Texas Woman's University and Houston Baptist University and the department heads, staff, and nurses at St.

Joseph Hospital. Finally, we must mention our colleagues who generously gave of their time to record the audio cassettes available as a supplement to this book: Dr. Carlos Monsanto, Dorothy Caram, and Diamantina Suárez.

J. J. T.

M. R. W.

B. V. M.

To the Student

Questions, answers, and conversations in which you participate actively will give you the necessary skills to function in everyday relationships with Spanish-speaking patients. The emphasis in this book is on practicing communication, not on why you say things a certain way. If you want an analytical explanation of the grammar or structures involved, either look up the structures listed at the end of each lesson in any basic Spanish text or ask questions after class.

Every language has different ways of saying the same thing, particularly when a language is spoken in many different countries, as are both Spanish and English. The Spanish structures given are the easiest correct ones for the speaker of English to learn and are selected to teach you to communicate at a basic level. While some of the answers may seem long and stilted for everyday conversation, repeating the whole answer gives you the practice necessary to master basic ways of saying things. When you use these in real-life situations, you will shorten them naturally. The English equivalents for the Spanish statements and questions are, as much as possible, what an English-speaking person would say in the same situation. In addition, you will be taught to recognize the much more complex and informal language that the native speaker may use.

Whether you have studied Spanish before is unimportant. By the end of each lesson you should be able to engage in a situation dialogue in the role of either patient or hospital staff member. By the end of the course you should be able to communicate with any Spanish-speaking person concerning his basic needs and wants. Then, we hope, you will want to continue to study Spanish in its broader aspects.

Contents

Introduction

THE FORMAT OF THE TEXT

Three main sections constitute the teaching material in the text: Pronunciation, the forty-one lessons (preceded by an introductory lesson of useful phrases), and Evaluation. In the lessons, question-and-answer drills for practicing conversations are supplemented by techniques for learning to understand the Spanish-speaking patient. Both the Pronunciation and the Evaluation sections are correlated with the lessons so that all three may be used together for classwork or separately for reference. Supplementary material at the end of the text includes lists of cognate words arranged by endings, tables of numbers and time units, Spanish-English and English-Spanish vocabularies, a list of suggested readings for cultural awareness, an index of grammar, and a communicator for quick reference in conveying basic phrases to a Spanish-speaking patient.

A set of two audio cassettes covering material from the book is available to supplement the text. These tapes, taken verbatim from text material, are intended to aid the student with his pronunciation of Spanish words and phrases.

PRONUNCIATION

In the Pronunciation section, Spanish sounds and the rules governing them are simply explained, one letter or diphthong at a time, with ample drill. Extensive practice on diphthongs is included since these are often difficult for English-speaking persons. The sounds are presented in order of frequency of use and of difficulty for the English speaker, rather than alphabetically; the index of pronunciation at the beginning of the section provides quick reference for drilling problems as they arise. As much as possible the pronunciation for a lesson is correlated with the vocabulary from previous lessons, so that when it is used as a warm-up drill at the beginning of each class the student is reviewing words he has already learned. Further practice on stress, accentuation, and syllabication of Spanish words completes the section.

LESSONS

In the lessons the student learns to communicate by practicing structures and vocabulary in situation dialogues between a medical staff member and a patient. These dialogues are divided into conversation blocks that are easy to practice. In the statements, the basic structures are underlined and the elements to be substituted for practice are listed below the main statements, slightly spaced; the student then repeats the underlined element with each alternative. In some cases, the student may choose from several alternative responses. If there are several ways to say the same thing, these are also grouped together but are single-spaced. The structure to be drilled may be in the hospital staff member's column, the patient's column, or both. However, the statement that is preceded by an open circle begins a conversation. These conversations are the drills that form the body of the text.

The dialogues are followed by an identification exercise in which the student practices decoding the language of a native speaker. This technique is based on the concept that, given the context of the medical situation, the student can be taught to understand more than he can probably say. The typical foreign language text depends on using graded material, but it is obvious that the Spanish-speaking patient will not limit his language in this way. Therefore, the identification exercises are designed to expose the student to language typical of the native speaker, without regard to previously studied vocabulary and structures. The student is taught to decipher at the patient's level, through listening for key words, recognizing verb forms for which he knows only the infinitive, and identifying the speaker's vocabulary. He thus captures the essence of the message even though he cannot understand every word and cannot express what the native speaker can. Perhaps most important, the student gains confidence in his ability to understand a Spanish-speaking person.

The structures and grammar drilled in each lesson are listed at the end of the lesson, with examples given the first time a new structure or point of grammar is introduced. By using this reference if he desires, the teacher can correlate the lesson with a standard text, or the interested student can look up an analytical explanation of the grammar drilled. A few basic points about Spanish are explained in nongrammatical terms in notes.

Although there is a gradual buildup of structures and vocabulary, the lessons need not be used sequentially. Because of the bilingual format and the repeated use of basic structures, lessons may be used in the order most suitable to a particular group. The lesson on physical characteristics and personality is placed at the end of the section since it does not deal with a medically oriented topic, but it may be taught at any time convenient since the vocabulary is easy and the distinction between _ser_ and _estar_ is important.

EVALUATION

The Evaluation section following the lessons provides additional practice in the form of self-checks, or tests, correlated with the material in each lesson. There are three exercises for each lesson, the first two dealing largely with the material in the lesson, and the third a systematic review of essential grammar and structures previously studied. A cumulative review replaces the evaluation exercises every fifth lesson, with a review of the first twenty lessons at Lesson 20 and a complete evaluation or mastery test of all lessons at the end of the section.

REFERENCE MATERIAL

Cognate words utilize knowledge the student already has, and they form an important part of medical vocabulary. Many of the Spanish cognates appearing in the lists toward the end of the book are within the vocabulary of the average person since Spanish is a direct descendant of Latin, from which most such vocabulary comes. (In English, many of these words are normally restricted to medical use because they have been replaced in everyday language by shorter Anglo-Saxon words.) Cognates are listed in both Spanish and English, alphabetized by Spanish, and grouped according to equivalent endings. Because they are helpful to the student, some cognate words which do not quite correspond in connotation or ending are included.

Medical personnel often need to refer to numbers and time units; therefore, following the cognates are bilingual lists of numbers, days of the week, months of the year, seasons, and cardinal points.

The Spanish-English and English-Spanish vocabularies include words from the lessons supplemented by additional vocabulary and verb forms. Many useful words have been added, especially to the English-Spanish vocabulary, in order to make the text a valuable reference tool in the hospital.

The grammar index is helpful to the advanced student or to the teacher who plans to correlate the material with that of a basic text.

The readings suggested for cultural awareness acquaint the student with Hispanic customs in broad perspective and as they affect the practice of medicine. This knowledge will enable the medical staff member to understand a patient's reactions as they relate to his customs.

The Minimum Spanish Communicator is an outline of essential communicating phrases and structures presented in the text. The student may use the communicator to learn to express himself in basic terms. In addition, these reference lists serve as a useful tool on the job.

HOW TO USE THIS BOOK

CLASS USE

In the first few sessions of beginning classes, the instructor gives an overview of the sounds and then reviews one or more sounds each class, or pronunciation problems may be drilled as they arise in class. The instructor always needs to insist on careful correction and repetition; this is especially true of medical vocabulary, with many long words that are difficult to pronounce. Pronunciation practice is always a good warm-up and review, and it is especially important for beginning students. Those who are not language oriented gain confidence from pronunciation practice.

The New Material contains the main conversation exercises, grouped in linguistic or subject matter segments of easy to practice length. With the instructor modeling correct pronunciation, the students repeat each question and answer. Then the instructor asks the questions and the students respond, and after that the roles are reversed. Next, the instructor questions the students individually. After they are familiar with the New Material, the students cover the English page and focus their total attention on the Spanish. As the students gain confidence in their ability to use the language, they will refer to the text less and less. This will vary according to the individual student's ability and background.

So that they truly have a chance to converse, at least part of each class period the students work in conversation groups of two to five, taking turns answering and asking each other questions in Spanish. An alternate method for a large class is to seat the students in conversation groups; after presentation of each conversation segment to the whole class, the students turn to their groups for a few minutes of practice. Then the class is called together for presentation of another new segment of conversation. Once taught the technique of the "conversation circle," students can work on their own with correction and supervision as needed. Grouping students in pairs and small groups according to background and ability in Spanish provides individualized study, and each student can progress at his own pace. Students are trained to use the English for reference only, never for oral practice.

Variety is important, and when students begin to tire of prolonged pronunciation and repetition, the instructor changes the emphasis to the communication aspect of the language. At this time it is particularly effective to let students play the role of hospital staff member and patient, asking each other questions at random. Original questions and unrehearsed answers may be used to review important aspects of the lesson content.

Generally, the instructor uses the Identification exercise as aural practice. Students hear the Spanish two or three times before they read it and are encouraged to guess what they do not know. Comprehension is checked in English for the most part, since the complex structures a native speaker will use are beyond the students' ability to handle at this stage, though not beyond their comprehension. However, if time permits, more of the Identification exercise can be handled in Spanish by having students ask "¿Qué quiere decir . . .?" The instructor answers, using synonyms and gestures, playing the role of a non-English-speaking person.

The Evaluation also can be used for additional oral practice as well as for checking mastery of vocabulary and structures. These exercises may be done as classwork or homework and then used orally with books closed at the next class session. Whether evaluation material is used as quizzes or exercises, students are encouraged to do it with the English translation covered and then to check their work.

A typical class session of an hour or an hour and a half may be planned as follows:

1. <u>Pronunciation practice</u> (5 to 10 minutes).

2. <u>Previous lesson</u> (10 to 15 minutes). Conversation to check mastery of previous lesson. This may use both the Lesson and the Evaluation. Students will have their books closed.

3. <u>New Material</u> (15 to 20 minutes). Section-by-section repetition; choral and individual response to practice the New Material.

4. <u>Small group conversation</u> (20 to 30 minutes). Conversation circles with two to five in a group, practicing New Material, referring to English as little as possible and to Spanish for guidance only. Role playing.

4a. <u>Alternate method</u>: New Material is interspersed with small group conversation (35 to 50 minutes).

5. <u>Identification</u> (10 to 15 minutes). Material is read orally by instructor two or three times. Further study of Identification exercise assigned for homework if needed.

While stress during class is totally on oral work, students are asked to do both written and oral assignments, as this reinforces learning. They may write answers to the Spanish questions, covering the English, or practice and check total mastery by writing Spanish for the English conversations. For oral practice, the student may tape the lesson in class on a cassette recorder. He will thus have a correct model to imitate when working on his own.

ADVANCED CLASSES

Complete mastery of the specialized vocabulary of this text is a challenge for advanced classes. In addition, there are many areas in which the instructor may expand the text material presented. Grammar and structures drilled in each lesson can be correlated with a standard text for amplified practice. An analysis of the New Material and Identification exercises reveals many complex structures that are suitable for more intense study and drill. In these classes, the instructor may change all questions in the Identification exercise to Spanish. And in the Evaluation section, advanced students may be asked to supply their own answers orally rather than choosing from the ones given. In fact, a variety of practice materials can be created from the exercises in the text. Students may be asked to rewrite sentences in different tenses, change person and number, and practice substituting more complex structures, such as commands, for simpler ones. Past participles can be formed from the cognate infinitives, and these may serve in practicing the use of _ser_ and _estar_ with adjectives. The cognate lists can be used in many ways, as can the vocabulary itself.

Most challenging to advanced students is the opportunity to do creative work. They may write and perform their own conversations, use the Identification exercises as models for original writing and conversations, and read and report on supplementary materials. The Health Services and Mental Health Administration of the U.S. Department of Health, Education, and Welfare distributes, free of charge, a bibliography listing materials in Spanish available through public agencies and private companies.*

IN-SERVICE TRAINING

The techniques suitable for teaching regular classes are also appropriate for in-service training sessions and workshops. However, since many programs will have only a few sessions, Useful Everyday Phrases and Lessons 1 to 7, 19, and 20 might be considered basic for any workshop. To these can be added, as time permits, whatever is of special interest to particular groups. Some lessons may be taught for mastery and some may be presented merely to acquaint the students with the material included. The order does not have to be sequential. Depending on the students' previous background in Spanish, a lesson will cover a session of an hour or a little more. If the workshop sessions involve several hours at a time, the basic lesson plan suggested can be changed for each hour to give more variety. Should the workshop have a large number of participants, native speakers recruited from the area can aid the instructor in small group practice and add valuable information concerning regional word usages.

While students in workshops are highly motivated, these adults have the problem of combining extra study with a demanding job. In addition, many in-service sessions meet only once a week. Students will learn more if the instructor divides the lessons drilled in class into six parts, one assigned to be practiced for fifteen to twenty minutes _each day_ until the next workshop session. Those who can bring a tape recorder or cassette recorder to class can record the lesson during class and then listen at odd moments during the week. Cassette recorders and tape decks can make commuting or driving valuable practice time. The instructor may ask each workshop participant to keep a log of time practiced to encourage the self-discipline necessary to profit most from noncredit language study.

SELF-STUDY

This text can be used by the student learning on his own, even if he has never studied Spanish. There is a high degree of correspondence in Spanish between the letters of the written language and the sounds of the spoken language. Once these correspondences are learned through the simple explanations of sounds, rules, and drills for practice, the motivated student can master the conversations on his own. There is a gradual buildup of pronunciation, vocabulary, and structures in each lesson that can be mastered sequentially. The format provides a variety of ways the student can practice and check for mastery. He can cover the entire page of English or Spanish and practice writing or saying the other; or he can cover one column and give answers to questions, or even give questions that correspond to

---

*Spanish-Language Health Communication Teaching Aids: A List of Printed Materials and Their Sources. DHEW Publication No. (HSM) 73-19, Office of Information, Public Inquiries, Rockville, Md. 20852.

answers. Even in self-study it is always a good technique to go over the drills, Identifications, and Evaluations orally as well as writing them. The Evaluations provide both exercises and self-testing. However, the final test of mastery for the nonsupervised student must be that he can correctly reproduce all of the New Material in Spanish. Then he knows he is ready to go on to the next lesson.

A WORD TO THE FOREIGN LANGUAGE TEACHER

Because of the pragmatic orientation of this text, the usage taught is quite different from what the teacher of the typical Spanish course is accustomed to. The attempt to integrate selected Spanish structures into a given medical topic, and to keep the text basic and nongrammatical, has resulted in difficult choices at times. We have felt that we must use easy yet idiomatic Spanish, but at the same time we have tried to include anything pertinent to a given subject, even if difficult. For this reason, where the subject requires a quantity of new vocabulary, we have tried to use fewer structures; where the vocabulary is more limited, or a repetition of that previously presented, we have included some complex but important structures. Some of the more complicated grammar is merely taught in phrases, with the understanding that for a more advanced class all structures can be analyzed and further drilled.

Verb forms are more limited than in a standard text; with a few basic verb-plus-infinitive constructions a broad range of expression can be covered. Emphasis is on the first and third persons singular of the verb, since these serve most conversational purposes between medical personnel and patient. Because relations between patient and staff member are basically more formal than informal, the second person familiar form has not been presented in the New Material except in Lesson 40, which is directed to dealing with children. The verbs ser and estar are used throughout, but they are not contrasted until late in the book. However, should the teacher wish to work with contrasting these verbs early in the course, Lesson 41 may be taught at any time.

Pronoun usage is different from that in a basic text. In order to keep the text material a useful reference for those not experienced in Spanish, the abbreviation for usted is not used in the Lessons. However, the abbreviated form Ud. is used beginning with Lesson 6 of the Evaluation, because the student needs to become familiar with this standard abbreviation. Object pronouns are introduced early and drilled extensively, particularly indirect object and reflexive pronouns, which are so necessary for discussing needs, wants, and procedures in terms of the patient.

Since the Identification exercises emphasize understanding highly idiomatic Spanish rather than correct handling of structures, comprehension is generally checked in English. Beginning with Lesson 30, though, the student is asked to answer in Spanish, as briefly as possible, questions designed to fall within his linguistic range.

Numbers are an important part of communicating in Spanish, and because the book will most commonly be taught to speakers of English, numbers are written out in Spanish; on the English pages, numerals are used instead of a verbal translation so that the student's attention is focused away from English. A reference table giving the Spanish, the numeral, and its English equivalent precedes the vocabularies.

In the Evaluation section, the directions for the Spanish exercises are given in English and those for the English exercises in Spanish, so that neither Spanish nor English students will have to look at the page opposite to understand directions — desirable since the translation is, in fact, the answer page.

We have tried to be idiomatic in both languages, but when idiomatic usage would have been too far removed from the literal meaning for the student to see a correspondence, we have used more formal language. When elements are given to substitute into longer sentences, the most natural shortened phrase in each language is used, even when the correspondence between languages is not exact. This is done so that each segment of the sentence can be used by itself as a natural conversational phrase. Examples are:

<u>Necesito</u>   cambiarle   la bata.
<u>I need to</u>   change   your gown.

<u>¿Qué va a hacer?</u>   Cambiarle la bata.
<u>What are you going to do?</u>   Change your gown.

<u>¿Qué va a cambiar?</u>   La bata.
<u>What are you going to change?</u>   Your gown.

While we have included regional vocabulary where it seemed useful for communication (eight Spanish words for bedpan), we have basically limited ourselves to standard usage in both Spanish and English.

Finally, we have attempted to write a text that is easy to teach and that does not demand technical knowledge in either language or medicine. Both Spanish teachers and medical personnel who know Spanish can present the lessons easily by following the simple guidelines given here. These same principles should make the material easy for any student to master.

Pronunciation Index

Pronunciation

LESSON <u>1</u>: <u>a</u>

to	you wash	room	buttocks
the	bed	lady	palm
the	you go in	chin	bad
you are going to	robe	you call	tomorrow
face	nothing	you calm	mama

LESSON <u>2</u>: <u>o</u>

no	I take	balloon, ball	mouth
it	little	elbow	insane
I	I eat	shoulder	little
eye	chicken	12	

Spanish	with	good	lung
please	pain	doctor	heart

Pronunciación

Vowels in Spanish are pronounced clearly and concisely, in contrast to English vowels, which tend to be drawn out. In English, unstressed vowels may become a kind of "uh" sound, as in "from the class," or "in a minute." In Spanish, even when the vowel does not receive the main emphasis in a word or phrase, the same clear, short sound is maintained. There is a longer vowel sound in Spanish, which is formed by the combination of two vowels. (See pp. 19 to 25 for further explanation.)

LECCION 1: a

Spanish a is similar to the English sound ah, as in father, but shorter.

a	lava	sala	nalgas
la	cama	dama	palma
las	pasa	barba	mal
va a	bata	llama	mañana
cara	nada	calma	mamá

LECCION 2: o

In syllables that end in o, Spanish o is similar to English o in pose but short and clipped.

no	tomo	globo	boca
lo	poco	codo	loco
yo	como	hombro	poco
ojo	pollo	doce	

In other syllables, Spanish o is similar to English o in for.

español	con	buenos	pulmón
por favor	dolor	doctor	corazón

LESSON 3: e

from, of	that, what	phlegm	you have
oneself	you see	chest	hair
faith	base	take	finger
me	come in	cure	chief
to you	fetus	I have	milk

the	you	to concede	to propose
he	paper	to dissolve	to see

LESSON 4: i

and	1,000,000	uncle	medicine
yes	to go	aunt	15
if	to hear	cold	infection
my	inner ear, hearing	difficult	nose
1000	day	5	sight

LESSON 5: u

one	wedge	I smoke	culture
one	grape	never	not any
nail	fight	girl	lung
moon	much	pleasure	pupil of the eye
cradle	many	Monday	October

LECCION 3: e

Spanish e is similar to English a in made in syllables that end in -e, and in some other syllables. You will hear many variations, depending on the region the speaker is from.

de	que	flema	tiene
se	ve	pecho	pelo
fe	base	tome	dedo
me	pase	cure	jefe
le	feto	tengo	leche

In most of the other syllables that do not end in -e, Spanish e is similar to English e in met.

el	usted	conceder	proponer
él	papel	disolver	ver

LECCION 4: i

Spanish i is similar to English i in unique. Y by itself, meaning "and," has the same sound.

y	millón	tío	medicina
sí	ir	tía	quince
si	oír	frío	infección
mi	oído	difícil	nariz
mil	día	cinco	vista

LECCION 5: u

Spanish u is similar to English oo in boot.

uno	cuña	fumo	cultura
una	uva	nunca	ninguno
uña	lucha	muchacha	pulmón
luna	mucho	gusto	pupila
cuna	muchos	lunes	octubre

LESSON 6: <u>b</u>, <u>v</u>

you're going	well	20	vagina
mouth	sight	arm	bladder
good	shoulder	gallbladder	pretty

lip	the bladder	let's see	2 babies
head	the vagina	please	the sight
the mouth	ankles	weak	
the chin	9	120	

mouth, the mouth   bladder, the bladder
chin, the chin   baby, pretty baby, 20 pretty babies
20, 120

LESSON 7: <u>r</u>, <u>rr</u>

hour	waist	insurance	calorie
face	yard	to operate	relative
nose	uterus	to prepare	divorced
ear	urethra	to separate	afternoon, late

knee	to breathe	religion	car
to reduce	to resolve	kidney	rapid
to remit	rich	the rectum	
to resist	relation	diarrhea	

LECCIÓN 6: b, v

In Spanish, b and v have the same sounds.

At the beginning of a word or breath group, or after m or n, b and v are similar to English b in but. Almost bite your lips together: there is no puff of air with this sound, as there is with English b.

va	bien	veinte	vagina
boca	vista	brazo	vejiga
bueno	hombro	vesícula	bonito

In all other positions, Spanish b and v are similar to English b, but with the lips not closed, allowing air to escape.

labio	la vejiga	a ver	dos bebés
cabeza	la vagina	por favor	la vista
la boca	tobillos	débil	
la barba	nueve	ciento veinte	

The following groups of words contrast the two sounds.

boca, la boca	vejiga, la vejiga
barba, la barba	bebé, bonito bebé, veinte bonitos bebés
veinte, ciento veinte	

LECCIÓN 7: r, rr

Spanish r between vowels, or before a consonant, is similar to the English d sound in Eddie, or the first t in cut it, said rapidly. The tongue taps once against the ridge above the front teeth.

hora	cintura	seguro	caloría
cara	vara	operar	pariente
nariz	útero	preparar	divorciado
oreja	uretra	separar	tarde

Spanish rr or r at the beginning of a word, or after l, n, or s, is heavily trilled, with several quick taps of the tongue against the ridge above the front teeth. If you have trouble making this trilled r sound, practice by saying cut it up rapidly.

rodilla	respirar	religión	carro
reducir	resolver	riñón	rápido
remitir	rico	el recto	
resistir	relación	diarrea	

LESSON 8: <u>d</u>

from	to give	back	to sleep
2	pain	you understand	division
12	the pain	diarrhea	description
10	in pain	to rest	address

nothing	life	mucus	father
doctor	knee	burning	you
medicine	liver	afternoon, late	city
elbow	sweat	mother	

finger	difficulty	weakness	pain, much pain

LESSON 9: <u>t</u>

cough	I have	14	stomach
3	ankle	20	another
30	heel	you feel	October
300	tension	fetus	Protestant
you have	7	intestine	Catholic

LESSON 10: <u>j</u>, <u>ge</u>, <u>gi</u>

eye	son	people	digestion
red	daughter	diligent	indigestion
eyebrows	George	bladder	religion
boss, head	girdle	vagina	Jewish
ear	general	pajamas	giant

LECCION 8: d

Spanish d at the beginning of a word or breath group, and after l or n, is similar to English d in dare.

de	dar	espalda	dormir
dos	dolor	comprende	división
doce	el dolor	diarrea	descripción
diez	con dolor	descansar	dirección

In all other cases, Spanish d is similar to English th in that. At the end of a word, Spanish d is a very weak th.

nada	vida	mucosidad	padre
médico	rodilla	ardor	usted
medicina	hígado	tarde	ciudad
codo	sudor	madre	

The two sounds are contrasted in the following words.

dedo	dificultad	debilidad	dolor, mucho dolor

LECCION 9: t

Spanish t is similar to English t in stock. Almost bite your tongue to keep the air from escaping.

tos	tengo	catorce	estómago
tres	tobillo	veinte	otro
treinta	talón	siente	octubre
trescientos	tensión	feto	protestante
tiene	siete	intestino	católico

LECCION 10: j, ge, gi

Spanish j, and ge, and gi are similar to German ach as in Bach. The sound is much harsher than English h.

ojo	hijo	gente	digestión
rojo	hija	diligente	indigestión
cejas	Jorge	vejiga	religión
jefe	faja	vagina	judío
oreja	general	pijama	gigante

LESSON 11: g, gue, gui

thank you	corpuscle	with pleasure	(surname)
grams	throat	I have	(surname)
pleasure, taste	blood	(surname)	(surname)

to swallow	I pay	inch	liver
insurance	buttock	glad to know you	stomach
then	water	giant	tingling

guitar	sting	turn off	wink
war	rinse	garland	pebble

LESSON 12: c, z

10	5	arm	(surname)
11	100	cup	(surname)
12	spleen	nose	(surname)

with	each	4	to eat
elbow	rectum	room	cramp
house	neck	married	kilometer

LECCION 11: g, gue, gui

Spanish g, when not before e or i, is similar to English g in go at the beginning of a breath group, or after n.

gracias	glóbulo	con gusto	Gómez
gramos	garganta	tengo	González
gusto	sangre	García	Gutiérrez

In other positions, Spanish g is much softer than English g. The back of the tongue does not touch the roof of the mouth, and there is a slight flow of air. (This is between vowels, before or after consonants other than n, and when not initial.)

tragar	pago	pulgada	hígado
seguro	nalga	mucho gusto	estómago
luego	agua	gigante	hormigueo

To keep the g sound hard before e or i, a u is inserted between the g and the vowel. In this case, the u has no sound of its own.

guitarra	aguijón	apague	guiño
guerra	enjuague	guirnalda	guijarro

LECCION 12: c, z, k

In Spanish America, c before e or i, and the letter z in any position, are similar to English s in saw. (In Castilian Spanish, these letters are similar to the th in thin.)

diez	cinco	brazo	López
once	ciento	taza	Martínez
doce	bazo	nariz	González

The Spanish c in all other positions (i.e., before a consonant, or before a, o, or u) is similar to the English k sound as in scan. Spanish k has the same sound.

con	cada	cuatro	comer
codo	recto	cuarto	calambre
casa	cuello	casado	kilómetro

LESSON 13: <u>h</u>, <u>ch</u>

there is, there are	hospital	brother	Hi!
you speak	son	sister	hotel
to do, make	daughter	now	there

much (m.)	many (f.)	date	80
many (m.)	boy	milk	check
much (f.)	girl	chocolate	jacket

LESSON 14: <u>s</u>

you are	nostril	permission	the intestines
they are	back	blood	anesthesia
6	cold (disease)	more	
7	until	the eyes	

the arms	the girls	slower	the glasses (drinking)
the hands	the buttocks	cosmetics	the glasses (eye)

LESSON 15: <u>n</u>

no	some (m.)	9	you need
in, on	some (f.)	90	nose
nothing	they are	100	nasal
a, an (m.)	well	900	to put
a, an (f.)	night	I need	condition

a glass	an arm	a little	1 meter
a poor person	a foot	immediately	

I have	blood	1 kilo	with Joseph
white	orange	1 gram	with George

LECCION 13: h, ch

Spanish h is always silent.

hay	hospital	hermano	¡Hola!
habla	hijo	hermana	hotel
hacer	hija	ahora	ahí

Spanish ch is similar to English ch in church.

mucho	muchas	fecha	ochenta
muchos	muchacho	leche	cheque
mucha	muchacha	chocolate	chaqueta

LECCION 14: s

Spanish s is usually similar to the English s in salt.

es	fosa nasal	permiso	los intestinos
son	espalda	sangre	anestesia
seis	resfriado	más	
siete	hasta	los ojos	

Before voiced consonants (b, v, d, g, l, m, n), Spanish s sounds more like English s in disease (like English z sound).

los brazos	las niñas	más despacio	los vasos
las manos	las nalgas	cosméticos	los lentes

LECCION 15: n

Spanish n is similar to English n in no, except as noted below.

no	unos	nueve	necesita
en	unas	noventa	nariz
nada	son	ciento	nasal
un	bien	novecientos	poner
una	noche	necesito	condición

Spanish n becomes an m sound before consonants formed with both lips (b, v, m, p).

un vaso	un brazo	un poco	un metro
un pobre	un pie	inmediatamente	

Spanish n is similar to English n in sing before c, qu, g, and j.

tengo	sangre	un kilo	con José
blanco	naranja	un gramo	con Jorge

LESSON 16: ñ

year	girl	pineapple	autumn
nail	signal	piñata	wrist
bath	man, Mr., sir	fist	company
bathtub	girl, miss, ma'am	tomorrow, morning	
boy	lady, Mrs., ma'am	Spain	

LESSON 17: l

the (m., singular)	flower	lip	wig
the (f., singular)	bad	skin	ice
the (m., plural)	to leave	glasses (eye)	lotion
the (f., plural)	book	skirt	armpit
pain	double	blouse	family

LESSON 18: ll

to call	stamps	washcloth	billfold
brush	rollers	knee	napkin
ring	neck	slippers	knife
ankle	towel	men's shorts	syringe

LESSON 19: y

I	yard (measure)	motionless	beach
already	son-in-law	jugular	ivy
yolk	iodine	American, yankee	legend
May	plaster cast	breakfast	

and	today	law	I'm going
there is, there are	very	flock	I am

LECCIÓN 16: ñ

Spanish ñ is similar to the English ny in canyon.

año	niña	piña	otoño
uña	señal	piñata	muñeca
baño	señor	puño	compañía
bañadera	señorita	mañana	
niño	señora	España	

LECCIÓN 17: l

Spanish l is similar to the English l in lit.

el	flor	labio	peluca
la	mal	piel	hielo
los	salir	lentes	loción
las	libro	falda	axila
dolor	doble	blusa	familia

LECCIÓN 18: ll

Spanish ll, as pronounced by most speakers, is similar to English y in yet. In some regions, however, there is an l sound with the y, similar to English lli in million. Sometimes, especially at the beginning of a word or breath group, the sound is similar to English j as in jargon.

llamar	sellos	toallita	billetera
cepillo	rollos	rodilla	servilleta
anillo	cuello	zapatillas	cuchillo
tobillo	toalla	calzoncillos	jeringuilla

LECCIÓN 19: y

Spanish y before a vowel is similar to English y in yet. In some regions the sound is similar to English j in jargon. The sound is usually the same as the ll.

yo	yarda	yerto	playa
ya	yerno	yugular	yedra
yema	yodo	yanqui	leyenda
mayo	yeso	desayuno	

At the end of a word, and in the word y ("and"), Spanish y is like Spanish i; that is, similar to English i in machine, though run together with the previous vowel. (See also diphthongs, pp. 19 to 25.)

y	hoy	ley	voy
hay	muy	grey	estoy

LESSON 20: f, m

phlegm	to sign	office	flower
fever	federal	scarf	vase
family	girdle	please	nostril

me	month	much, a lot	bad
my	less	many	bed
more	mama	very	cream

LESSON 21: p

for	dish	papa, daddy	problem
pear	turkey	pork	worried
weight	chicken	fish	to lose
chest	potato	celery	measles
pie	potato (in Spain)	to operate	Pap test

LESSON 22: qu

that, what	quiet	jacket	chemist
who	tranquil	one must	to take away
I want	here	check	X (letter in the alphabet)
you want	bronchial tubes	cake	
cheese	headache	razor	

LECCION 20: f, m

Spanish f is similar to English f in fit.

flema	firmar	oficina	flor
fiebre	federal	bufanda	florero
familia	faja	por favor	fosa nasal

Spanish m is similar to English m in mist.

me	mes	mucho	mal
mi	menos	muchos	cama
más	mamá	muy	crema

LECCION 21: p

Spanish p is similar to English p in spot, but there is no puff of air with this sound as there is in an English p.

para	plato	papá	problema
pera	pavo	puerco	preocupado
peso	pollo	pescado	perder
pecho	papa	apio	sarampión
pastel	patata	operar	examen de Papanicolaou

LECCION 22: qu

Spanish qu (always in this combination) is pronounced like English k, as in kit.

que	quieto	chaqueta	químico
quien	tranquilo	hay que	quitar
quiero	aquí	cheque	equis
quiere	bronquios	queque	
queso	jaqueca	máquina de afeitar	

LESSON 23: x, w

examination	lifeless	expectoration	extension
to examine	oxide	excrement	strange
armpit	to exhibit	to exclaim	stranger
taxi	extensive	to express	extreme
success	exterior	to excuse	to explain

(name)	Wagnerian

LESSON 24: Diphthongs

oh	dance	traitor	landscape
there is, there are	to dance	vanilla	playing card
one must	I fall	alligator	pheasant
air	I bring	sheath	Jim

LESSON 25: ia

thanks	pharmacy	to change	spices
family	diarrhea	cold (disease)	hives
half	anesthesia	divorced	pepper
blond	emergency	student	carrot
material, matter	to travel	social	infancy

LECCION 23: x, w

Spanish x is usually similar to a weak English gs as in wigs. Before a consonant, it often becomes like an s. In some regions of Spanish America, x is almost like the English x in exam or the cs in ecstasy.

examen	exánime	expectoración	extensión
examinar	óxido	excremento	extraño
axila	exhibir	exclamar	extranjero
taxi	extenso	expresar	extremo
éxito	exterior	excusar	explicar

There is no w in Spanish except in a few foreign words, or words of foreign origin.

Washington   wagneriano

LECCION 24: Diptongos

In Spanish a diphthong is a combination of two vowels, one of which is unstressed i or u. The two vowels become one syllable. A y may replace i.

Spanish ai (ay) is similar to English aye.

ay	baile	traidor	paisaje
hay	bailar	vainilla	naipe
hay que	caigo	caimán	faisán
aire	traigo	vaina	Jaime

LECCION 25: ia

The Spanish diphthong ia is similar to English ya as in yard. (See also the cognates that end in ia on pp. 529 and 531. All end in this sound.)

gracias	farmacia	cambiar	especias
familia	diarrea	resfriado	urticaria
media	anestesia	divorciado	pimienta
rubia	emergencia	estudiante	zanahoria
materia	viajar	social	infancia

LESSON 26: ie

well	you feel	foot	conscious
who	I feel	100	September
you come	ice	patient	November
tooth	old	parent	December
you have	10	it's appropriate	left

LESSON 27: ei (ey)

comb	26	razor	king
to comb	20th	law	to reign
6	30	deity	kingdom
20	to shave	baseball	

LESSON 28: io

good-bye	nervousness	exercise	lotion
God	slow	ovary	air conditioning
several	laboratory	polio	motion
clean	insomnia	pressure	explanation
nervous	tapioca	infection	

LESSON 29: oi (oy)

today	I give	thyroid
I'm going	I hear	hemorrhoids
I am	beret	to boycott
I am	typhoid	

LECCION 26: ie

The Spanish diphthong ie is similar to English ye as in yet.

bien	siente	pie	conciente
quien	siento	cien	septiembre
viene	hielo	paciente	noviembre
diente	viejo	pariente	diciembre
tiene	diez	conviene	izquierda

LECCION 27: ei (ey)

The Spanish diphthong ei (ey) is similar to English ei in vein.

peine	veintiséis	máquina de afeitar	rey
peinar	veintavo	ley	reinar
seis	treinta	deidad	reino
veinte	afeitar	béisbol	

LECCION 28: io

The Spanish diphthong io is similar to English yo as in yo-yo. (See also the list of -ión cognates on pp. 527 and 529. All have this diphthong in the last syllable.)

adiós	nerviosidad	ejercicio	loción
Dios	despacio	ovario	aireacondicionado
varios	laboratorio	poliomielitis	moción
limpio	insomnio	presión	explicación
nervioso	tapioca	infección	

LECCION 29: oi (oy)

The Spanish diphthong oi (oy) is similar to English oy in toy.

hoy	doy	tiroide
voy	oigo	hemorroides
soy	boina	boicotear
estoy	tifoidea	

LESSON 30: <u>au</u>

car	nausea	to howl	cage
automobile	abundance	gaucho	baptism
cause	authorization	author	to meow
pause	audio-	daring	

LESSON 31: <u>ua</u>

water	4	avocado	John
when?	room, <u>or</u> quarter	slip (lingerie)	(surname)
how much?	40	to rinse	(surname)
how many?	tongue	evacuation	(city and state in Mexico)

LESSON 32: <u>ue</u>

good	neck	strong	father-in-law
good morning	9	serum	mother-in-law
good afternoon	egg	cord	glasses (eye)
later	scrambled eggs	50	strength
bill	bone	daughter-in-law	lunch

ointment	shame	find out

LESSON 33: <u>eu</u>

neuter, neutral	debtor	reunification	euthanasia
neutral	Europe	reunion	regular pulse
pseudo-	European	to reunite	euphoria
pseudonym	rheumatic	Eustachian	eucalyptus
debt	rheumatism	eugenics	euphemism

LECCION 30: au

The Spanish diphthong au is similar to English ou as in ouch.

auto	náuseas	aullar	jaula
automóvil	caudal	gaucho	bautizo
causa	autorización	autor	maullar
pausa	audio-	audaz	

LECCION 31: ua

The Spanish diphthong ua is similar to English wa in water.

agua	cuatro	aguacate	Juan
¿cuándo?	cuarto	enagua	Juárez
¿cuánto?	cuarenta	enjuagar	Suárez
¿cuántos?	lengua	evacuación	Chihuahua

LECCION 32: ue

The Spanish diphthong ue is similar to English wa in way.

bueno	cuello	fuerte	suegro
buenos días	nueve	suero	suegra
buenas tardes	huevo	cuerda	espejuelos
luego	huevos revueltos	cincuenta	fuerza
cuenta	hueso	nuera	almuerzo

Spanish üe in the combination güe has the same sound.

ungüento	vergüenza	averigüe

LECCION 33: eu

The Spanish diphthong eu is similar to English e and u in educate: drop the d and combine the e and u into one sound.

neutro	deudor	reunificación	eutanasia
neutral	Europa	reunión	euritmia
seudo	europeo	reunir	euforia
seudónimo	reumático	Eustaquio	eucalipto
deuda	reumatismo	eugenesia	eufemismo

LESSON 34: ui (uy)

very	to flee	rhubarb	Louise
care	noise	vile	suicide
to care for	noisy	ruins	to commit suicide
careful	judgment	vulture	Swiss

LESSON 35: iu (yu)

city	citizenry	widowhood
citizen (m.)	widower	jugular
citizen (f.)	widow	diurnal

LESSON 36: uo

continuous	virtuous	fluoridation	dues
individual	greasy	fluorescent	
oblique	sinuous, winding	fluoroscope	12th
sumptuous	hydrofluoric	duodenum	

LECCION 34: ui (uy)

The Spanish diphthong ui (uy) is similar to the English word we.

muy	huir	ruibarbo	Luisa
cuidado	ruido	ruin	suicidio
cuidar	ruidoso	ruinas	suicidarse
cuidadoso	juicio	buitre	suizo

LECCION 35: iu (yu)

The Spanish diphthong iu (yu) is similar to English you.

ciudad	ciudadanía	viudez
ciudadano	viudo	yugular
ciudadana	viuda	diurno

LECCION 36: uo

The Spanish diphthong uo is similar to English wo in won't.

continuo	virtuoso	fluorización	cuota
individuo	untuoso	fluorescente	
oblicuo	sinuoso	fluoroscopio	duodécimo
suntuoso	fluorhídrico	duodeno	

LESSON 37: Emphasis, Accents

robe	bed	they take	lavatory
brother	friend	you eat	scissors
hour	friends	they eat	blanket
hours	you take	we eat	nurse

paper	to leave	to take	mucus
you	to come in	to eat	sweat
watch, clock	to rest	hospital	burning

doctor	description	vomit	liver
bedpan	telephone	machine	cosmetics
lotion	good-bye	stomach	here

LECCION 37: Enfasis, acentos

There are three simple rules that tell you which syllable in a Spanish word to emphasize.

Words that end in a vowel, n, or s are stressed on the next to the last syllable.

ba-ta	ca-ma	to-man	la-va-ma-nos
her-ma-no	a-mi-go	co-me	ti-je-ras
ho-ra	a-mi-gos	co-men	fra-za-da
ho-ras	to-ma	co-me-mos	en-fer-me-ra

Words that end in a consonant other than n or s are stressed on the last syllable.

pa-pel	sa-lir	to-mar	mu-co-si-dad
us-ted	pa-sar	co-mer	su-dor
re-loj	des-can-sar	hos-pi-tal	ar-dor

Any words that are exceptions to these two rules have a written accent mark over the stressed vowel.

mé-di-co	des-crip-ción	vó-mi-to	hí-ga-do
ba-cín	te-lé-fo-no	má-qui-na	cos-mé-ti-cos
lo-ción	a-diós	es-tó-ma-go	a-quí

LESSON 38: Accents, Breaking Diphthongs

he, the (m.)	yes, if	I know, oneself	more, but

Who? (singular)	When?	Which? (What?) (plural)
Who? (plural)	How much?	What!
What?	How many?	How?
Why?	Which? (What?) (singular)	

day	fall, drop	watermelon	yet
uncle	country	surgery	casket
aunt	corn	radiology	Saul
cold	nursing	dysentery	Ralph
ear (hearing)	company	police	(surname)

lotion	nausea	antibiotic	he suffered
motion	position	emotion	he wrote

LECCION 38: Acentos, separación de diptongos

Accents are also used to differentiate words that are spelled the same but have different meanings.

él, el   sí, si   sé, se   más, mas

In addition, an accent is used on the stressed syllable of an interrogative or exclamatory word.

¿Quién?	¿Cuándo?	¿Cuáles?
¿Quiénes?	¿Cuánto?	¡Qué!
¿Qué?	¿Cuántos?	¿Cómo?
¿Por qué?	¿Cuál?	

A diphthong is broken into two separate syllables when an accent mark is placed on the i or u. The stress of the word is on the accented vowel.

día	caída	sandía	aún
tío	país	cirugía	ataúd
tía	maíz	radiología	Saúl
frío	enfermería	disentería	Raúl
oído	compañía	policía	García

If the accent is on the other vowel of the diphthong (a, e, or o), it is kept as one syllable and the whole syllable is stressed.

loción	náuseas	antibiótico	sufrió
moción	posición	emoción	escribió

LESSON 39: Dividing Words into Syllables

no
brother
well
I feel
specialization

face	hour	bed	scissors	lavatory

brother	30		curable	central
until	afternoon		you speak	to declare
you (plural)	50		progress	
permission	frequent (plural)			

LECCION 39: División de palabras en sílabas

Dividing words into syllables will help you pronounce readily any Spanish word. If you learn to pronounce each letter, you can sound out whole words syllable by syllable. A Spanish word has as many syllables as it has vowels and diphthongs. A diphthong is a combination of an unstressed <u>i</u> or <u>u</u> with another vowel. (See pp. 19 to 25 for further practice on diphthongs.) For example:

<u>no</u>	1 vowel, 1 syllable
her-<u>ma</u>-<u>no</u>	3 vowels, 3 syllables
<u>bien</u>	1 diphthong, 1 syllable
<u>sien</u>-<u>to</u>	1 diphthong and 1 vowel, 2 syllables
es-<u>pe</u>-<u>cia</u>-<u>li</u>-<u>za</u>-<u>ción</u>	4 vowels and 2 diphthongs, 6 syllables

There are a few basic rules for dividing into syllables.

Begin a syllable with a consonant if there is one.

<u>ca</u>-ra   <u>ho</u>-ra   <u>ca</u>-ma   ti-<u>je</u>-ras   la-va-<u>ma</u>-nos

When there are two consonants together, divide between them. However, <u>l</u> or <u>r</u> as a second consonant usually forms an inseparable cluster which goes with the following syllable.

her-<u>ma</u>-no	<u>trein</u>-ta	But:	cu-<u>ra</u>-ble	cen-<u>tral</u>
<u>has</u>-ta	<u>tar</u>-de		<u>ha</u>-bla	de-cla-<u>rar</u>
us-<u>te</u>-des	cin-<u>cuen</u>-ta		pro-<u>gre</u>-so	
per-<u>mi</u>-so	fre-<u>cuen</u>-tes			

When there are more than two consonants together, you can usually tell as you sound out each syllable which one they are most naturally said with.

LESSON 40: Linking and Rhythm

It's here. (he's here, etc.)
You are going to do. (he is going to do, etc.)

in this
the eyes

It's here.
What's this?
the eyes
You have an eye infection.
He's a friend.
It's a symptom.
It's being done.
That's serious.
Who is your husband?
Do you have children?

LECCION 40: Enlace y ritmo

In Spanish, several words are linked together without pause as one breath group. When the same or similar vowel sounds begin and end a word, the sounds run together.

Está‿aquí.

Va‿a‿hacer.

The rules on p. 31 about division of words into syllables also apply from word to word within the same breath group. That is, where there is a consonant, it begins a syllable, even if that consonant is part of the previous word.

en‿este

los‿ojos

Spanish syllables are rather evenly and rhythmically stressed. Repeat the following phrases and sentences, keeping the rhythm and syllabification indicated.

Está aquí.   (es - taa - quí)

¿Qué es esto?   (quée - ses - to)

los ojos   (lo - so - jos)

Tiene infección en los ojos. (tie - nein - fec - cio - nen - lo - so - jos)

Es un amigo.   (e - su - na - mi - go)

Es un síntoma.   (e - sun - sín - to -ma)

Se está haciendo. (sees - táƴa - cien - do)

Eso es serio.   (e - soe - se - rio)

¿Quién es su esposo?   (quié - ne - ssues - po - so)

¿Tiene usted hijos?   (tie - neus - te - dƴi - jos)

Useful Everyday Phrases

°Good morning.   Good morning.

Good afternoon.   Good afternoon.

Good evening.   Good evening.
Good night.   Good night.

How are you?   Very well.
                                        Very well, thanks.
                                        Fine, thanks, and you?
                                        Not very well.

How do you feel today?   I feel bad.
                                             good.
                                             better.
                                             worse.

How's it going?

What's the matter with you?

I hope you feel better.   Thanks.
           get

Hi!   Hi!

How's everything?   So-so.
                                        As usual.

Until tomorrow.   Until later.

See you later.   Good-bye.

Tell your family hello.   Thanks. Same to yours.
(Give my regards to your family.)

34

Frases útiles

Buenos días.	Buenos días.
Buenas tardes.	Buenas tardes.
Buenas noches.	Buenas noches.
¿Cómo está usted?	Muy bien. Muy bien, gracias. Bien, gracias, ¿y usted? No muy bien.
¿Cómo se siente hoy?	Me siento mal. bien. mejor. peor.
¿Cómo le va?	Bien, gracias.
¿Qué le pasa?	Me siento mejor.
¡Qué se mejore!	Gracias.
¡Hola!	¡Hola!
¿Qué tal?	Así así. Regular.
Hasta mañana.	Hasta luego.
Hasta la vista.	Adíos.
Saludos a la familia.	Gracias. Igualmente.

Courtesy

^oThanks.

You're welcome.
Don't mention it.

Excuse me.
May I come in?

Come in.
You may.

Pardon.
Forgive me.

It's nothing.

I'm sorry.

Thank you.

My deepest sympathy.

Please.

Gladly.

Communication

^oDo you understand?

Yes, sir, I understand.
    ma'am
    miss
    doctor
No, sir, I don't understand.

Do you speak English?
          Spanish?

Yes, a little.
No, very little.

Do you understand Spanish?
                English?

Repeat, please.

Yes, sir, gladly.

Please speak more slowly.

How do you say "nurse"?
             "bathroom"?
             "hall"?
             "bed"?

You say "enfermera."
        "baño."
        "pasillo."
        "cama."

What does "póngase" mean?
        "quítese"
        "siéntese"

It means "put on."
        "take off."
        "sit down."

Cortesía

°Gracias.

Con permiso.

Perdón.

Lo siento.

Mi sentido pésame.

Por favor.

De nada.
No hay de qué.

Pase.
Adelante.

Usted lo tiene.

No es nada.

Gracias.

Con mucho gusto.

Comunicación

°¿Comprende?

¿Habla usted inglés?
           español?

¿Comprende usted español?
                inglés?

Repita, por favor.

Favor de hablar más despacio.
Hable más despacio, por favor.

¿Cómo se dice "enfermera"?
          "baño"?
          "pasillo"?
          "cama"?

¿Qué quiere decir "put on"?
          "take off"?
          "sit down"?

Sí, señor, comprendo.
    señora
    señorita
    doctor
No, señor, no comprendo.

Sí, un poco.
No, muy poco.

Sí, señor, con mucho gusto.

Se dice "nurse."
      "bathroom."
      "hall."
      "bed."

Quiere decir "póngase."
         "quítese."
         "siéntese."

Exclamations

°I feel bad.

What a shame!
Poor thing! (m.)
Poor thing! (f.)

I feel very good.

Stupendous!
Marvelous!
Fantastic!

The food is just delicious.

Thanks a lot!
Thanks a million!

very good.

Good luck.

Thanks. Same to you.

Useful Phrases

°Where's the bathroom?

It's here.
right there.
there.

Tell me, please.

Yes, of course.
Yes, gladly.

Sit down,

Get up,

Go to bed,

Take this off,

Put this on,

Do you need something?

Nothing, thanks.

Do you want something?

May I help you?
What can I do for you?

No, thank you.

If you need something, tell me.

Okay.

What's the matter?

I don't know.
This thing isn't working.

You should take care of yourself.

You are right.

Exclamaciones

°Me siento mal.

¡Qué lástima!
¡Pobrecito!
¡Pobrecita!

Me siento muy bien.

¡Estupendo!
¡Maravilloso!
¡Fantástico!

La comida está deliciosa.
(muy rica)
(muy sabrosa)
muy buena.

¡Mil gracias!
¡Un millón de gracias!
Muchas gracias.

Buena suerte.

Gracias. Igualmente.

Frases útiles

°¿Dónde está el baño?

Está aquí.
ahí.
allí.

Dígame, por favor.

Sí, cómo no.
Sí, con mucho gusto.

Siéntese,

Levántese,

Acuéstese,

Quítese esto,

Póngase esto,

¿Necesita algo?

Nada, gracias.

¿Desea algo?

¿En qué puedo servirle?

En nada, gracias.

Si necesita algo, dígame.

Muy bien, gracias.

¿Qué pasa?

No sé.
El aparato está malo.

Debe cuidarse.

Usted tiene razón.

Lesson 1
The Human Body: Parts of the Body

NEW MATERIAL

On the Anatomical Chart

Instructor	Student
°What is this?	
Is it the cranium?	It's the cranium.
(the skull)	(the skull)
the hair?	
the eye?	
the eyeball?	
the eyelid?	
the lip?	
the neck?	
°What is this?	
Is it the breast?	It's the breast.
the chest?	
(the breast)	
the bust?	
(the breast)	
the shoulder?	
the stomach?	
the abdomen?	
the trunk?	
°What is this?	
Is it the arm?	It's the arm.
the elbow?	
the finger?	
the fist?	
the ankle?	
the foot?	
the toe?	
the heel?	

Lección 1
El cuerpo humano: Partes del cuerpo

En la carta anatómica

Profesor   Estudiante

°¿Qué es esto?

   ¿Es el cráneo?   Es el cráneo.

     el pelo?
     (el cabello)

     el ojo?

     el globo del ojo?

     el párpado?

     el labio?

     el cuello?

°¿Qué es esto?

   ¿ Es el seno?   Es el seno.

     el pecho?

     el busto?

     el hombro?

     el estómago?

     el abdomen?

     el tronco?

°¿Qué es esto?

   ¿Es el brazo?   Es el brazo.

     el codo?

     el dedo?

     el puño?

     el tobillo?

     el pie?

     el dedo del pie?

     el talón?

Instructor	Student

^o<u>What is this</u>?

   <u>Is it</u> the bone?   <u>It's</u> the bone.

       the nerve?

       the muscle?

       the thigh?

       the diaphragm?

^o<u>What is this</u>?

   <u>Is it</u> the head?   <u>It's</u> the head.

       the face?

       the forehead?

       the pupil?

       the eyebrow?

       the eyelash?

       the mouth?

       the tongue?

       the nose?

       the nostril?

       the cheek?

       the chin?
     (the beard)

       the jaw?

       the ear (outer)?

^o<u>What is this</u>?

   <u>Is it</u> the skin?   <u>It's</u> the skin.

       the back?

       the rib?

       the spinal column?

       the waist?

       the buttock?

       the hip?

       the pelvis?

       the groin?

Profesor	Estudiante

°¿Qué es esto?

    ¿Es el hueso?   Es el hueso.
        el nervio?
        el músculo?
        el muslo?
        el diafragma?

°¿Qué es esto?

    ¿Es la cabeza?   Es la cabeza.
        la cara?
        la frente?
        la pupila?
        la ceja?
        la pestaña?
        la boca?
        la lengua?
        la nariz?
        la fosa nasal?
        la mejilla?
        la barba?

        la mandíbula?
        la oreja?

°¿Qué es esto?

    ¿Es la piel?   Es la piel.
        la espalda?
        la costilla?
        la columna vertebral?
        la cintura?
        la nalga?
        la cadera?
        la pelvis?
        la ingle?

Instructor	Student

^o_What is this_?

  _Is it_ the wrist?   _It's_ the wrist.

       the hand?

       the palm of the hand?

       the nail?

       the armpit?

^o_What is this_?

  _Is it_ the leg?   _It's_ the leg.

       the crotch?

       the knee?

       the joint?

       the sole of the foot?

^o _Are they_ the eyes?   _They're_ the eyes.

         the eyelids?

         the lips?

         the breasts?

         the shoulders?

         the arms?

         the elbows?

         the fingers?

         the ankles?

         the feet?

         the toes?

         the heels?

         the bones?

^o _Are they_ the cheeks?   _They're_ the cheeks.

         the ears?

         the nostrils?

         the buttocks?

         the ribs?

         the hips?

         the wrists?

Profesor	Estudiante
º¿<u>Qué es esto</u>?	
¿<u>Es</u> la muñeca?	<u>Es</u> la muñeca.
la mano?	
la palma de la mano?	
la uña?	
la axila?	
º¿<u>Qué es esto</u>?	
¿<u>Es</u> la pierna?	<u>Es</u> la pierna.
la entrepierna?	
la rodilla?	
la articulación? (la coyuntura)	
la planta del pie?	
º¿<u>Son</u> los ojos?	<u>Son</u> los ojos.
los párpados?	
los labios?	
los senos?	
los hombros?	
los brazos?	
los codos?	
los dedos?	
los tobillos?	
los pies?	
los dedos de los pies?	
los talones?	
los huesos?.	
º¿<u>Son</u> las mejillas?	<u>Son</u> las mejillas.
las orejas?	
las fosas nasales?	
las nalgas?	
las costillas?	
las caderas?	
las muñecas?	

Instructor	Student

°<u>Are they</u> the hands?   <u>They're</u> the hands.

              the palms of the hands?

              the nails?

              the legs?

              the knees?

              the soles of the feet?

              the joints?

1. Nutrition is important.

2. The operation is necessary.

3. It's polio (poliomyelitis).

4. The situation is serious.

5. Are the attacks frequent?

Profesor	Estudiante
°¿<u>Son</u> las manos?	<u>Son</u> las manos.
¿Son las palmas de las manos?	
¿Son las uñas?	
¿Son las piernas?	
¿Son las rodillas?	
¿Son las plantas de los pies?	
¿Son las articulaciones?	

IDENTIFICATION

Cover the English opposite, and pronounce the following sentences aloud. Then check to see if you have understood.

1. La nutrición es importante.

2. La operación es necesaria.

3. Es poliomielitis.

4. La situación es seria.

5. ¿Son frecuentes los ataques?

NOTES

COGNATES

Cognates are words that look similar and have similar meanings in two languages. Some Spanish words sound even more similar to the English cognates than they look. Often, if a cognate is not immediately clear, you can see what it means if you cover the first or the last part of the word.

NOUNS

In Spanish all nouns (names of things) are either masculine or feminine. This is usually a matter of grammatical form, not identifiable with sex except in the case of human beings and higher animals. Generally, nouns that end in -o are masculine, and nouns that end in -a are feminine. Those that end in consonants or -e are variable, and you will learn them by use. In this text the abbreviations m. and f. are used where helpful.

THE

In Spanish there are four words for the English word "the":

el brazo -- the arm	la pierna -- the leg
los brazos -- the arms	las piernas -- the legs

These articles (el, la, los, las) have forms that correspond to the nouns in gender (masculine or feminine) and in number (singular -- one, or plural -- more than one).

GRAMMAR AND STRUCTURES DRILLED IN LESSON 1

verbs

es -- it is, is it?

son -- they are, are they?

definite articles

el, la, los, las -- agreement with noun

plurals of nouns

pronouns

neuter demonstrative pronoun esto

¿Qué es esto?   What is this?

Lesson 2
The Human Body: Organs

On the Anatomical Chart

NEW MATERIAL

Instructor	Student
°What is this?	
Is it the brain?	It's the brain.
the heart?	
the intestine?	
the colon?	
the kidney?	
the liver?	
the stomach?	
the stomach? (the abdomen)	
the spleen?	

°What is this?

    Is it the ear (inner)?　　　　It's the ear (inner).
　　　　　　　　　　　　　　　　　　　It's not the ear.

        the pancreas?

        the lung?

        the rectum?

        the anus?

        the uterus? (the womb)

        the cervix?

        the testicle?

        the penis?

Lección 2
El cuerpo humano: Organos

En la carta anatómica

MATERIA NUEVA

Profesor	Estudiante
°¿Qué es esto?	
¿Es el cerebro?	Es el cerebro.
el corazón?	
el intestino?	
el colon?	
el riñón?	
el hígado?	
el estómago?	
el vientre?	
el bazo?	
(el esplín)	
°¿Qué es esto?	
¿Es el oído?	Es el oído.
	No es el oído.
el páncreas?	
el pulmón?	
el recto?	
el ano?	
el útero?	
el cuello uterino?	
(el cuello de la matriz)	
el testículo?	
el pene?	

Instructor	Student

^O<u>What is this</u>?

    <u>Is it</u> the throat?   <u>It's</u> the throat.

            the skin?

            the bladder?

            the gallbladder?

            the vagina?

            the uterus?

^O<u>What are these</u>?

    <u>Are they</u> the bronchial tubes?   <u>They're</u> the bronchial tubes.

               the intestines?

               the kidneys?

               the lungs?

               the genitals?

               the ovaries?

^O<u>What is</u> the heart?   <u>It's an organ</u> of the circulatory system.

        the stomach?   of the digestive system.

        the kidney?   of the genitourinary system.

        the brain?   of the nervous system.

^O<u>What are</u> the lungs?   <u>They're organs</u> of the respiratory system.

Hospital	Patient

<u>Yes, you have</u> a throat infection.   ^O<u>Do I have</u> a throat <u>infection</u>?

                                    a tonsil

                                    an eye

                                    a bronchial

                                    a skin

                                    a mouth

Profesor	Estudiante
°¿Qué es esto?	
¿Es la garganta?	Es la garganta.
la piel?	
la vejiga?	
la vesícula?	
la vagina?	
la matriz?	
°¿Qué son éstos?	
¿Son los bronquios?	Son los bronquios.
los intestinos?	
los riñones?	
los pulmones?	
los genitales?	
los ovarios?	
°¿Qué es el corazón?	Es un órgano del aparato circulatorio.
el estómago?	del aparato digestivo.
el riñón?	del aparato génitourinario.
el cerebro?	del sistema nervioso.
°¿Qué son los pulmones?	Son órganos del aparato respiratorio.

Hospital	Paciente
Sí, tiene infección en la garganta.	°¿Tengo infección en la garganta?
	las amígdalas?
	los ojos?
	los bronquios?
	la piel?
	la boca?

Hospital	Patient

Yes, you have an intestinal infection.   ^oDo I have an intestinal infection?

a kidney

a gallbladder

a liver

a stomach

an inner ear

a vaginal

a finger

a hand

a toe

1. The doctor prohibited my working.
2. Did you notice the symptoms?
3. I wish the doctor would stop the injections.
4. Did you decide to proceed with the operation?
5. I don't know if he will use a general anesthesia.
6. Be calm, ma'am. Don't worry about the child.
7. Let me examine your ears.
8. What does this medicine contain?
9. Have you noticed whether your stomach hurts before you eat?
10. We will consult the surgeon and other doctors.

Hospital

Paciente

Sí, tiene infección en los intestinos.   °¿Tengo infección en los intestinos?

los riñones?

la vesícula?

el hígado?

el estómago?

el oído?

la vagina?

el dedo?

la mano?

el dedo del pie?

IDENTIFICATION

Consult the list of cognate infinitives on pp. 525 and 527 and practice pronouncing some of them. The following sentences contain cognate verbs that have been changed from the infinitive form to show time and person. Underline the cognate verb or verbs in each sentence, and then guess at the general idea of what is being said. Check the English opposite to see how close you were.

1. El médico me prohibió trabajar.

2. ¿Notaste los síntomas?

3. Ojalá que el médico suspenda las inyecciones.

4. ¿Resolvió usted proceder con la operación?

5. No sé si usará anestesia general.

6. Cálmese, señora. No hay que preocuparse por el niño.

7. Permítame examinarle los oídos.

8. ¿Qué contiene esta medicina?

9. ¿Ha observado usted si le duele el estómago antes de comer?

10. Consultaremos con el cirujano y otros médicos.

NOTES

INFINITIVES

Infinitives are names of actions without beginning or end. They are verbs that have no time or person with them, and thus in a sense are infinite. In Spanish all infinitives end in -ar, -er, or -ir. In English such forms are usually given with "to," as in "to examine," or sometimes simply "examine" will be a better translation for the Spanish.

Infinitives are important forms for students of Spanish to know. There are many things you can say by combining a few set verb forms with various infinitives, even though you cannot use verbs the way a native speaker does. However, it is not difficult to learn to recognize the basic verb, even when it is used in other forms.

GRAMMAR AND STRUCTURES DRILLED IN LESSON 2

verbs

| ser -- to be | es -- it is, is it? | son -- they are, are they? |
| tener -- to have | tengo -- I have | tiene -- you have, do you have? |

definite articles

el, la, los -- the

agreement with noun

contraction de + el -- del

plurals of nouns

simple negation

Es la piel. It's the skin.

No es la piel. It's not the skin.

Lesson 3
The Human Body: Functions and Complications

<u>NEW MATERIAL</u>

Hospital	Patient

° <u>Do you have</u> a cough?
     coughing?
	<u>Yes, I have</u> a cough.
	     a little coughing.
	     a lot of coughing.

° <u>Do you have</u> phlegm?
     dizziness?
     nausea?
     tingling?
     diarrhea?
     sinus trouble?
     cramps?
     belching?
     sweating?
     fever?
     chills?
     hives?
     mucus?
	<u>Yes, I have</u> phlegm.

° <u>Are you</u> weak? (<u>Do you feel</u>) nervous?	<u>I'm always</u> weak. <u>I'm never</u>

° <u>Do you have</u> itching?
     a good appetite?
     yellowish skin?
     indigestion?
     constipation?
	<u>No, I don't have</u> itching.

Lección 3
El cuerpo humano: Funciones y complicaciones

MATERIA NUEVA

Hospital	Paciente
°¿Tiene usted tos?	Sí, yo tengo tos.
	un poco de tos.
	mucha tos.

Hospital	Paciente
°¿Tiene usted flema?	Sí, yo tengo flema.
mareo?	
náuseas?	
hormigueo?	
diarrea?	
sinusitis?	
calambres?	
eructos?	
sudores?	
fiebre?	
escalofríos?	
urticaria?	
mucosidad?	

Hospital	Paciente
°¿Tiene usted debilidad?	Siempre tengo debilidad.
	Nunca tengo
nerviosidad?	

Hospital	Paciente
°¿Tiene usted picazón?	No, no tengo picazón.
buen apetito?	
la piel amarilla?	
indigestión?	
constipación?	
(estreñimiento)	

Hospital	Patient

°<u>Do you have</u> frequent bowel movements?   <u>No, I don't have</u> frequent bowel movements.
many colds?   <u>Yes, I have</u>
hemorrhoids?
piles?

°<u>Do you have</u> expectoration when you   <u>Yes, I have</u> expectoration when I cough.
cough?   a lot of expectoration.
                                                                            a little expectoration.

a bad taste in your mouth?

a bad odor in your saliva?
obstruction in the esophagus?
blood in the urine?
burning in the urethra?

°<u>Do you have pain</u> in your legs?   <u>No, I don't.</u>
in your muscles?
in your chest?
in your waist?
in your arm?

°<u>Do you have</u> a stomachache?
a headache?

frequent colds?

°<u>Do you feel</u> burning when you urinate?   <u>When I urinate?</u> Yes, doctor.
irritation when you urinate?
pain when you urinate?

°<u>Do you have</u> difficulty when you swallow? When I swallow? Yes, doctor.

Hospital	Paciente

° ¿Tiene usted evacuaciones frecuentes?   No, no tengo evacuaciones frecuentes.
              muchos resfriados?   Sí, tengo

              hemorroides?

              almorranas?

° ¿Tiene expectoración al toser?   Sí, tengo expectoración al toser.
                                           mucha saliva.
                                           poca saliva.

              mal sabor en la boca?
             (mal gusto en la boca)

              mal olor en la expectoración?

              obstrucción en el esófago?

              sangre en la orina?

              ardor en la uretra?

° ¿Tiene dolor en las piernas?   No, no tengo.
                  en los músculos?

                  en el pecho?

                  en la cintura?

                  en el brazo?

° ¿Tiene dolor de estómago?
              dolor de cabeza?
             (jaqueca)

              catarros con frecuencia?

° ¿Siente ardor al orinar?   ¿Al orinar? Sí, doctor.
                irritación al orinar?

                dolor al orinar?

° ¿Tiene dificultad al tragar?   ¿Al tragar? Sí, doctor.

1. The doctor visited the sick woman.
2. Dissolve this medicine in water.
3. I ate a lot, and I suffered from indigestion.
4. The nurse will watch to see if you cough a lot.
5. The patient has not eliminated since the operation.
6. The doctor will examine the patient.
7. The patient was breathing with difficulty.
8. He decided to operate on the patient tomorrow.
9. He will recuperate from the operation soon.
10. The intestinal obstruction will cause problems for him.

IDENTIFICATION

Review the list of cognate infinitives on pp. 525 and 527. In the following sentences, some of these verbs are used in different tenses (times) and persons. Pronounce each sentence aloud two or three times, underline the cognate verbs you recognize, and then try to determine the general idea of each sentence.

1. El médico visitó a la enferma.

2. Disuelva esta medicina en agua.

3. Comí mucho y sufrí una indigestión.

4. La enfermera observará si usted tose mucho.

5. El paciente no ha eliminado después de la operación.

6. El médico examinará al enfermo.

7. El enfermo respiraba con dificultad.

8. Decidió operar al paciente mañana.

9. Se recuperará de la operación pronto.

10. La obstrucción intestinal le causará problemas.

GRAMMAR AND STRUCTURES DRILLED IN LESSON 3

verbs

tener -- to have   tengo -- I have   tiene -- you have, do you have?

tener plus noun of physical condition -- to feel

Tengo debilidad.   I feel weak.

sentir -- to feel   siente -- you feel, do you feel?

negation

nunca -- never, ever

Nunca tengo indigestión.   I never have indigestion. (I don't ever have --)

definite article

contraction of el + a -- al

al + infinitive = when + verb

¿Tiene dificultad al tragar?   Do you have difficulty when you swallow?

to show possession with parts of the body:

¿Tiene dolor en el pecho?   Do you have pain in your chest?

subject pronoun   yo -- I

Lesson 4
Numbers: Time

Hospital	Patient
At 1:00.	°When do I take the medicine? At 1:00?
At 2:00.	At 2:00?
	3:00
	4:00
	5:00
	6:00
	7:00
	8:00
	9:00
	10:00
	11:00
	12:00
At noon.	°Do I take the medicine at noon?
At midnight.	at midnight?
Every 2 hours.	When do I take the medicine?
3 hours.	
4 hours.	
6 hours.	
Before meals.	
After meals.	
With meals.	
Before bedtime.	
Now.	
In the morning.	°In the morning?
In the afternoon.	In the afternoon?
At night.	At night?

Lección 4
Números: Las horas

Hospital	Paciente
A la una.	°¿Cuándo tomo la medicina? ¿A la una?
A las dos.	¿A las dos?
	las tres
	las cuatro
	las cinco
	las seis
	las siete
	las ocho
	las nueve
	las diez
	las once
	las doce
Al mediodía.	°¿Tomo la medicina al mediodía?
A medianoche.	a medianoche?
Cada dos horas.	¿Cuándo tomo la medicina?
tres horas.	
cuatro horas.	
seis horas.	
Antes de las comidas.	
Después de las comidas.	
Con las comidas.	
Antes de acostarse.	
Ahora.	
Por la mañana.	°¿Por la mañana?
Por la tarde.	¿Por la tarde?
Por la noche.	¿Por la noche?

	Hospital		Patient
It's 1:00.		°What time is it? 1:00?	
2:00.		2:00?	
2:12.			
3:00.		3:00?	
3:13.			
4:00.		4:00?	
4:14.			
5:00.		5:00?	
5:15.			
6:00.		6:00?	
6:16.			
7:00.		7:00?	
7:17.			
8:00.		8:00?	
8:18.			
9:00.		9:00?	
9:19.			
10:00.		10:00?	
10:20.			
11:00.		11:00?	
11:21.			
12:00.		12:00?	
12:22.			

Hospital		Paciente
<u>Es</u> la una.	°¿<u>Qué hora es</u>?	¿<u>La una</u>?
<u>Son</u> las dos.		¿<u>Las dos</u>?
las dos y doce.		
las tres.		¿<u>Las tres</u>?
las tres y trece.		
las cuatro.		¿<u>Las cuatro</u>?
las cuatro y catorce.		
las cinco.		¿<u>Las cinco</u>?
las cinco y quince.		
las seis.		¿<u>Las seis</u>?
las seis y dieciséis.		
las siete.		¿<u>Las siete</u>?
las siete y diecisiete.		
las ocho.		¿<u>Las ocho</u>?
las ocho y dieciocho.		
las nueve.		¿<u>Las nueve</u>?
las nueve y diecinueve.		
las diez.		¿<u>Las diez</u>?
las diez y veinte.		
las once.		¿<u>Las once</u>?
las once y veintiuno.		
las doce.		¿<u>Las doce</u>?
las doce y veintidós.		

Hospital	Patient
It's 3:00.	°What time is it? 3:00?
3:23.	
4:00.	4:00?
4:24.	
5:00.	5:00?
5:25.	
6:00.	6:00?
6:26.	
7:00.	7:00?
7:27.	
8:00.	8:00?
8:28.	
9:00.	9:00?
9:29.	
It's 2:30.	°What time is it? 2:00?
3:31.	3:00?
3:32.	
4:40.	4:00?
4:41.	
4:42.	
No, it's 5 till 5:00.	°What time is it? Is it 5:00 already?
16 till 6:00.	6:00
20 till 7:00.	7:00
quarter till 12:00. (15 till 12:00)	12:00
4 till 11:00.	11:00
22 till 10:00.	10:00

Hospital	Paciente
<u>Son</u> las tres.	^o¿<u>Qué hora es</u>? ¿<u>Las tres</u>?
las tres y veintitrés.	
las cuatro.	¿<u>Las cuatro</u>?
las cuatro y veinticuatro.	
las cinco.	¿<u>Las cinco</u>?
las cinco y veinticinco.	
las seis.	¿<u>Las seis</u>?
las seis y veintiséis.	
las siete.	¿<u>Las siete</u>?
las siete y vientisiete.	
las ocho.	¿<u>Las ocho</u>?
las ocho y veintiocho.	
las nueve.	¿<u>Las nueve</u>?
las nueve y veintinueve.	
<u>Son</u> las dos y media. (las dos y treinta)	^o¿<u>Qué hora es</u>? ¿<u>Las dos</u>?
las tres y treinta y uno.	¿<u>Las tres</u>?
las tres y treinta y dos.	
las cuatro y cuarenta.	¿<u>Las cuatro</u>?
las cuatro y cuarenta y uno.	
las cuatro y cuarenta y dos.	
<u>No, son</u> las cinco menos cinco.	^o¿<u>Qué hora es</u>? ¿Son ya las cinco?
las seis menos dieciséis.	las seis?
las siete menos veinte.	las siete?
las doce menos cuarto. (las doce menos quince)	las doce?
las once menos cuatro.	las once?
las diez menos veintidós.	las diez?

	Hospital			Patient

Hospital

It's 8:00 A.M.
    8:00 P.M.
At   8:00 A.M.
    5:00 P.M.
    9:00 P.M.
Yes, it's time.
Yes, it's time to take the medicine.
            to eat.
            to leave.

Patient

○What time is it?

○When do I take the medicine?

○Is it time?

Circulation

Blood circulates through the arteries and veins. The arteries carry pure blood to all parts of the body. The veins collect the impure blood and carry it to the heart. From the heart the blood goes to the lungs. In the lungs the blood is purified with the oxygen of the air we breathe. In the laboratory the blood is examined to see the condition of the red and white corpuscles.

Hospital	Paciente

<u>Son</u> las ocho de la mañana. °¿Qué hora tiene?

    las ocho de la noche.

<u>A</u>   las ocho de la mañana. °¿Cuándo tomo la medicina?

    las cinco de la tarde.

    las nueve de la noche.

<u>Sí, es hora.</u>   °¿Es hora?

<u>Sí, es hora de</u> tomar la medicina.

         comer.

         salir.

IDENTIFICATION

KEY WORDS

Much of understanding a language depends on being able to pick out the important words that give clues to what is being said. Many of these <u>key</u> <u>words</u> are nouns (names of things) and verbs (action words). You really don't have to know every word to understand what a native speaker is saying.

Read the following passage aloud. Then reread it, underlining what you think are the key words, many of which are cognates. Then write the English above each word you have underlined. Some new words you can determine from the context. If you aren't sure, guess. Now read just the English you have written, and check to see if you have the basic information about the circulatory system.

La circulación

La sangre circula por las arterias y las venas. Las arterias llevan

la sangre pura a todas partes del cuerpo. Las venas recogen la sangre

impura y la llevan al corazón. Del corazón la sangre va a los pulmones.

En los pulmones la sangre se purifica con el oxígeno del aire que se

respira. En el laboratorio se examina la sangre para ver la condición

de los glóbulos rojos y blancos.

GRAMMAR AND STRUCTURES DRILLED IN LESSON 4

verbs

    tomar -- to take   tomo -- I take, do I take?

telling time

    ¿Qué hora es?   What time is it?

    Es la una.   It's 1:00.
    Son las dos.   It's 2:00.

numbers to 40 (see also list, pp. 242 to 243)

interrogative words

    ¿cuándo?   when?
    ¿qué?   what?

Lesson 5
Numbers: Weights and Measures

Hospital	Patient
It weighs 10 grams.	°How many grams does this weigh?
Yes, it weighs 20 grams.	Does it weigh 20 grams?
	21 grams?
	21?
	30 grams?
	40 grams?
	50 grams?
	60 grams?
	70 grams?
	80 grams?
	90 grams?
Yes, it weighs 100 grams.	°Does it weigh 100 grams?
	110 grams?
	120 grams?
	200 grams?
	221 grams?
	221?
	300 grams?
	331 grams?
	331?

Lección 5
Números: Pesos y medidas

<u>MATERIA NUEVA</u>

Hospital	Paciente

Hospital

<u>Pesa</u> diez <u>gramos</u>.

<u>Sí, pesa</u> veinte <u>gramos</u>.

Paciente

° ¿<u>Cuántos gramos</u> pesa esto?

¿<u>Pesa</u> veinte gramos?

     veintiún gramos?

     veintiuno?

     treinta gramos?

     cuarenta gramos?

     cincuenta gramos?

     sesenta gramos?

     setenta gramos?

     ochenta gramos?

     noventa gramos?

<u>Sí, pesa</u> cien <u>gramos</u>.

° ¿<u>Pesa</u> cien gramos?

     ciento diez gramos?

     ciento veinte gramos?

     doscientos gramos?

     doscientos veintiún gramos?

     doscientos veintiuno?

     trescientos gramos?

     trescientos treinta y un gramos?

     trescientos treinta y uno?

Hospital	Patient

Hospital

Yes, it weighs 400 grams.

Patient

Does it weigh 400 grams?

444 grams?

444?

500 grams?

555 grams?

600 grams?

666 grams?

700 grams?

777 grams?

800 grams?

888 grams?

900 grams?

999 grams?

1000 grams?

1,000,000 grams?

2,000,000 grams?

How many calories does this have?

Yes, 100 calories.

100 calories?

110 calories?

121 calories?

121?

200 calories?

222 calories?

300 calories?

333 calories?

400 calories?

444 calories?

500 calories?

555 calories?

Hospital	Paciente
<u>Sí, pesa</u> cuatrocientos <u>gramos</u>.	°¿<u>Pesa</u> cuatrocientos gramos?

Paciente

°¿<u>Pesa</u> cuatrocientos gramos?
   cuatrocientos cuarenta y cuatro gramos?
   cuatrocientos cuarenta y cuatro?
   quinientos gramos?
   quinientos cincuenta y cinco gramos?
   seiscientos gramos?
   seiscientos sesenta y seis gramos?
   setecientos gramos?
   setecientos setenta y siete gramos?
   ochocientos gramos?
   ochocientos ochenta y ocho gramos?
   novecientos gramos?
   novecientos noventa y nueve gramos?
   mil gramos?
   un millón de gramos?
   dos millones de gramos?

°¿<u>Cuántas calorías tiene esto</u>?
  ¿Cien calorías?
  ¿Ciento diez calorías?
  ¿Ciento veintiuna calorías?
  ¿Ciento veintiuna?
  ¿Doscientas calorías?
  ¿Doscientas veintidós calorías?
  ¿Trescientas calorías?
  ¿Trescientas treinta y tres calorías?
  ¿Cuatrocientas calorías?
  ¿Cuatrocientas cuarenta y cuatro calorías?
  ¿Quinientas calorías?
  ¿Quinientas cincuenta y cinco calorías?

<u>Sí</u>, cien calorías.

Hospital	Patient
	^oHow many calories does this have?
<u>Yes</u>, 600 calories.	600 calories?
700 calories.	700 calories?
800 calories.	800 calories?
900 calories.	900 calories?
^oIt has 1000 calories.	1000 calories?
1200 calories.	
2222 calories.	
millions of calories.	

Instructor	Student
^o<u>How much is</u> a dram?	1 teaspoonful.
1 cubic centimeter (cc)?	1 milliliter.
1 liter?	1000 cubic centimeters.
1/2 liter?	500 cubic centimeters.
1 gram?	1000 milligrams.
1 kilogram?	1000 grams.
1 pound?	16 ounces.
1 gallon?	4 quarts.
1 cup?	8 ounces.
	(1/2 pint)
1 pint?	2 cups.
	(1/2 quart)
1 meter?	100 centimeters.
1 centimeter?	10 millimeters.
1 foot?	12 inches.
1 yard?	3 feet.
1 vara?	Almost a yard.

Hospital	Paciente
	° ¿Cuántas calorías tiene esto?
Sí, seiscientas calorías.	¿Seiscientas calorías?
setecientas calorías.	¿Setecientas calorías?
ochocientas calorías.	¿Ochocientas calorías?
novecientas calorías.	¿Novecientas calorías?
° Tiene mil calorías.	¿Mil calorías?
mil doscientas calorías.	
dos mil doscientas veintidós calorías.	
millones de calorías.	

Profesor	Estudiante
° ¿Cuánto es un dracma?	Una cucharadita.
un centímetro cúbico?	Un mililitro.
un litro?	Mil centímetros cúbicos.
medio litro?	Quinientos centímetros cúbicos.
un gramo?	Mil miligramos.
un kilogramo?	Mil gramos.
una libra?	Dieciséis onzas.
un galón?	Cuatro cuartos.
una taza?	Ocho onzas. (Media pinta)
una pinta?	Dos tazas. (Medio cuarto)
un metro?	Cien centímetros.
un centímetro?	Diez milímetros.
un pie?	Doce pulgadas.
una yarda?	Tres pies.
una vara?	Casi una yarda.

Patient: Oh, miss!

Nurse: What's the matter with you, sir?

Patient: The thing is I feel really bad.

Nurse: Why? Is it your head? Is it your throat? Do you have a

         stomachache?

Patient: It's more than that. I'm weak, nervous, and I have chills.

Nurse: Now just be calm, sir. I'll ask the doctor about it.

Patient: Just a moment. I have pain in the area of my heart, too.

Nurse: Your condition is serious. When do you have these symptoms?

Patient: Let's see -- when I see you.

IDENTIFICATION

To understand conversation in a language you are not thoroughly familiar with, it is helpful to keep in mind the context, that is, what you know about the situation and the people who are speaking. Imagine that the following conversation takes place between a pretty young nurse and an amiable older man who likes to tease.

Read the conversation aloud, picking out key words and cognate words. Can you understand the general ideas, except perhaps the last line? From the context given, try to guess the last line before checking the English.

Paciente: ¡Ay, señorita!

Enfermera: ¿Qué le pasa, señor?

Paciente: Es que me siento muy mal.

Enfermera: ¿Por qué? ¿Es la cabeza? ¿Es la garganta? ¿Tiene dolor en el

estómago?

Paciente: Es más que eso. Tengo debilidad, nerviosidad, y escalofríos.

Enfermera;   ¡Cálmese, señor! Tengo que consultar con el médico.

Paciente: Un momento. También tengo dolor en el corazón.

Enfermera: Su condición es seria. ¿Cuándo tiene esos síntomas?

Paciente: A ver . . . cuando la veo a usted.

NOTES

An adjective tells something about a noun. Unlike English, adjectives in Spanish have forms that correspond to nouns.

un gramo   1 gram
una caloría   1 calorie

¿Cuántos gramos?   How many grams?
¿Cuántas calorías?   How many calories?

GRAMMAR AND STRUCTURES DRILLED IN LESSON 5

verbs

tener -- to have   tiene -- it has, has it?, does it have?
pesar -- to weigh   pesa -- it weighs, does it weigh?

numbers   10 to 1,000 (see also list, pp. 242 to 243)

agreement of hundreds with nouns

doscientos gramos   -- 200 grams
doscientas calorías -- 200 calories

units of measure

interrogative words

¿Cuántos?   How many (m.)?
¿Cuántas?   How many (f.)?
¿Cuánto es?   How much is it?

pronouns

neuter demonstrative   esto -- this

Lesson 6
In the Hospital: Admission and the Family

<u>NEW MATERIAL</u>

Hospital	Patient
°<u>Is it</u> your father?	<u>Yes, it's</u> my father.
your mother?	my mother.
your stepfather?	my stepfather.
your stepmother?	my stepmother.
your husband?	my husband.
your wife?	my wife.
your son?	my son.
your daughter?	my daughter.
your brother?	my brother.
your sister?	my sister.
your father-in-law?	my father-in-law.
your mother-in-law?	my mother-in-law.
your grandfather?	my grandfather.
your grandmother?	my grandmother.
your grandson?	my grandson.
your granddaughter?	my granddaughter.
your uncle?	my uncle.
your aunt?	my aunt.
your cousin (m.)?	my cousin (m.).
your cousin (f.)?	my cousin (f.).
your nephew?	my nephew.
your niece?	my niece.
your brother-in-law?	my brother-in-law.
your sister-in-law?	my sister-in-law.
your son-in-law?	my son-in-law.
your daughter-in-law?	my daughter-in-law.
your fiancé?	my fiancé.
your fiancée?	my fiancée.

Lección 6
En el hospital: Admisión y la familia

MATERIA NUEVA

Hospital	Paciente
°¿Es su padre?	Sí, es mi padre.
su madre?	mi madre.
su padrastro?	mi padrastro.
su madrastra?	mi madrastra.
su esposo?	mi esposo.
su esposa?	mi esposa.
su hijo?	mi hijo.
su hija?	mi hija.
su hermano?	mi hermano.
su hermana?	mi hermana.
su suegro?	mi suegro.
su suegra?	mi suegra.
su abuelo?	mi abuelo.
su abuela?	mi abuela.
su nieto?	mi nieto.
su nieta?	mi nieta.
su tío?	mi tío
su tía?	mi tía.
su primo?	mi primo.
su prima?	mi prima.
su sobrino?	mi sobrino.
su sobrina?	mi sobrina.
su cuñado?	mi cuñado.
su cuñada?	mi cuñada.
su yerno?	mi yerno.
su nuera?	mi nuera.
su novio?	mi novio.
su novia?	mi novia.

Hospital	Patient
°Are they your parents?	Yes, they're my parents
your children?	my children.
your brothers and sisters?	my brothers and sisters.
your grandparents?	my grandparents.
°How many children do you have?	I have 3 children.
	1 son and 3 daughters.
How many brothers and sisters do you have?	I have 3 brothers and sisters.
	2 brothers and 1 sister.
How many aunts and uncles do you have?	I have 5 aunts and uncles.
	5 uncles and 2 aunts.
How many cousins do you have?	I have many cousins.
	I don't have any cousins.
	I have 1 cousin (f.).
Do you have any family here?	Yes, I have family here.
°Are you married (m.)?	Yes, I'm married.
married (f.)?	
a widower?	
a widow?	
divorced (m.)?	
divorced (f.)?	
a friend (m.)?	
a friend (f.)?	
a neighbor (m.)?	
a neighbor (f.)?	
a relative?	
°Are you separated (m.) now?	Yes, I'm separated.
separated (f.)	

Hospital	Paciente

Hospital	Paciente
°¿<u>Son</u> sus padres?	<u>Sí, son</u> mis padres.
sus hijos?	mis hijos.
sus hermanos?	mis hermanos.
sus abuelos?	mis abuelos.
°¿Cuántos hijos tiene usted?	<u>Tengo</u> tres hijos.
	un hijo y tres hijas.
<u>¿Cuántos hermanos tiene usted?</u>	<u>Tengo</u> tres hermanos.
	dos hermanos y una hermana.
<u>¿Cuántos tíos tiene usted?</u>	<u>Tengo</u> cinco tíos.
	cinco tíos y dos tías.
<u>¿Cuántos primos tiene usted?</u>	Tengo muchos primos.
	No tengo primos.
	Tengo una prima.
¿Tiene usted familia aquí?	Sí, tengo familia aquí.
°¿<u>Es usted</u> casado?	<u>Sí, soy</u> casado.
casada?	casada.
viudo?	
viuda?	
divorciado?	
divorciada?	
amigo?	
amiga?	
vecino?	
vecina?	
pariente?	
°¿<u>Está usted</u> separado <u>ahora</u>?	<u>Sí, estoy</u> separado.
separada	separada.

Hospital	Patient

Hospital

°What is your father's name?
     your mother's
     your son's
     your daughter's
     your neighbor's

What is your name?
Glad to know you.

°I want to introduce the doctor to you.
           the nurse

Patient

My father's name is Juan Gómez.
My mother's name is María Gómez.
        name is

My name is Carmen Romero.
°I want you to meet my father.
            my mother.
Glad to know you.

Hospital	Paciente

°¿Cómo se llama su padre?
           su madre?
           su hijo?
           su hija?
           su vecino?

Mi padre se llama Juan Gómez.
Mi madre se llama María Gómez.
           se llama

¿Cómo se llama usted?
Mucho gusto.

Me llamo Carmen Romero.
°Quiero presentarle a mi padre.
                a mi madre.

°Quiero presentarle al doctor.
           a la enfermera.

Mucho gusto.

IDENTIFICATION

There are many cognate nouns that end in -ion in both Spanish and English. In general, English -tion is equivalent to -ción in Spanish, and -sion to -sión. To approximate the sound of this ending in Spanish-American pronunciation, say yo (as in yo-yo), put an s in front, and add n: syon. Avoid putting in the sh sound that the English equivalents of these word endings have. Now turn to the list of these cognates on pp. 527 and 529 and practice pronouncing some of them.

Doctor: What's the matter with you, ma'am?

Patient: I have difficulty with digestion.

Doctor: How long have you had this problem?

Patient: I had an operation three months ago because I was having difficulty
with elimination, and constipation gave me so many problems that
I had to take a lot of laxatives.

Doctor: You need attention. We'll admit you to the hospital. I'm going
to call the admissions office. We'll put you under observation
for a few days.

The following conversation has several _-ión_ cognates. Read through the Spanish aloud, underlining these and other key words. Then, before you check the English, try to answer these questions: What does the patient complain about? What is the doctor going to do?

Doctor: Señora, ¿qué le pasa?

Paciente: Tengo dificultad con la digestión.

Doctor: ¿Desde cuándo tiene esa condición?

Paciente: Tuve una operación hace tres meses porque tenía bastante dificultad

con la eliminación y la constipación me daba tantos problemas que

tenía que tomar muchos laxantes.

Doctor: Usted necesita atención. La admitiremos en el hospital. Voy a

llamar a la oficina de admisiones. La pondremos en observación por

unos días.

GRAMMAR AND STRUCTURES DRILLED IN LESSON 6

verbs

ser -- to be   soy -- I am   es -- it is, is it?   son -- they are,
                                 you are, are you?   are they?
tener -- to have   tengo -- I have   tiene -- you have, do you have?
llamarse -- to be named   me llamo -- my name is   se llama -- (his, her)
                                                                  name is

gender of nouns and adjectives

Es mi primo.   It's my cousin (m.).
Es mi prima.   It's my cousin (f.).

¿Es usted casado?   Are you married (m.)?
¿Es usted casada?   Are you married (f.)?

possessive adjectives

su primo   your cousin   mi primo   my cousin
sus primos   your cousins   mis primos   my cousins

Lesson 7
In the Hospital: Admission and Forms

NEW MATERIAL

Hospital	Patient
°Are you the patient (m.)?	Yes, I'm the patient.
the patient (f.)?	
Yes, I'm the doctor.	°Are you the doctor?
Yes, I'm the nurse.	Are you the nurse?
°Sit down, please.	Thanks.
Tell me, please.	Yes?
Tell me, what is the patient's name?	His name is Juan Gómez.
your father's	
your mother's	Her
Tell me, what is your name?	My name is Pablo Romero.
Tell me, do you have family here?	Yes, I have family here.
children?	
insurance?	
°What's the matter with you?	They're going to operate on me.
What do you feel?	A pain here.
What age is your father?	He's 50 years (old).
your son?	
(are) you?	I'm
°What number is your house?	The number of my house is 1320.
your apartment?	my apartment
your telephone?	my telephone
What work do you do?	I work in an office.
	in a factory.
	in a store.

92

Lección 7
En el hospital: Admisión y formas

<u>MATERIA NUEVA</u>

<table>
<tr><td align="center">Hospital</td><td align="center">Paciente</td></tr>
<tr><td>°¿Es usted el paciente?
      (la paciente)</td><td>Sí, soy el paciente.
      (la paciente)</td></tr>
<tr><td>Sí, soy el médico.</td><td>°¿Es usted el médico?</td></tr>
<tr><td>Sí, soy la enfermera.</td><td>¿Es usted la enfermera?</td></tr>
<tr><td>°Siéntese, por favor.</td><td>Gracias.</td></tr>
<tr><td><u>Dígame</u>, por favor.</td><td>¿Sí?</td></tr>
<tr><td><u>Dígame</u>, ¿<u>cómo se llama</u> el paciente?</td><td><u>Se llama</u> Juan Gómez.</td></tr>
<tr><td>   su padre?</td><td></td></tr>
<tr><td>   su madre?</td><td></td></tr>
<tr><td><u>Dígame</u>, ¿<u>cómo se llama</u> usted?</td><td><u>Me llamo</u> Pablo Romero.</td></tr>
<tr><td><u>Dígame</u>, ¿<u>tiene usted</u> familia aquí?</td><td><u>Sí, tengo</u> familia aquí.</td></tr>
<tr><td>   hijos?</td><td></td></tr>
<tr><td>   seguro?</td><td></td></tr>
<tr><td>°¿<u>Qué</u> le pasa?</td><td>Me van a operar.</td></tr>
<tr><td>¿Qué siente?</td><td>Un dolor aquí.</td></tr>
<tr><td>¿Qué <u>edad tiene</u> su padre?</td><td><u>Tiene</u> cincuenta años.</td></tr>
<tr><td>   su hijo?</td><td></td></tr>
<tr><td>   usted?</td><td>Tengo</td></tr>
<tr><td>°¿Qué <u>número tiene</u> su casa?</td><td><u>El número de</u> mi casa <u>es</u> trece veinte.</td></tr>
<tr><td>   su apartamento</td><td>mi apartamento</td></tr>
<tr><td>   su teléfono?</td><td>mi teléfono</td></tr>
<tr><td>¿<u>Qué trabajo hace</u>?
¿<u>En qué trabaja usted</u>?</td><td><u>Trabajo</u> en una oficina.</td></tr>
<tr><td></td><td>en una fábrica.</td></tr>
<tr><td></td><td>en una tienda.</td></tr>
</table>

Hospital	Patient
°What <u>work does</u> your husband <u>do</u>?	He's a businessman.
	a student.
your wife	(She's) a housewife.
<u>What</u> is his relationship to you?	He's my son.
<u>How</u> is he related to you?	
Is he your son?	Yes, he's my son.
<u>What is your religion</u>?	I'm Protestant.
	Catholic (m.).
	Catholic (f.).
	Jewish (m.).
	Jewish (f.).
<u>What is</u> your husband's <u>religion</u>?	He's Catholic.
	Jewish.
	Protestant.
	He has no preference.
What insurance company do you have?	The General Insurance Company.
What kind of room do you want, private or double?	Private.
°<u>Who is</u> the doctor?	Dr. Smith.
the patient?	Mrs. Gómez.
the responsible party?	Mr. Gómez.
Who is going to pay the hospital bill?	
Whom should we notify in case of emergency?	

Hospital	Paciente
°¿Qué <u>trabajo hace</u> su esposo?	Es hombre de negocios.
	estudiante.
su esposa?	ama de casa.
¿Qué parentesco tiene con usted?	Es mi hijo.
¿Qué es de usted? ¿Es su hijo?	Sí, es mi hijo.
¿Qué <u>religión tiene</u>?	Soy protestante.
	católico.
	católica.
	judío.
	judía.
¿Qué <u>religión tiene</u> su esposo?	Es católico.
	judío.
	protestante.
	No tiene preferencia.
¿Qué compañía de seguros tiene?	La Compañía Seguros Generales.
¿Qué cuarto quiere, privado o doble?	Privado.
°¿Quién es el doctor?	El doctor Smith.
el paciente?	La señora Gómez.
el responsable?	El señor Gómez.
¿Quién va a pagar el hospital?	
¿A quién se notifica en caso de emergencia?	Al señor Gómez.

Hospital	Patient

Hospital   Patient

ºWhere were you born?   In Mexico.

       do you live?   Here, in the United States.

Where are you from?   From Puerto Rico.

What is your address?   22 Washington Street.

What is your zip code?
           postal zone?   60010.

What is your address at work?   1206 Main Street.

What is your Social Security number?   465-13-1342.

       your insurance policy?   98760.

What is your date of birth?   April 2, 1938.

What is your occupation?   I'm a mechanic.

                             carpenter.

                             lawyer.

ºWhy have you come to the hospital?   They're going to operate on me.

Is this your first time in the hospital? Yes, sir.   No, sir.
                                      ma'am.   ma'am.
                                      miss.   miss.

| | | |
| Hospital | Paciente | |

°¿<u>Dónde</u> nació? — En México.

      vive? — Aquí, en los Estados Unidos.

¿De dónde viene? — De Puerto Rico.

¿Cuál es la dirección de su casa? — Calle Washington veintidós.

¿Cuál es la zona postal? — Seis cero cero diez.

¿Cuál es la dirección de su trabajo? — Calle Main doce cero seis.

¿<u>Cuál es el número</u> de su seguro social? — Cuatro seis cinco -- trece -- uno tres
                                                 cuatro dos.

   de su póliza de seguro? — Nueve ocho siete seis cero.

¿Cuál es la fecha de su nacimiento? — El dos de abril de mil novecientos
                                                treinta y ocho.

¿<u>Cuál es su ocupación</u>? — <u>Soy</u> mecánico.

                                  carpintero.

                                  abogado.

°¿Por qué viene al hospital? — Me van a operar.

¿Es ésta la primera vez en el hospital? — Sí, señor.   No, señor.
                                       señora.   señora.
                                       señorita.   señorita.

<u>General Hospital</u>

<u>Admission Information</u>

Name_____

Address_____

City_____

State_____

Telephone_____ Age_____ Religion_____

Social Security No._____ Occupation_____

Place of Employment_____

Insurance Company_____ Policy or Medicare No._____

Nearest Relative_____ Address_____

_____

Responsible Party_____ Address_____

_____

Diagnosis_____ Previous Admission_____

Family Doctor_____ Consulting Physician_____

Room No._____	Date_____	Time_____
Discharged_____	Date_____	Time_____
Deceased_____	Date_____	Time_____

IDENTIFICATION

Understanding a foreign language often involves applying what you already know to new words. The following form for admission to the hospital uses mainly vocabulary from Lesson 7. Create a fictitious patient and fill out the form, using as much Spanish as possible. Guess the words that are new to you before checking the English.

Hospital General

Información para admisión

Nombre_____

Domicilio_____

Ciudad_____

Estado_____

Teléfono_____ Edad_____ Religión_____

Seguro social núm._____ Ocupación_____

Lugar de empleo _____

Compañía de seguros_____ Póliza núm. o Medicare_____

Pariente más cercano_____ Direoción_____

_____

Persona responsable_____ Dirección_____

_____

Diagnóstico_____ Admisión previa_____

Médico de la familia_____ Médico de consulta_____

Cuarto núm. _____	Fecha_____	Hora_____
De alta _____	Fecha_____	Hora_____
Fallecido _____	Fecha_____	Hora_____

NOTES

Interrogative words are the keys to answering as well as asking questions, since all questions except those that can be answered yes or no begin with interrogatives. You will want to learn these interrogatives in Spanish.

¿Qué?	What?
¿Cuál? (sing.) ¿Cuáles? (pl.)	Which? (or What? in the sense of which)
¿Quién? (sing.) ¿Quiénes? (pl.)	Who?
¿A quién? (sing.) ¿A quiénes? (pl.)	Whom?
¿Por qué?	Why?
¿Cómo?	How?
¿Cuándo?	When?
¿Dónde?	Where?
¿Adónde?	Where (to)?
¿De dónde?	Where (from)?
¿Cuánto? (m.) ¿Cuánta? (f.)	How much?
¿Cuántos? (m.) ¿Cuántas? (f.)	How many?

GRAMMAR AND STRUCTURES DRILLED IN LESSON 7

verbs

ser -- to be   soy -- I am   es -- you are, he is, she is
tener -- to have tengo -- I have tiene -- you have, he has, she has

interrogative words

numbers in addresses, dates, etc.

Lesson 8
In the Hospital: Signatures and Payments

NEW MATERIAL

Hospital	Patient
It's a private hospital.	°What kind of hospital is it?
public	
general	
military	
federal	
specialized	
state	
county	
city	
county and city	
charity	
maternity	
psychiatric	
pediatric	
orthopedic	
It's a hospital for cancer.	
hospital for mental illnesses.	
It's a clinic.	
°Do you have hospitalization insurance?	Yes, I have insurance.
	No, I don't have insurance.
Yes, of course.	°Can I have a private room?
No, there aren't any vacant.	a double
No, I'm sorry. You can't.	a ward
It costs $75.	How much does a private room cost?
	a double
	a ward

Lección 8
En el hospital: Firmas y pagos

Hospital	Paciente

Es un hospital privado.   °¿ Qué tipo de hospital es?

                  público.

                  general.

                  militar.

                  federal.

                  especializado.

                  del estado.

                  del condado.

                  de la ciudad.

                  del condado y la ciudad.

                  de caridad.

                  de maternidad.

                  de psiquiatría.

                  de pediatría.

                  de ortopedia.

Es un hospital de cáncer.

                  de enfermedades mentales.

Es una clínica.

°¿ Tiene usted seguro de hospitalización?   Sí, tengo seguro.

                                            No, no tengo seguro.

Sí, como no.   °¿ Puedo tener un cuarto privado?

No, no hay vacante.   doble?

No, lo siento. No puede.   múltiple?

Cuesta setenta y cinco dólares.   ¿Cuánto cuesta un cuarto privado?

                                                         doble?

                                                         múltiple?

Hospital	Patient

^o__Please__ come with me.
  go to the emergency room.

  go to the laboratory.
  sign here.

You must sign the authorization.
(One)

 ^oWhat must I sign?
     (one)

__The authorization__ for the operation.
     for the anesthesia.
     for the doctor.

 __For what__?

You must have the doctor's permission.
(One)

 ^oWhat must I have?
     (one)

__To__ leave.
 be discharged.
  (dismissed)

 __For what__?

You don't have to pay cash.
(One doesn't)

 Must I pay cash?
   (one)

__You must pay__ a minimum deposit.
(__One__)

 ^o__How much must I pay__?
       (__one__)

  the rest.
  what the insurance doesn't
   pay.
  100 dollars deposit.

  200 dollars deposit.

  300 dollars deposit.

  400 dollars deposit.

  500 dollars deposit.

Hospital	Paciente

Hospital / Paciente

°Favor de venir conmigo. — Gracias.

      ir a la sala de emergencia.
              (urgencia)

      ir al laboratorio.

      firmar aquí.

Hay que firmar la autorización. — °¿Qué hay que firmar?

La autorización para la operación. — ¿Para qué?

             para la anestesia.

             para el médico.

Hay que tener el permiso del médico. — °¿Qué hay que tener?

Para salir. — ¿Para qué?

    darle de alta.

No hay que pagar al contado. — ¿Hay que pagar al contado?

Hay que pagar un depósito mínimo. — °¿Cuánto hay que pagar?

        el resto.

        lo que no paga el seguro.

        cien dólares de depósito.

        doscientos dólares de
          depósito.

        trescientos dólares de
          depósito.

        cuatrocientos dólares de
          depósito.

        quinientos dólares de
          depósito.

Hospital	Patient
You must pay in the office. (One)	°Where must I pay? (one)
at the cashier's office.	
the cashier.	
Yes, you can pay on terms.	°Can I pay on terms?
	by the month?
	in January?
	in February?
	in March?
	in April?
	in May?
	in June?
	in July?
	in August?
	in September?
	in October?
	in November?
	in December?
°You can pay 50 dollars in January.	In January?
25 dollars in February.	In February?
You must enter on Sunday. (One)	°When must I enter the hospital? (one)
on Monday.	
on Tuesday.	
on Wednesday.	
on Thursday.	
on Friday.	
on Saturday.	

Hospital   Paciente

Hay que pagar en la oficina.   °¿Dónde hay que pagar?

        en la caja.

        a la cajera.

Sí, usted puede pagar a plazos.   °¿Puedo pagar a plazos?

                        por meses?

                        en enero?

                        en febrero?

                        en marzo?

                        en abril?

                        en mayo?

                        en junio?

                        en julio?

                        en agosto?

                        en septiembre?

                        en octubre?

                        en noviembre?

                        en diciembre?

°Usted puede pagar cincuenta dólares
   en enero.   ¿En enero?

   veinticinco dólares en febrero.   ¿En febrero?

Hay que entrar el domingo.   °¿Cuándo hay que entrar en el hospital?

       el lunes.

       el martes.

       el miércoles.

       el jueves.

       el viernes.

       el sábado.

General Hospital

Authorization for the Surgeon to Operate

Date_____ 19_____ Hour_____

I, _____, hereby give my consent for the surgical
        (name of patient)

procedure known as _____.
                        (type of operation or procedure)

I certify that the reasons such a procedure is considered necessary, its

advantages and possible complications, as well as alternate treatments,

have been explained to me by _____, and in view
                              (name of doctor or surgeon)

of this information, I the undersigned authorize _____
                                                  (name of surgeon)

to perform under whatever anesthesia he believes necessary the

above-mentioned operation and also to do any additional procedures that

may be therapeutically necessary, based on what is discovered in the course

of the operation. I also authorize the surgeon, or the hospital, to dis-

pose of the tissues removed surgically in the usual manner in such cases.

Witness_____ Signed_____
                                        (patient or nearest relative)

Witness_____ _____
                                        (relationship)

The authorization must be signed by the patient, or by the nearest relative

if the patient is a minor or is physically or mentally incapacitated.

IDENTIFICATION

By using your knowledge of medical consent forms and picking out key words and cognate words, analyze what the following consent form says.

<u>Hospital General</u>

<u>Autorización al cirujano para operar</u>

Fecha_____ 19_____ Hora_____

Yo,_____, por este medio doy mi
       (nombre de paciente)

consentimiento para el procedimiento quirúrgico conocido como

_____.
          (tipo de operación o procedimiento)

Certifico que las razones por las cuales tal procedimiento se considera

necesario, sus ventajas y posibles complicaciones, así como los tratamientos

alternos, me han sido explicados por _____,
                              (nombre del médico o del cirujano)

y en vista de esta información, el firmante autoriza a _____
                                           (nombre de cirujano)

para efectuar bajo la anestesia que crea necesaria la operación arriba

mencionada y también para efectuar los procedimientos adicionales que

puedan ser terapéuticamente necesarios basados en lo que se descubra en

el curso de la operación. También autorizo que el cirujano, o el hospital,

disponga de los tejidos removidos quirúrgicamente del modo acostumbrado en

tales casos.

Testigo_____ Firmado_____
                                     (paciente o pariente más cercano)

Testigo_____ _____
                                     (relación de parentesco)

La autorización tiene que ser firmada por el paciente o por el pariente

más cercano en caso de ser el paciente menor de edad o cuando el paciente

esté física o mentalmente incompetente o incapacitado.

GRAMMAR AND STRUCTURES DRILLED IN LESSON 8

verbs

    hay que + infinitive -- one must + verb

        Hay que pagar.   One must pay. (In English, often I or you is more
                      conversational.)

    favor de + infinitive -- please + verb

        Favor de ir.   Please go.

    poder + infinitive -- can + verb

        Puedo pagar aquí.   I can pay here.
        Sí, usted puede pagar aquí.   Yes, you can pay here.

months of the year

days of the week

Lesson 9
In the Hospital: Clothing

NEW MATERIAL

Hospital	Patient
^o<u>What are you going to take to the</u> <u>hospital</u>?	<u>I'm going to take</u> my robe.
	my slippers.
	my nightgown.
	my pajamas.
^o<u>What are you going to put on today</u>? (<u>wear</u>)	<u>I'm going to put on</u> my dress. (<u>wear</u>)
	my skirt.
	my pants suit.
	my blouse.
	my bra.
	my girdle.
	my slip.
	my panties.
	my hose. (stockings)
	my shoes.
	my coat.
	my scarf.
	my rings.
	my earrings.
	my wig.

Lección 9
En el hospital: La ropa

MATERIA NUEVA

Hospital

¿Qué va a llevar al hospital?

°¿Qué va a ponerse hoy?

Paciente

Voy a llevar la bata.

las zapatillas.

la camisa de noche.

las pijamas.
(las piyamas)

Voy a ponerme el vestido.

la falda.

el traje pantalón.

la blusa.

el sostén.

la faja.

la enagua.

el pantalón.
(los calzones)
(las pantaletas)

las medias.

los zapatos.

el abrigo.

la bufanda.

los anillos.

los aretes.

la peluca.

Hospital	Patient

Hospital   Patient

^oSir, are you going to put on your suit?   No, I'm not going to put on my suit.
                    (wear)   (wear)

    your tie?

    your belt?

    your shorts?

    your undershirt?

    your sweater?

    your shirt?

    your vest?

^oSir, are you going to put on   Yes, I'm going to put on
                    (wear)   (wear)

    your pants?   my pants.
     (slacks)   (my slacks)

    your socks?

    your shoes?

    your jacket?

    your watch?

^oPlease put on your robe.   My robe? Right away.

       your slippers.

       your shoes.

       your pajamas.

       your sweater.

Your watch? Gladly.   ^oPlease put away my watch.

                                 my ring.

                                 my jeweled ring.

                                 my billfold.

                                 my handbag.
                                  (purse)

                                 my money.

Hospital	Paciente
°Señor, ¿va usted a ponerse el traje?	No, no voy a ponerme el traje.

la corbata?

el cinturón?

los calzoncillos?

la camiseta?

el suéter?

la camisa?

el chaleco?

°Señor, ¿va usted a ponerse	Sí, voy a ponerme

los pantalones?
(el pantalón)

los calcetines?

los zapatos?

la chaqueta?

el reloj?

los pantalones.
(el pantalón)

°Favor de ponerse la bata.	¿La bata? Ahora mismo.

las zapatillas.

los zapatos.

las pijamas.

el suéter.

¿El reloj? Con mucho gusto.	°Favor de guardar el reloj.

el anillo.

la sortija.

la cartera.
(la billetera)

la bolsa.
(el bolso)
(la cartera)

el dinero.

Hospital	Patient
Your bracelet? <u>Gladly</u>.	^o<u>Please put away</u> my bracelet.
	my glasses.
	my contact lenses.
	my documents.
	my checkbook.
^o<u>Please</u> take the medicine.	<u>Very well</u>. Right away.
wear your robe.	
sign here.	
go to the bathroom.	

Mrs. López is going to the emergency room of a local hospital. She says that she has sharp pains in the abdomen. The doctor has diagnosed acute appendicitis and has ordered that she be admitted for an operation.

But Mrs. López doesn't want to go to the hospital because her husband is out of town and she has two children in elementary school. What a problem!

Hospital	Paciente
¿La pulsera? Con mucho gusto.	°Favor de guardar la pulsera.

°Favor de guardar la pulsera.
                        (el brazalete)

                 los lentes.
                 (los anteojos)
                 (los espejuelos)

                 los lentes de contacto.

                 los documentos.

                 el libro de cheques.

°Favor de tomar la medicina.   Muy bien. Ahora mismo.
       usar la bata.
       firmar aquí.
       ir al baño.

IDENTIFICATION

La señora López va a la sala de emergencia de un hospital local. Dice que tiene fuertes dolores en el abdomen. El médico diagnostica apendicitis aguda y ordena que sea admitida para operarla.

Pero la señora López no quiere ingresar en el hospital porque su esposo no está en la ciudad y tiene dos hijos en la escuela elemental. ¡Qué problema!

In the first paragraph, underline these key words:

señora López	diagnostica
sala de emergencia	apendicitis
hospital	ordena
dolores	admitida
abdomen	operarla
médico	

In the second paragraph, underline these key words:

señora López	no está
no	dos hijos
ingresar	escuela
hospital	problema
esposo	

<u>IDENTIFICATION</u> (continued)

Now, write the English beside each word you know in the above lists. Then guess the ones you don't know. Summarize in English what you think each paragraph says. Notice that <u>no</u> is always an important key word.

<u>GRAMMAR AND STRUCTURES DRILLED IN LESSON 9</u>

verbs

<u>ir</u> -- to go   <u>voy</u> -- I go, I'm going   <u>va</u> -- you go, you're going

<u>ir a</u> + infinitive -- to be going to + verb

<u>Voy a llevar el traje.</u>   I'm going to take my suit.

<u>favor de</u> + infinitive -- please + verb

<u>Favor de guardar mi anillo.</u>   Please put away my ring.

<u>ponerse</u> -- to put on, wear

¿<u>Va usted a ponerse la falda</u>?   Are you going to put on your skirt?
<u>Sí, voy a ponerme la falda.</u>   Yes, I'm going to put on my skirt.

definite article as possessive with articles of clothing (see examples with <u>ponerse</u>)

simple negation

subject pronoun <u>usted</u>

Lesson 10
In the Hospital: Articles for Personal Use

NEW MATERIAL

Hospital	Patient

Hospital

The bathroom is here.

Patient

°Where is the bathroom?

the closet?

The bed is near.

Where is the bed?

the table?

the stationery?

the magazine?

the newspaper?

the vase?

the pen?

the thermometer?

The lavatory is there.
is far.

°Where is the lavatory?

the washbowl?

The toilet is far.
(The commode)

Where is the toilet?
(the commode)

the shower?

the tub?

Lección 10
En el hospital: Artículos de uso personal

Hospital	Paciente
El baño está aquí.	°¿Dónde está el baño?
	el closet?
	(el gabinete para la ropa)
	(el ropero)
	(el armario)
La cama está cerca.	¿Dónde está la cama?
	la mesa?
	el papel para escribir?
	la revista?
	el periódico?
	(el diario)
	el florero?
	la pluma?
	el termómetro?
El lavamanos está allí. está lejos.	°¿Dónde está el lavamanos?
	el lavabo?
	la palangana?
El excusado está lejos. (El inodoro)	¿Dónde está el excusado?
	(el inodoro)
	la ducha?
	(la regadera)
	la bañandera?
	(la tina)

Hospital

^OWhere is the thermometer?

the basin for vomit?
(the emesis basin)

the basin for a bed bath?

the bedpan?

the urinal?

The books are here.

Patient

The thermometer? Here.

The basin for vomit? Here.

^OWhere are the books?

the flowers?

the stamps?

the magazines?

^OWhat do you need, sir?

Soap?

Deodorant?

Toothpaste?

Your toothbrush?

Your hairbrush?

Your comb?

Your razor?

Some razor blades?

Some scissors?

A pitcher?

Lotion?

Water?

Ice?

A glass?

Yes, I need soap.

Hospital	Paciente
°¿Dónde está el termómetro?	¿El termómetro? Aquí.
el tazón de vómito? (la vasija para vomitar)	¿El tazón de vómito? Aquí.
la bandeja para el baño?	
el bacín? (el bidet) (la cuña) (la chata) (la taza) (la paleta) (la silleta) (el pato)	
el orinal?	

Los libros están aquí.

°¿Dónde están los libros?

las flores?

los sellos?
(las estampillas)

las revistas?

° ¿Qué necesita usted, señor?

¿El jabón?

¿El desodorante?

¿La pasta de dientes?

¿El cepillo de dientes?

¿El cepillo de cabeza?

¿El peine?

¿La máquina de afeitar?

¿Unas cuchillas de afeitar?

¿Unas tijeras?

¿Una jarra?

¿Loción?

¿Agua?

¿Hielo?

¿Un vaso?

Sí, necesito el jabón.

Hospital	Patient
^o<u>Do you need</u> talcum powder, ma'am?	<u>Yes, I need</u> talcum powder.
perfume	
cream	
cosmetics	
makeup	
rollers	
a mirror	
^o<u>What do you need, ma'am</u>?	<u>I need</u> tampons.
	sanitary napkins.
	tissues.
	bathroom tissue.
	the towel.
	the washcloth.
<u>What do you need, miss</u>?	<u>I need</u> a blanket.
	a pillow.
	my robe.
	my slippers.

Hospital   Paciente

°¿Necesita usted talco, señora?   Sí, necesito talco.
              perfume
              crema
              cosméticos
              maquillaje
              rollos
              un espejo

°¿Qué necesita usted, señora?   Necesito tampones.
                                              (tapones)

                                              servilletas sanitarias.
                                              (kotex)

                                              pañuelos de papel.
                                              (kleenex)

                                              papel para el baño.

                                              la toalla.

                                              la toallita.

¿Qué necesita usted, señorita?   Necesito una frazada.
                                              (una manta)

                                              una almohada.

                                              la bata.

                                              las zapatillas.

They took my neighbor to the hospital in an ambulance. It was an emergency. Luckily her sister-in-law was visiting her, and she called my neighbor's husband at work to tell him. The woman is suffering from heart trouble, and they had to take her to the intensive care unit.

You know that the intensive care unit is only for patients who are critically ill and need special attention and equipment. The patients are admitted by a doctor's orders. Special nurses watch these patients carefully. There is oxygen available for every patient in case it is needed in an emergency, and a hospital doctor is available at all hours.

I would like to visit my neighbor, but only one person can visit a patient when he's in intensive care.

Her husband took her a suitcase with clothing. She doesn't need a nightgown right now, but she wants her toothbrush, makeup, a comb, and a hairbrush. She can only have a few things there.

IDENTIFICATION

Consult the list of cognates that end in -ia on pp. 529, 531. Generally, Spanish words that end in -ancia or -encia correspond to English words that end in -ance or -ence. Most of the others that end in -ia have the same ending in English. Practice pronouncing these words.

Some of these cognates, as well as new vocabulary and other cognates, are used in the following paragraphs. Read the Spanish aloud, and then try to answer the questions before looking at the translation.

A mi vecina la llevaron al hospital en una ambulancia. Fue un caso de emergencia. Afortunadamente su cuñada estaba de visita en su casa y llamó al esposo de mi vecina al trabajo para darle la información. La señora padece del corazón y la han tenido que llevar a la unidad de cuidados intensivos.

Usted sabe que la unidad de cuidados intensivos es sólo para pacientes en estado crítico que necesitan atención y equipo especiales. Los pacientes son admitidos por orden médica. Enfermeras especializadas vigilan con cuidado a estos pacientes. Hay oxígeno disponible para cada enfermo en caso de que se necesite de urgencia, y un médico del hospital está disponible a todas horas.

Me gustaría visitar a mi vecina, pero sólo una persona puede entrar a visitar a un enfermo cuando está en la sala de cuidados intensivos.

Su esposo le llevó una maleta con su ropa. Ella no necesita una bata de dormir inmediatamente, pero quiere su cepillo de dientes, maquillaje, un peine y un cepillo de cabeza. Sólo muy pocas cosas puede tener allí.

1. What happened to the neighbor, and where is she now?

2. What is available in this unit?

3. What does the neighbor need?

GRAMMAR AND STRUCTURES DRILLED IN LESSON 10

verbs

<u>estar</u> -- to be   <u>está</u> -- (it) is   <u>están</u> -- (they) are

to show place where something is

<u>El baño está aquí.</u>   The bathroom is here.

<u>necesitar</u> -- to need   <u>necesito</u> -- I need   <u>necesita</u> -- you need, do you
                                                      need?

Lesson 11
In the Hospital: Rules and Rooms

NEW MATERIAL

Hospital	Patient
^oWhat do you need?	I need a private room.
	a special nurse.
	the bedpan.
You need to sign here.	All right. I'm going to sign here.
go to the bathroom.	
pay in the office.	
buy the medicine.	
sleep.	
close your eyes.	
leave now.	
wait outside.	
go to the laboratory now.	
ring the bell.	
You need to write your address.	All right. I'm going to write my address.
call your husband.	call my husband.
call your mother.	call my mother.
call your daughter.	call my daughter.
I need to change the bed.	^oWhat do you need?
close the door.	
raise the head of the bed.	
the foot	
lower the head of the bed.	
the foot	

130

Lección 11
En el hospital: Reglamentos y cuartos

MATERIA NUEVA

Hospital	Paciente

°¿Qué necesita usted?

Necesito un cuarto privado.

una enfermera especial.

el bacín.
(la chata)

Usted necesita firmar aquí.

Muy bien. Voy a firmar aquí.

    ir al baño.

    pagar en la oficina.

    comprar la medicina.

    dormir.

    cerrar los ojos.

    salir ahora.

    esperar afuera.

    ir al laboratorio ahora.

    tocar el timbre.

Usted necesita escribir su dirección.

Muy bien. Voy a escribir mi dirección.

    llamar a su esposo.

    llamar a mi esposo.

    llamar a su madre.

    llamar a mi madre.

    llamar a su hija.

    llamar a mi hija.

Necesito cambiar la cama.

°¿Qué necesita usted?

    cerrar la puerta.

    levantar la cabecera de la cama.
        los pies

    bajar la cabecera de la cama.
        los pies

Hospital	Patient
^o<u>What do you need?</u>	<u>I need to</u> use the telephone.
	turn on the light.
	turn off the light.
	turn on the television.
	turn off the television.
Open the drapes? <u>Gladly</u>.	^o<u>Please</u> open the drapes.
(blinds)	(blinds)
Close the door?	close the door.
	turn on the air conditioning.
	change the bed.
	put the flowers on the table.
	put the flowers on the dresser.
	put the flowers outside.
<u>You may visit</u> from 2:00 to 4:00.	^o<u>When may I visit</u>?
(One)	(one)
from 7:00 to 9:00.	
after 8:00.	
at any time.	
in the afternoon.	
You may not visit in the morning.	
<u>You may see the patient</u> now.	When may I see the patient?
(One)	(one)
after 2:00.	
later.	
<u>You may</u> visit <u>now</u>.	When may I visit?
(One)	(one)
	eat?
	pay?
	leave?

Hospital	Paciente
°¿Qué necesita usted?	Necesito usar el teléfono.
	encender la luz.
	apagar la luz.
	poner el televisor.
	apagar el televisor.
¿Abrir la cortina? Con mucho gusto.	°Favor de abrir la cortina.
¿Cerrar la puerta?	
	cerrar la puerta.
	poner el aireacondicionado.
	cambiar la cama.
	poner las flores en la mesa.
	poner las flores en el tocador.
	poner las flores afuera.
Se puede visitar de dos a cuatro.	°¿Cuándo se puede visitar?
de siete a nueve.	
después de las ocho.	
a todas horas. (a cualquier hora)	
por la tarde.	
No se puede visitar por la mañana.	
Se puede ver al paciente ahora.	¿Cuándo se puede ver al paciente?
después de las dos.	
más tarde.	
Se visita ahora.	¿Cuándo se visita?
	se come?
	se paga?
	se sale?

Hospital

<u>Breakfast is served</u> now.
early.
right away.
late.
soon.

^o<u>When is</u> breakfast <u>served</u>?

lunch?

dinner?
(the meal)

supper?

They're flexible.

One person can stay with the patient at night.

Children under 15 years of age can't visit.

The patient can receive visitors.

<u>What are the rules</u>?

Hospital	Paciente

<u>Se sirve el</u> desayuno ahora.
       temprano.
       en seguida.
       tarde.
       pronto.

° ¿<u>Cuándo se sirve</u> el desayuno?

        el almuerzo?

        la comida?

        la cena?

Son flexibles.

¿<u>Cuáles son las reglas</u>?

Una persona puede estar con el paciente
  de noche.

Menores de quince años no pueden visitar.

El paciente puede recibir visitas.

PART A

Mrs. M.:   I'm going to have to go to the hospital, and I need information.

Hospital: What information would you like?

Mrs. M.:   What are the rooms like?

Hospital: They're large, they have a comfortable bed, telephone and television. The bed is beside the window.

Mrs. M.:   How much does a private room cost?

Hospital: About $65 a day.

Mrs. M.:   And a semi-private room?

Hospital: About $53 a day.

PART B·

Mrs. M.:   Is it necessary to pay cash?

Hospital: No, it isn't necessary if you have insurance.

Mrs. M.:   And if I don't have insurance?

Hospital: Then you do have to pay cash.

Mrs. M.:   May I have visitors?

Hospital: At certain hours, if you feel well enough.

IDENTIFICATION

First read through the entire conversation below for general meaning. Then reread Part A, reading only the underlined words. Notice that these underlined key words are ones that you have already studied, or they are cognates. They tell you everything important about the conversation up to this point. In Part B there are some new words, such as en efectivo, which you can figure out. Look at the context of questions and answers in the first four lines in Part B. Keep in mind the no. Also, Si means if. (Sí, with accent, means yes.) Of course, when you hear them, they sound the same, but you can usually tell what is meant by the context. Now, in Part B, if you cannot figure out line 1, look at line 2:

Key words in answer, line 2:

No,   si   tiene   seguro.
No,   if   you have insurance.

Now go back to the question, line 1:

¿Es necesario   pagar   en efectivo?
Is it necessary   to pay   _____?

You should now be able to guess correctly what en efectivo means.

Mrs. Martínez is calling the hospital:

PART A

Mrs. M.: Voy a tener que ir al hospital y necesito información.

Hospital: ¿Qué información desea?

Mrs. M.: ¿Cómo son los cuartos?

Hospital: Son amplios, tienen una cama cómoda, teléfono y televisor. La cama está al lado de la ventana.

Mrs. M.: ¿Cuánto cuesta un cuarto privado?

Hospital: Como sesenta y cinco dólares diarios.

Mrs. M.: ¿Y un cuarto semi-privado?

Hospital: Unos cincuenta y tres dólares diarios.

PART B

Mrs. M.: ¿Es necesario pagar en efectivo?

Hospital: No, no es necesario si usted tiene seguro.

Mrs. M.: ¿Y si no tengo seguro?

Hospital: Entonces sí tiene que pagar en efectivo.

Mrs. M.: ¿Puedo tener visitas?

Hospital: A ciertas horas, si usted se siente bien.

GRAMMAR AND STRUCTURES DRILLED IN LESSON 11

verbs

    necesitar + infinitive -- to need to + verb

        Necesito dormir.   I need to sleep.
        Necesita esperar afuera.   You need to wait outside.

    ir a + infinitive -- to be going to + verb

    favor de + infinitive -- please + verb

reflexive pronoun se as impersonal subject

    ¿Cuándo se come?   When does one (may I) eat?
    Se come ahora.   One (you) may eat now.

Lesson 12
Laboratory: Examinations

<u>NEW MATERIAL</u>

Hospital	Patient
Yes, you need a complete examination.	°Do I need a physical examination?
°<u>Please</u> make a fist.	A fist? <u>All right.</u> <u>Like this</u>? <u>What else</u>?
open your hand.	My hand?
bend your arm.	My arm?
roll up your sleeve.	
go to the bathroom.	
urinate in this receptacle.	
<u>I'm going to do</u> a urinalysis.	°<u>What are you going to do</u>? A urinalysis?
<u>an analysis</u> of your blood.	<u>An analysis</u> of my blood?
	of the smear?
	of the sputum?
	of the vomit?
	of the excrement?
<u>I'm going to</u> take an x-ray.	°<u>What are you going to do</u>? <u>Are you going to</u> take an x-ray?
	take a count?
	take blood?
	take a sample?
	take a smear?
<u>I'm going to</u> measure the albumin.	°<u>Are you going to</u> measure the albumin?
	measure the coagulation?
	measure my metabolism?
	analyze my blood?
	analyze my urine?
	analyze my sputum?

Lección 12
Laboratorio: Exámenes

MATERIA NUEVA

Hospital	Paciente
Sí, usted necesita un reconocimiento completo.	°¿Necesito un reconocimiento médico?

°Favor de cerrar el puño.	¿El puño? Bien.
	        ¿Así?
	        ¿Qué más?

abrir la mano.	¿La mano?
doblar el brazo.	¿El brazo?
levantarse la manga.	
ir al baño.	
orinar en este recipiente.	
Le voy a hacer un urinálisis.	°¿Qué va a hacer? ¿Un urinálisis?
un análisis de sangre.	¿Un análisis de sangre?

del unto.
        (del frotis)
	del unto?
	        (del frotis)

	del esputo?
	del vómito?
	del excremento?
Le voy a hacer una radiografía.	°¿Qué me va a hacer? ¿Me va a hacer una radiografía?
	hacer un conteo? (un recuento globular)
	sacar sangre?
	tomar una muestra?
	tomar un unto? (un frotis)
Le voy a medir la albúmina.	°¿Me va a medir la albúmina?
	medir la coagulación?
	medir el metabolismo?
	analizar la sangre?
	analizar la orina?
	analizar el esputo?

Hospital   Patient

We're going to do the rabbit test.   °What test are you (plural) going to do?

  a test for Rh factor.
  a test to see if you're pregnant.

  a blood test.
  a test for sugar in the blood.
  Pap smears.

°Do you have the written order for the
  blood count?   Yes. Here.

Yes, I have many instruments.   °Do you have various instruments?
                                                      various syringes?
                                                      various tubes?
                                                      various microscopes?
                                                      various things?

°Do you have much pain?   No. I have little pain.
        much work?   Yes. I have a lot of work.
        many relatives?   No. I have few relatives.
        many friends?

I'm going to examine you (m.).   °What are you going to do?
        examine you (f.).

°Please get up on the table.   Yes, of course.
     get down.
     open your arms.
     put your legs apart.
     take a deep breath.

     hold your breath.

Hospital	Paciente

Hospital

Vamos a hacer <u>el examen</u> del conejo.

    del factor Rhesus.

    para saber si está embarazada.
    (para saber si está encinta)
    (para saber si está en estado de
      gestación)

    de sangre.

    de azúcar en la sangre.

    los untos de Papanicolaou.
    (los frotis)

º¿Tiene usted la orden escrita para el
    recuento globular?

<u>Sí, tengo</u> muchos instrumentos.

Paciente

º¿Qué examen van a hacer?

Sí. Aquí.

º¿<u>Tiene usted</u> varios instrumentos?

              varias jeringuillas?

              varios tubos?

              varios microscopios?

              varias cosas?

º¿<u>Tiene usted</u> mucho dolor?

           mucho trabajo?

           muchos parientes?

           muchos amigos?

No. <u>Tengo poco</u> dolor.

<u>Sí. Tengo</u> mucho trabajo.

No. <u>Tengo pocos</u> parientes.

Voy a examinarlo.
      examinarla.

º¿Qué va a hacer?

º<u>Favor de</u> subir a la mesa.

        bajar.

        abrir los brazos.

        separar las piernas.

        hacer una inspiración profunda.
      (respirar profundamente)

        sostener la respiración.

<u>Sí, cómo no.</u>

Patient: I have to go to the laboratory. The technician is going to take
some samples for analysis.

Hospital: What analyses does he have to do?

Patient: I don't know. All the doctor wants. I think they're a urinalysis,
a blood count, and a chest x-ray.

Hospital: You're lucky. Those are routine examinations. Sometimes the tests
are very bothersome and complicated.

Patient: And also very expensive.

Hospital: That's always true. But it's necessary to go to the doctor and
follow his directions in order to have good health.

Patient: You're right.

Hospital: Let's go to the laboratory now.

Patient: I hope the technician doesn't pinch my finger or arm.

Hospital: It won't hurt.

IDENTIFICATION

In the conversation below, key words, cognate words, and words that you have just learned in this lesson are underlined once. See if you can get the general meaning of the conversation by looking at them. Other words are double underlined. See how many of these you can guess. Look at the words around them, or consider what might be the gist of a conversation involving the words you do know. You may miss several, but with intelligent guessing, you may be surprised how many you can figure out.

The patient is talking with a nurse at the hospital:

Paciente: Tengo que ir al laboratorio. El técnico va a tomar unas muestras

para los análisis.

Hospital: ¿Qué análisis tiene que hacer?

Paciente: No sé. Todos los que el médico quiera. Creo que son un análisis

de orina, un recuento globular y una radiografía del tórax.

Hospital: Usted tiene suerte. Esos son exámenes de rutina. A veces los

exámenes son muy molestos y complicados.

Paciente: Y también muy caros.

Hospital: Eso siempre. Pero es necesario ir al médico y seguir sus órdenes

para tener buena salud.

Paciente: Usted tiene razón.

Hospital: Vamos al laboratorio ahora.

Paciente: Ojalá que el técnico no me pinche el dedo, o el brazo.

Hospital: No va a tener dolor.

GRAMMAR AND STRUCTURES DRILLED IN LESSON 12

verbs

   ir -- to go

   ir a + infinitive -- to be going to + verb

   voy a -- I'm going to   va a -- you're going to
   vamos a -- we're going to   van a -- you're going to (plural)
                                         they're going to

   favor de + infinitive -- please + verb

adjectives

   mucho -- much, a lot of   poco -- little   varios -- various
   muchos -- many   pocos -- few

   agreement with nouns

      Tiene varias cosas. You have various things.

   indirect object pronoun to show personal involvement

      Le voy a hacer un análisis de sangre. I'm going to do an analysis of
                                             your blood.

Lesson 13
Diagnostics: Symptoms

NEW MATERIAL

| Hospital | Patient |

○How long have you had indigestion?   For 1 hour.
    constipation?   1 day.
    diarrhea?   some days.
    little appetite?   1 week.
    belching?   1 month.
    sweating?   some months.
    fever?   1 year.
    hives?
    yellowish skin?
    many colds?

○How long have you had a cough?   For 2 hours I've had a cough.
    expectoration when you cough?   2 days
    bad odor in the expectoration?   2 weeks
    asthma?   2 months
    sinus trouble?
    phlegm?
    mucus?

○How long have you had cramps?
    weakness?
    dizziness?
    tingling?
    nervousness?
    obstruction in the esophagus?

○You have dizziness? For how long?   For 3 days I've had dizziness.
                               3 hours
                                 3 weeks
                                 3 months
                                 3 years

Lección 13
Diagnóstico: Síntomas

MATERIA NUEVA

<table>
<tr><td align="center">Hospital</td><td align="center">Paciente</td></tr>
</table>

°¿Desde cuándo tiene usted indigestión?   Hace una hora.

    constipación?   un día.

    diarrea?   unos días.

    poco apetito?   una semana.

    eructos?   un mes.

    sudores?   unos meses.

    fiebre?   un año.

    urticaria?

    la piel amarilla?

    muchos resfriados?

°¿Desde cuándo tiene usted tos?   Hace dos horas que tengo tos.

    expectoración al toser?   dos días

    mal olor en la expectoración?   dos semanas

    asma?   dos meses

    sinusitis?   dos años

    flema?

    mucosidad?

°¿Desde cuándo tiene usted calambres?

    debilidad?

    mareo?

    hormigueo?

    nerviosidad?

    obstrucción en el esófago?

°¿Usted tiene mareo? ¿Desde cuándo?   Hace tres días que tengo mareo.

                                           tres horas

                                         tres semanas

                                         tres meses

                                         tres años

Hospital	Patient

°<u>You have</u> difficulty swallowing? <u>For how long</u>?

    shortness of breath?

    burning when you urinate?

    burning in the urethra?

    hemorrhaging?

    fainting?

    cramps?

    colic?

    convulsions?

<u>For</u> 2 days <u>I've had</u> difficulty swallowing.

    shortness of breath.

    burning when I urinate.

    burning in the urethra.

    hemorrhaging.

    fainting.

    cramps.

    colic.

    convulsions.

°<u>How long have you had</u> headaches?

    insomnia?

    vomiting of blood?

    nausea?

    weakness?

    an ear infection?

<u>I've had</u> headaches <u>for</u> a week.

°<u>How long have you had</u> suppuration?
                (discharge of pus)

    this pimple?

    itching?

    a rash?

    a stuffy nose?

    numbness in your arm?

°<u>How long have you had</u> a sore throat?

    backache?

    low back pain?
   (pain in back at the waist)

    headache?

<u>I've had</u> a sore throat <u>for</u> 3 days.

Hospital	Paciente

°¿Usted tiene dificultad al tragar? ¿Desde cuándo?

Hace dos días que tengo dificultad al tragar.

falta de aire?

falta de aire.

ardor al orinar?

ardor al orinar.

ardor en la uretra?

ardor en la uretra.

hemorragia?

hemorragia.

desmayos?

desmayos.

calambres?

calambres.

cólicos?

cólicos.

convulsiones?

convulsiones.

°¿Desde cuándo tiene usted jaqueca?

Hace una semana que tengo jaqueca.

insomnio?

vómitos de sangre?

náuseas?

debilidad?

infección del oído?

°¿Desde cuándo tiene usted supuración?
                          (pus)

este grano?

picazón?

erupción?

la nariz tupida?
          (tapada)

el brazo entumecido?

°¿Desde cuándo tiene usted dolor de garganta?

Hace tres días que tengo dolor de garganta.

dolor de espalda?

dolor de cintura?

dolor de cabeza?

Hospital	Patient
°Is <u>your</u> urine concentrated?	Yes, it's concentrated.
Do <u>you</u> have any vision difficulties?	No, <u>I</u> don't have any vision difficulties.
Do <u>you</u> see dark spots?	No, <u>I</u> don't see dark spots.
Do <u>you</u> see well?	Yes, <u>I</u> see well.
Do <u>you</u> eliminate well?	No, <u>I</u> don't eliminate well.
Do <u>you</u> urinate frequently?	
Are <u>your</u> bowel movements normal?	
Do <u>you</u> chew well?	
Do <u>you</u> drink enough water?	
milk?	
Do <u>you</u> walk much?	
Do <u>you</u> eat well?	
Do <u>you</u> rest well?	
Do <u>you</u> sleep well?	
Do <u>you</u> cough frequently?	

Hospital	Paciente
^o¿Tien<u>e</u> usted la orina concentrada?	Sí, ten<u>go</u> la orina concentrada.
¿Tien<u>e</u> usted trastornos en la vista?	No, no ten<u>go</u> trastornos en la vista.
¿V<u>e</u> usted obscuro?	No, no ve<u>o</u> obscuro.
¿V<u>e</u> usted bien?	Sí, ve<u>o</u> bien.
¿Elimin<u>a</u> usted bien?	No, y<u>o</u> no elimin<u>o</u> bien.
¿Orin<u>a</u> usted con frecuencia?	
¿Defec<u>a</u> usted normalmente?	
¿Mastic<u>a</u> usted bien?	
<u>¿Toma usted bastante</u> agua?	
leche?	
¿Camin<u>a</u> usted mucho?	
¿Com<u>e</u> usted bien?	
¿Descans<u>a</u> usted bien?	
¿Duerm<u>e</u> usted bien?	
¿Tos<u>e</u> usted con frecuencia?	

Nurse: Let's see the patient in Room 214, Mrs. Reyes.

Doctor: May I have the information?

Nurse: Gladly. Here it is.

Doctor: I see that the patient is resting well and eliminates well.

Nurse: Yes, doctor.

Doctor: She doesn't have any more bleeding?

Nurse: She hasn't had any bleeding for six hours, but she coughs a lot and
        is weak. She eats little, and she's nervous.

Doctor: Has she had convulsions or fainting?

Nurse: She hasn't fainted for two days.

Doctor: I need to examine the patient tomorrow and observe other symptoms.
        Have her continue the same diet one or two more days. She can get
        up and walk.

Nurse: The lady does walk from the bed to the bathroom. Today she's going
        to walk in the hallway.

Doctor: Very well, nurse. Thanks a lot.

Nurse: You're welcome, doctor. Let's go to see Mr. Gómez.

IDENTIFICATION

MEANING OF VERBS

One of the things that can make learning Spanish easy for you is the verb endings. In Spanish, the verb ending can indicate the subject (person or thing that does the action), whereas in English the subject must be supplied by another word. In the following conversation, notice that the underlined verbs all end in -a or -e. These endings can be understood to refer to different individuals. For example, va means "you are going," but it can also be understood to mean all of the following: "he is going," "she is going," "it is going." If se is added in front of va, then se va refers to "one" or "you" or "they" in a general sense (see Lesson 11).

The following conversation is between a doctor and a nurse about a patient, but all these things could be said directly to the patient, using the same underlined verbs. Read through the conversation, first referring to the woman patient; that is, think of all the underlined verbs as meaning she. Next, go back to the underlined verb phrases and read each one, saying usted (you) before it. The usted is not necessary to the meaning, but it is often more polite. Imagine you are stating these facts directly to the patient. For example, Usted descansa bien -- You are resting well.

Enfermera: Vamos a ver a la paciente en el cuarto 214, la señora Reyes.

Doctor: ¿Me permite la información?

Enfermera: Con mucho gusto. Aquí la tiene.

Doctor: Veo que la enferma descansa bien y elimina bien.

Enfermera: Sí, doctor.

Doctor: ¿Ya no tiene hemorragia?

Enfermera: Hace seis horas que no tiene hemorragia pero tose mucho y

tiene debilidad. Come poco y está nerviosa.

Doctor: ¿Ha tenido convulsiones o desmayos?

Enfermera: Hace dos días que no se desmaya.

Doctor: Necesito examinar a la paciente mañana y observar otros síntomas.

Que continúe con la misma dieta uno o dos días más. Puede

levantarse y caminar.

Enfermera: La señora camina de la cama al baño. Hoy va a caminar en los

pasillos.

Doctor: Muy bien, señorita. Muchas gracias.

Enfermera: De nada, doctor. Vamos a ver al señor Gómez.

GRAMMAR AND STRUCTURES DRILLED IN LESSON 13

verbs

-ar and -er verbs, first and third person of present tense

masticar -- to chew   mastico -- I chew   mastica -- you chew
(he chews)
(she chews)

comer -- to eat   como -- I eat   come -- you eat
(he eats)
(she eats)

hace + time + que + present tense -- length of time something has gone on

Hace dos días que tengo tos. I've had a cough for two days.

¿Desde cuándo + present tense . . . ? How long have (has) . . . ?

¿Desde cuándo tiene usted tos? How long have you had a cough?

Lesson 14
Diagnostics: Medical History

<u>NEW MATERIAL</u>

Hospital	Patient

°<u>Do you have</u> tonsilitis?

No, doctor, <u>I don't have</u> tonsilitis.

    diabetes?

    cancer?

    paralysis?

    high blood pressure?

    difficulty in breathing?

    shortness of breath?

    pain in the chest?

    pain in the region of the heart?

    palpitations?

    bluish lips and nails?

    swelling in the legs?

    swelling in the feet?

    swelling in the hands?

    swelling around the eyes?

<u>Do you</u> tire easily when you walk?

°<u>Do you suffer from</u> heart trouble?
    (<u>have</u>)

No, doctor, <u>I don't suffer from</u> heart
              (<u>have</u>)
trouble.

    kidney disease?

    liver disease?

    nervous disorders?

    throat problems?

    rheumatism?

    epilepsy?

    colitis?

    anemia?

Lección 14
Diagnóstico: Historia médica

<u>MATERIA NUEVA</u>

Hospital	Paciente
º¿<u>Tiene usted</u> amigdalitis? (tonsilitis)	<u>No</u>, doctor, <u>no tengo</u> amigdalitis. (tonsilitis)

diabetes?

cáncer?

parálisis?

alta presión?

dificultad al respirar?

la respiración corta?

dolor en el pecho?

dolor en la región del corazón?

palpitaciones?

los labios y las uñas azules?

hinchazón en las piernas?

hinchazón en los pies?

hinchazón en las manos?

hinchazón en los ojos?

¿<u>Tiene usted</u> cansancio al caminar?

º¿<u>Padece usted</u> del corazón?   No, doctor, no padezco del corazón.

de los riñones?

del hígado?

de los nervios?

de la garganta?

de reumatismo?

de epilepsia?

de colitis?

de anemia?

Hospital	Patient

O<u>Do you suffer from</u> acne?

<u>No, doctor, I don't suffer from</u> acne.

    bursitis?

    diabetes?

    hoarseness?

    asthma?

O<u>Have you had</u> tonsilitis?

                    No, doctor, <u>I have</u> not <u>had</u> tonsilitis.

    blood diseases?

    childhood illnesses?

    scarlet fever?

    measles?

    German measles?

    diphtheria?

    whooping cough?

    rheumatic fever?

    epilepsy?

    anemia?

    jaundice?

    diverticulitis?

    colitis?

    appendicitis?

O<u>What have you had</u>? Paralysis?

                    <u>I've had</u> paralysis.

    Diabetes?

    Cancer?

    High blood pressure?

    A heart attack?

    Difficulty in breathing?

    Pain in the chest?

    Pain in the region of the heart?

    Palpitations?

    Shortness of breath?

    Tiredness when you walk?

    Bluish lips and nails?

    Swelling in the legs?

    Swelling in the feet?

Hospital	Paciente
º¿Padece usted de acné?	No, doctor, no padezco de acné.
de bursitis?	
de diabetes?	
de ronquera?	
de asma?	

º¿Ha tenido usted amigdalitis?	No doctor, no he tenido amigdalitis.
(tonsilitis)	(tonsilitis)
enfermedades de la sangre?	
enfermedades de la infancia?	
escarlatina?	
sarampión?	
rubéola?	
difteria?	
tos ferina?	
fiebre reumática?	
epilepsia?	
anemia?	
ictericia?	
diverticulitis?	
colitis?	
apendicitis?	

º¿Qué ha tenido usted? ¿Parálisis?	He tenido parálisis.
¿Diabetes?	
¿Cáncer?	
¿Alta presión?	
¿Un ataque de corazón?	
¿Dificultad al respirar?	
¿Dolor en el pecho?	
¿Dolor en la región del corazón?	
¿Palpitaciones?	
¿La respiración corta?	
¿Cansancio al caminar?	
¿Los labios y las uñas azules?	
¿Hinchazón en las piernas?	
¿Hinchazón en los pies?	

Hospital	Patient
°What <u>have you felt</u>?	<u>I've felt</u> pain in my legs.
	pains in the chest.
	weakness.
	tiredness when I walk.
<u>Have you</u> slept <u>well</u>?	Yes, <u>I've</u> slept <u>well</u>.
eaten	
rested	
eliminated	
chewed	

Hospital	Paciente

°¿Qué <u>ha sentido usted</u>?

<u>He sentido</u> dolor en las piernas.

dolores en el pecho.

debilidad.

cansancio al caminar.

¿<u>Ha</u> dormido <u>bien</u>?

comido

descansado

eliminado

masticado

Sí, <u>he</u> dormido <u>bien</u>.

Doctor: How do you feel today?

Patient: Not very well. I have a terrible cold. My whole body aches,
            my back and my throat, and I have a stuffy nose and congestion
            in my chest. It's hard for me to breathe, and I cough a lot.

Doctor: That's too bad. Do you have fever?

Patient: No, luckily.

Doctor: Well, you need to take these pills for your chest congestion and
            this medicine for your cough. Also, you should stay in bed and
            rest, and take a lot of liquids. Call my office Thursday to let
            me know how you are.

Patient: When do I have to take the medicine?

Doctor: Every four hours during the day.

Patient: Thanks a lot, doctor. See you Thursday.

Doctor: Until Thursday, sir.

IDENTIFICATION

Read the following conversation aloud. Try to get a general idea of what is being said.

Doctora: ¿Cómo se siente usted hoy?

Paciente: No muy bien. Tengo un resfriado terrible. Me duele todo el

cuerpo, la espalda, la garganta y tengo congestión en las fosas

nasales y en el pecho. Tengo dificultad para respirar, y toso

mucho.

Doctora: ¡Qué malo! ¿Tiene fiebre?

Paciente: No, afortunadamente.

Doctora: Pues, necesita usted tomar estas píldoras para la congestión en

el pecho y esta medicina para la tos. También debe descansar en

cama y tomar muchos líquidos. Debe llamar a mi oficina el jueves

para decir cómo está.

Paciente: ¿Cuándo tengo que tomar la medicina?

Doctora: Cada cuatro horas durante el día.

Paciente: Muchas gracias, doctora. Hasta el jueves.

Doctora: Hasta el jueves, señor.

Now, notice the following: (1) The word duele (in line 2) is one you have not studied, but you can probably figure it out from the context, or understand the symptoms without it. (2) The beginning and end of the conversation are merely social amenities and contain no important information. (3) The double-underlined words are not key words; they are what might be called signal words. They are usually right before, or right after, key words. Key words that you did not understand may be clarified by asking the person speaking such questions as:

¿terrible qué?   terrible what?
¿mucho qué?   much what?

Summarize in English what the conversation says before you look at the translation.

GRAMMAR AND STRUCTURES DRILLED IN LESSON 14

verbs

padecer -- to suffer, to have (disease)

usted padece -- you suffer   padezco -- I suffer

present perfect tense, regular verbs, first and third person

¿Ha tenido usted escarlatina?   Have you had scarlet fever?
He tenido escarlatina.   I have had scarlet fever.

Lesson 15
Foods: Drinks, Soup, Bread, Cheese, Seasonings, Fruit

NEW MATERIAL

Hospital   Patient

Hospital   Patient

Drinks

°<u>Do you like</u> coffee?   <u>Yes, I like</u> coffee.
       (black coffee)

     instant coffee?

     tea?

     iced tea?

     milk?

     chocolate milk?

     coffee with milk?

     coffee with cream?

     cola?

     hot chocolate?

     lemonade?

     juice?

     orange juice?

     tomato juice?

     grapefruit juice?

     water?

     soda pop?

°<u>Do you like</u> hot drinks?   <u>Yes, I like</u> hot drinks.

     cold drinks?

     wine?

     beer?

     cocktails?

Lección 15
Comidas: Bebidas, sopa, pan, queso, condimentos, fruta

Hospital	Paciente

Bebidas

Hospital	Paciente
°¿Le gusta el café?	Sí, me gusta el café.
(el café solo)	
el nescafé?	
el té?	
el té helado?	
la leche?	
la leche con chocolate?	
el café con leche?	
el café con crema?	
la coca?	
el chocolate?	
(el chocolate caliente)	
la limonada?	
el jugo?	
el jugo de naranja?	
el jugo de tomate?	
el jugo de toronja?	
el agua?	
la soda?	
°¿Le gusta la bebida caliente?	Sí, me gusta la bebida caliente.
la bebida fría?	
el vino?	
la cerveza?	
el coctel?	

169

Hospital   Patient

Soup

°Do you like soup?   No, I don't like soup.
  broth?

Bread

°Do you like bread?   No, I don't like bread.
  white bread?
  dark bread?
  toast?
  sweet rolls?
  soda crackers?
  cereal?
  oatmeal?

Cheese, Butter

°Do you like cheese?   I love cheese!
                                      I don't like cheese at all!
  white cheese?
  cream cheese?
  cottage cheese?
  yellow cheese?
  butter?
  peanut butter?

  jam?
  (preserves)
  honey?

Hospital   Paciente

Sopa

°¿Le gusta la sopa?   No, no me gusta la sopa.

  el caldo?

Pan

°¿Le gusta el pan?   No, no me gusta el pan.

  el pan blanco?

  el pan moreno?

  el pan tostado?

  el pan dulce?

  la galleta blanca?

  el cereal?

  la avena?

Queso, mantequilla

°¿Le gusta el queso?   ¡Me encanta el queso!
                                  ¡No, no me gusta nada el queso!

  el queso blanco?

  el queso crema?

  el queso requesón?

  el queso amarillo?

  la mantequilla?

  la crema de cacahuete?
          (cacahuate)

  la mermelada?

  la miel?

Hospital   Patient

Spices, Seasonings

^oDo you like salt?   Yes, I like salt.

    pepper?

    sugar?

    saccharin?

    vinegar?

    oil?
    (salad oil)

    sauce?

    salad dressing?

    catsup?

    hot sauce?

    hot peppers?

    mayonnaise?

    onions?

    garlic?

Do you like spices?   Yes, I like them.

Fruit

^oDo you like fruit?   Yes, I like fruit.

    apples?

    oranges?

    grapefruit?

    lemons?

    limes?

    pears?

Hospital   Paciente

Especias, condimentos

^o¿Le gusta la sal?   Sí, me gusta la sal.

    la pimienta?

    el azúcar?

    la sacarina?

    el vinagre?

    el aceite?

    la salsa?

    la salsa de ensalada?

    la salsa de tomate?

    la salsa picante?

    el chile picante?

    la mayonesa?

    la cebolla?

    el ajo?

¿Le gustan las especias?   Sí, me gustan.

Frutas

^o¿Le gustan las frutas?   Sí, me gustan las frutas.

    las manzanas?

    las naranjas?

    las toronjas?

    los limones?

    las limas?

    las peras?

Hospital	Patient
^o<u>Do you like</u> grapes?	<u>I love them</u>! <u>I love</u> grapes!
peaches?	
apricots?	
bananas?	
pineapple?	
melons?	
watermelon?	
cherries?	
strawberries?	
^o<u>Do you like</u> raspberries?	<u>No, I don't like them at all</u>.
mangos?	<u>Yes, I like them</u> a little
	a lot.
	very much.
papayas?	
plums?	
prunes?	
raisins?	

Hospital	Paciente
º¿<u>Le gustan</u> las uvas?	¡<u>Me encantan</u>!
	¡<u>Me encantan</u> las uvas!
los duraznos?	
(los melocotones)	
los albaricoques?	
los plátanos?	
las piñas?	
los melones?	
las sandías?	
(los melones de agua)	
las cerezas?	
las fresas?	
º¿<u>Le gustan</u> las frambuesas?	No, no me gustan nada.
los mangos?	Sí, me gustan un poco.
	mucho.
	muchísmo.
las papayas?	
las ciruelas?	
las ciruelas pasas?	
las pasas?	

Saccharin

People who want to lose weight can sweeten their drinks with saccharin.

The National Academy of Science has a contract to evaluate the safety of using saccharin in the treatment of certain metabolic disorders.

The government considers that the limited use of saccharin is not harmful, and recommends that one should not take more than one gram per day.

One gram is equal to 60 small tablets (1/4 grain).

Studies are being made to see whether saccharin produces cancer, genetic changes, or birth defects.

In 1970 four and a half million pounds of saccharin were manufactured for use by diabetics and people with high blood pressure.

Saccharin is 300 to 500 times sweeter than sugar, and 10 times sweeter than cyclamates.

IDENTIFICATION

Read the following selection through for general meaning. Then reread sentence by sentence. Check your understanding by answering a question about each sentence.

La sacarina

Las personas que desean perder peso pueden endulzar sus bebidas con sacarina.

La Academia Nacional de Ciencias tiene un contrato para evaluar la seguridad del uso de la sacarina en el tratamiento de ciertas enfermedades del metabolismo.

El gobierno considera que el uso limitado de la sacarina no hace daño y recomienda que no se debe tomar más de un gramo al día.

Un gramo es equivalente a 60 tabletas pequeñas (1/4 grano).

Se hacen investigaciones para saber si la sacarina puede producir cáncer, cambios genéticos o defectos de nacimiento.

En 1970 se fabricaron 4.5 millones de libras de sacarina para uso de diabéticos y personas que tengan la presión alta.

La sacarina es de trescientas a quinientas veces más dulce que el azúcar y diez veces más que los ciclamatos.

1. What can people do if they want to lose weight?

2. What is the National Academy of Sciences going to do?

3. What should be the limit of saccharin taken in one day?

4. How much are 60 small tablets?

5. What is being investigated concerning saccharin?

6. How many pounds of saccharin were manufactured in 1970?

7. How sweet is saccharin?

GRAMMAR AND STRUCTURES DRILLED IN LESSON 15

verbs of reverse construction

    gustar -- to like (to be pleasing)
    encantar -- to like a lot, to love

Me gusta la carne.	I like meat.
Me gustan las manzanas.	I like apples.
¿Le gusta la carne?	Do you like meat?
¿Le gustan las manzanas?	Do you like apples?

definite article used with nouns in a general sense, to indicate a kind or class (see above examples)

indirect object pronoun before verb of reverse construction (see above examples)

Lesson 16
Foods: Meats and Vegetables

NEW MATERIAL

<table>
<tr><td>Hospital</td><td>Patient</td></tr>
</table>

Meats

°<u>Do you want</u> meat?

       roast beef?

       beef?

       veal?

       lamb?

       barbecue?

       hamburger?

       steak?

<u>Yes, I want a slice of</u> meat.

<u>Yes, I want</u> barbecue.

<u>How do you want your steak?</u>

Rare.
Medium.
Well done.

°<u>Do you want</u> kid?

       pork?

       ribs?

       barbecued ribs?

       baked ribs?

       ham?

       bacon?

       sausage?

<u>Yes, I want</u> kid.

°<u>Do you want</u> chicken?

       fried chicken?

       roast chicken?

       stuffed chicken?

       chicken soup?

       turkey?

<u>No, I don't want</u> chicken.

Lección 16
Comidas: Carnes y vegetales

Hospital	Paciente

Carnes

°¿Quiere usted carne?   Sí, quiero una tajada de carne.

        rosbif?
        (carne asada)

        carne de res?

        carne de ternera?

        carne de cordero?

        barbacoa?   Sí, quiero barbacoa.

        hamburguesa?

        bistec?
        (biftec)
        (filete)

¿Cómo quiere el bistec?   Poco asado.
                                  Medio asado.
                                  Bien asado.

°¿Quiere usted cabrito?   Sí, quiero cabrito.

        carne de puerco?

        costillas asadas?

        costillas a la parrilla?

        costillas al horno?

        jamón?

        tocino?

        salchicha?
        (chorizo)

°¿Quiere usted pollo?   No, no quiero pollo.

        pollo frito?

        pollo asado?

        pollo relleno?

        pollo en caldo?

        pavo?
        (guajalote)

	Hospital	Patient

°<u>Do you want</u> fish?   <u>Yes, I want</u> fish.

              sardines?

              salmon?

              tuna?

              shrimp?

              clams?

              shellfish?

              oysters?

              crabs?

              lobster?

              anchovies?

°<u>Do you want</u> eggs?   <u>No, I don't want</u> eggs.

              soft-boiled eggs?

              hard-boiled eggs?

              poached eggs?

              scrambled eggs?

              bacon and eggs?

              ham and eggs?

°<u>Do you want</u> stuffed pepper?   <u>Yes, I want</u> a stuffed pepper.

              a serving of casserole?

              a serving of stew?

Hospital	Paciente
°¿Quiere usted pescado?	Sí, quiero pescado.
sardinas?	
salmón?	
atún?	
camarones?	
almejas?	
mariscos?	
ostras?	
cangrejos?	
langosta?	
anchoas?	
°¿Quiere usted huevos?	No, no quiero huevos.
huevos pasados por agua?	
huevos duros?	
huevos hervidos en agua?	
huevos revueltos?	
huevos con tocino?	
huevos con jamón?	
°¿Quiere usted chile relleno?	Sí, quiero chile relleno.
una porción de cacerola?	
una porción de cocido?	
(guisado)	

Hospital   Patient

Vegetables

°Do you want vegetables?   Yes, I want a small portion of vegetables.

        salad?
        lettuce?
        tomato?
        green beans?

        white beans?
        peas?

        corn?

        corn on the cob?
        potatoes?

        mashed potatoes?
        fried potatoes?
        (French fried potatoes)
        baked potatoes?
        rice?

°Do you want beets?   Yes, I want a double portion of beets.

        eggplant?
        squash?
        (pumpkin)
        carrots?
        avocado?

        beans?
        cabbage?

        cauliflower?
        Brussels sprouts?
        asparagus?
        spinach?
        onion?

Hospital   Paciente

Vegetales

°¿Quiere usted vegetales?   Sí, quiero una porción pequeña de
          (verduras)   vegetales.
          (legumbres)

          ensalada?

          lechuga?

          tomate?

          habichuelas?
          (ejotes)

          habas?

          chícharos?
          (guisantes)

          maíz?
          (maíz tierno)

          elote?

          papas?
          (patatas)

          puré de papas?

          papas fritas?

          papas asadas?

          arroz?

°¿Quiere usted remolacha?   Sí, quiero una porción doble de remolacha.
          (betabel)

          berenjena?

          calabaza?

          zanahorias?

          aguacate?
          (palta)

          frijoles?

          repollo?
          (col)

          coliflor?

          coles de Bruselas?

          espárragos?

          espinaca?

          cebolla?

Hospital	Patient
^o<u>Do you want</u> celery?	<u>No, I don't like</u> celery (sing.).
mushrooms?	<u>No, I don't like</u> mushrooms (pl.).
bell pepper?	
cucumber?	
pickles?	
parsley?	
broccoli?	
radishes?	

	Hospital	Paciente
°¿Quiere usted	apio?	No, no me gusta el apio.
	hongos? (champiñones)	No, no me gustan los hongos.
	pimiento?	
	pepino?	
	pepinillos?	
	perejil?	
	bróculi?	
	rábanos?	

IDENTIFICATION

Imagine you are helping a Spanish-speaking patient select a meal from the menu printed below. The patient points to a word and says: "¿Qué quiere decir . . .?" ("What does . . . mean?") Give each food in Spanish as best you can. If you don't know a word, try to say it in some similar way, or make up a cognate.

Supper

Check items desired. Double check for double portions.

Soup:	____ Vegetable	____ Chicken	
Meat:	____ Baked chicken	____ Chopped sirloin	
Vegetables:	____ Tossed salad	____ Mashed potatoes	
	____ Green beans	____ Creamed corn	
	____ Broccoli		
Dessert:	____ Fruit salad	____ Tapioca	
Beverage:	____ Coffee	____ Tea	____ Milk

GRAMMAR AND STRUCTURES DRILLED IN LESSON 16

verb

querer -- to want, wish   quiero -- I want   quiere -- you want, do you want?

Lesson 17
Foods: Desserts and Dishes

<u>NEW MATERIAL</u>

Hospital		Patient	
Dessert?	<u>I don't know.</u>	^o<u>May I have</u> dessert?	
		ice cream?	
		ice milk?	
		(sherbet)	
		(ice)	
		pudding?	
		custard?	
		tapioca?	
		rice pudding?	
		gelatin?	
		fruit gelatin?	
		fruit cocktail?	
<u>We</u> <u>must ask</u> the doctor.		^o<u>May I have</u> pie?	
(<u>One</u>) the dietitian.		(pastry)	
the nurse.		(cake)	
the specialist.		lemon pie?	
		apple pie?	
		cherry pie?	
		cake?	
		cookies?	
		wafers or sweet biscuits?	
The tray?	<u>Of course!</u>	^o<u>May I have</u> the tray?	
	<u>Certainly!</u>	the cup?	
		the glass?	
		the plate?	
		the small plate?	
		(the saucer)	
		the soup bowl?	

Lección 17
Comidas: Postres y utensilios

<u>MATERIA NUEVA</u>

Hospital		Paciente

Hospital   Paciente

¿Postre? <u>No sé</u>.

°<u>¿Me permite tomar</u> postre?

         helado?

         nieve?
         (sorbete)

         pudín?

         flan?

         tapioca?

         arroz con leche?

         gelatina?

         gelatina con fruta?

         coctel de fruta?

<u>Hay que preguntarle</u> al médico.
         al dietista.
         a la enfermera.
         al especialista.

°<u>¿Me permite tomar</u> pastel?

         pastel de limón?

         pastel de manzana?

         pastel de cereza?

         queque?
         (torta)

         galletas?
         (galleticas)

         bizcochos?

¿La bandeja? ¡<u>Claro</u>!
            ¡<u>Cómo no</u>!

°<u>¿Me permite</u> la bandeja?

         la taza?

         el vaso?

         el plato?

         el platillo?

         el sopero?

Hospital	Patient

The fork? <u>Of course</u>!

^o<u>May I have</u> the fork?

the knife?

the spoon?

the teaspoon?

the napkin?

<u>At about</u> 6:00.
7:00.
11:00.
12:00.
5:00.
5:30.

^o<u>When is</u> the meal <u>served</u>?
(dinner)
(food)

breakfast

lunch

supper

Whenever you want.

a snack

^o<u>You need to</u> choose your menu.

<u>All right</u>. <u>Thanks</u>.

select your lunch.

select your meal.

select your snack.

select your supper.

mark the dish you want.

^o<u>Do you like</u> fresh <u>fruit</u>?

<u>It's delicious</u>!

frozen

canned

dried

cooked

^o<u>Do you like</u> fresh <u>vegetables</u>?

<u>They're delicious</u>!

frozen

dried

cooked

canned

Hospital	Paciente
¿El tenedor? ¡Claro! ¡Cómo no!	O¿Me permite el tenedor? el cuchillo? la cuchara? la cucharita? (la cucharilla) la servilleta?
A eso de las seis. las siete. las once. las doce. las cinco. las cinco y media.	O¿Cuándo se sirve la comida? el desayuno? el almuerzo? la cena? la merienda?
Cuando usted quiera.	

OUsted necesita escoger su menú.
        seleccionar su almuerzo.

Muy bien. Gracias.

        seleccionar su comida.

        seleccionar su merienda.

        seleccionar su cena.

        marcar el plato preferido.

O¿Le gusta la fruta fresca?

¡Es deliciosa!

          congelada?

        en lata?
       (enlatada)

        seca?

        cocida?

O¿Le gustan los vegetales frescos?

¡Son deliciosos!

          congelados?

          secos?

          cocidos?

          en lata?
        (enlatados)

Diseases and Nutrition

With the development of medical sciences, man today controls many infectious diseases that were once fatal. There are vaccines against typhoid, rabies, whooping cough, smallpox, poliomyelitis, and other serious diseases. There are antibiotics that can rapidly cure diseases such as syphilis and tuberculosis. Nevertheless, there are a great number of diseases that exist today that are related to nutrition. These may be caused by deficiency, excess, or the use of a diet that does not contain adequate basic foods.

It is necessary to have a balanced diet to maintain physical and mental health. Modern research has found more and more concrete evidence of the relationship that exists between mental illness and food. The use of a correct diet can prevent or retard certain degenerative diseases, such as arteriosclerosis.

IDENTIFICATION

Most of the key words in the following selection are either cognates or words you have studied previously. New words that also are important to the meaning are: desarrollo -- development; enfermedad -- disease; vacuna -- vaccine. Read each paragraph twice and summarize in English what it says.

Enfermedades y la nutrición

Con el desarrollo de las ciencias médicas el hombre controla hoy muchas enfermedades infecciosas que antes eran fatales. Hay vacunas contra la tifoidea, la rabia, la tos ferina, la viruela, la poliomielitis y otras enfermedades graves. Hay antibióticos que pueden curar rápidamente enfermedades como la sífilis y la tuberculosis. Sin embargo, hay un gran número de enfermedades que existen hoy que se relacionan con la nutrición. Pueden ser causadas por deficiencia, exceso, o por el uso de una dieta que no contiene los alimentos básicos adecuados.

Es necesario tener una dieta balanceada para mantener la salud física y mental. Las investigaciones modernas encuentran cada vez más evidencia concreta de la relación que existe entre las enfermedades mentales y la alimentación. El uso de una dieta apropiada puede prevenir o retardar la aparición de ciertas enfermedades degenerativas como la arterioesclerosis.

Using the lists of cognate words on pp. 527-541, make a list of other diseases related to nutrition.

GRAMMAR AND STRUCTURES DRILLED IN LESSON 17

verbs

necesitar + infinitive

pronouns

indirect object pronoun with gustar, permitir

reflexive pronoun se as impersonal subject

Lesson 18
Foods: Diets

NEW MATERIAL

Hospital	Patient
Yes, you should follow a special diet.	°Should I follow a special diet?
a strict diet.	
a salt-free diet.	
a fat-free diet.	
a diet low in roughage.	
a high-protein diet.	
a high-carbohydrate diet.	
a diet rich in protein.	
a diet rich in vitamins.	
a diet rich in iron.	
a diet rich in minerals.	
a low-carbohydrate diet.	
a balanced diet.	
a diet for diabetics.	
a diet for ulcers.	
°You should follow a diet for the baby.	What diet? For the baby?
for the baby until he's 1 or 2.	
for controlling weight.	
for losing weight.	
for gaining weight.	
for those who have high cholesterol.	
for those who have gallbladder trouble.	
for those who have liver trouble.	
for those who have heart trouble.	

Lección 18
Comidas: Dietas

Hospital	Paciente

Sí, debe seguir una dieta especial.

    una dieta estricta.

    una dieta sin sal.

    una dieta sin grasa.

    una dieta de residuo bajo.

    una dieta con mucha proteína.

    una dieta con muchos carbohidratos.

    una dieta rica en proteína.

    una dieta rica en vitaminas.

    una dieta rica en hierro.

    una dieta rica en minerales.

    una dieta baja en carbohidratos.

    una dieta balanceada.

    una dieta para los diabéticos.

    una dieta para las úlceras.

°**Debe seguir una dieta** para el bebé.

    para el bebé hasta uno o dos años.

    para controlar el peso.

    para perder peso.

    para aumentar de peso.

    para los que tienen
      el colesterol alto.
     (la colesterina alta)

    para los que padecen de la vesícula.

    para los que padecen del hígado.

    para los que padecen del corazón.

°¿**Debo seguir** una dieta especial?

¿Qué dieta? ¿Para el bebé?

Hospital	Patient

You should follow the diet.   °What should I do?
       follow the instructions.
       get weighed every day.
       drink milk before bedtime.
       drink a lot of water.
       drink a lot of liquids.
       exercise.
       eat more.
       eat less.
       eat one slice.

       eat one portion.
       eat one piece.
       lose weight.

You shouldn't have alcoholic beverages.   °What should I not have?
           stimulants.
           fried foods.
           greasy foods.

You shouldn't eat many sweets.   °What should I not eat?
         (much candy)
         fried foods.
         chocolate.

You should not use many spices.   °What should I not use?
         many sauces.
         many fats.
         much salt.

°You shouldn't drink that water.   Why?
        eat that food.

It'll make you (m.) sick.   It'll make me sick?
      you (f.)

It's spoiled.   Oh? Is it spoiled?
    bad.
    contaminated.

It's not potable.   (drinking water)

Hospital	Paciente
	°¿ Qué debo hacer?

Debe seguir la dieta.

    seguir las instrucciones.

    pesarse todos los días.

    tomar leche antes de dormir.

    tomar mucha agua.

    tomar muchos líquidos.

    hacer ejercicios.

    comer más.

    comer menos.

    comer una tajada.
        (rebanada)

    comer una porción.

    comer un pedazo.

    perder peso.

No debe tomar bebidas alcohólicas.   °¿Qué no debo tomar?

       estimulantes.

       alimentos fritos.

       alimentos grasosos.

No debe comer muchos dulces.   °¿Qué no debo comer?

       alimentos fritos.

       chocolate.

No debe usar muchas especias.   °¿Qué no debo usar?

       muchas salsas.

       muchas grasas.

       mucha sal.

°**No debe** tomar esa agua.   ¿Por qué?

      comer esa comida.

Lo enferma.   ¿Me enferma?
La

Está corrompida.   ¿Sí? ¿Está corrompida?

    mala.

    contaminada.

No es potable.

Hospital	Patient

Hospital

You shouldn't lose much weight.
    lose much weight rapidly.
    eat much before going to bed.
    drink much coffee.

You should lose 10 pounds.
             20 pounds.
             25 pounds.
             30 pounds.
             40 pounds.
             1 pound per week.
             2 pounds
             3 pounds
             5 pounds a month.
             6 pounds
             7 pounds

°How much have you lost?

Patient

°What should I not do?

°How much should I lose?

I've lost 5 pounds.
         9 pounds.

Hospital	Paciente

No debe perder mucho peso.
        perder mucho peso rápidamente.
        comer mucho antes de acostarse.
        tomar mucho café.

°¿Qué no debo hacer?

Debe perder diez libras.
        veinte libras.
        veinticinco libras.
        treinta libras.
        cuarenta libras.
        una libra a la semana.
        dos libras
        tres libras
        cinco libras al mes.
        seis libras
        siete libras

°¿Cuánto debo perder?

°¿Cuánto ha perdido usted?

He perdido cinco libras.
        nueve libras.

Foods in Diet for Lowering Cholesterol Count

Drinks: Coffee, tea, and carbonated drinks

Bread: White, whole wheat, rye, soda or bran crackers, and breads made with fats
   permitted on the diet but without milk or egg yolks

Cereals: Cooked or dry but with skim milk

Cheese: Cottage cheese made with skim milk

Eggs: Egg white has no fat or cholesterol. One or two eggs a week prepared in
   the fat that is permitted on the diet

Milk: Skim milk, powdered (skim) milk, evaporated skim milk, curds and whey,
   yogurt

Fats: Olive oil, margarine (artificial butter), sesame oil, cottonseed oil,
   salad dressings made without egg yolk or milk or cream

Soups: Vegetable soup, creamed soups made with skim milk, consommé

Meat, fish, chicken: Lean beef, lamb or mutton, veal, ham or pork, chicken,
   tongue, turkey, dried meat, fresh or frozen fish (nothing fried)

Potatoes or substitutes: Potatoes or sweet potatoes, macaroni, noodles,
   spaghetti, rice (all made without eggs)

Vegetables: Fresh, frozen, dry, canned -- prepared only with the fats permitted

Fruits: Fresh, canned, dried, or frozen fruits and fruit juices

Desserts: Meringue, sherbet, gelatin, fruit ices, pudding made with skim milk
   but without egg yolk, cookies and cakes made with the fats allowed and with
   skim milk

Sweets: Honey, syrups, sugar syrups, bonbons, caramel candy

Miscellaneous: Salt, spices, seasonings, lemon, lime, vinegar, pickles, popcorn

Not permitted: Cornbread, hot breads such as biscuits, creamed cheese
   and creamed cottage cheese, commercial pastries, butter, lard

IDENTIFICATION

By combining your knowledge of Spanish names for foods and what you know about diets, see if you can explain the following diet. Try to guess what you don't know.

Alimentos en la dieta para bajar el nivel de colesterol

Bebidas: Café, té, y bebidas gaseosas

Pan: Blanco, de trigo entero, de centeno, galletas saladas o de acemite, y panes hechos con las grasas que se permitan en la dieta, pero sin leche o yema de huevo

Cereales: Cocidos o secos pero con leche descremada

Quesos: Requesón hecho de leche descremada

Huevos: La clara del huevo no contiene grasa o colesterol. Uno o dos huevos a la semana en grasa que se permita en la dieta

Leche: Leche descremada, leche en polvo (descremada), leche descremada evaporada, leche de suero o leche cuajada, yogurt

Grasas: Aceite de oliva, margarina (mantequilla artificial), aceite de sésame (ajonjolí), aceite de semillas de algodón, salsas hechas para ensaladas sin yema de huevo o leche o crema

Caldos: Caldo de vegetales, caldos de crema con leche descremada, consomé

Carne, pescado, pollo: Carne de res sin grasa, carnero, ternera, jamón o puerco, pollo, lengua, pavo, carne seca, pescado fresco o congelado (nada frito)

Papas o substitutos: Papas o camotes, macarrón, fideos, tallarín, arroz (todos hechos sin huevos)

Vegetales: Frescos, congelados, secos, o en lata -- preparados solamente con grasas permitidas

Frutas: Frutas frescas, en lata, secas, o congeladas y jugos de fruta

Postres: Merengues, sorbete, gelatina, helados de fruta, pudín hecho de leche descremada pero sin la yema del huevo, galletas y tortas hechas con las grasas que se permitan y con leche descremada

Dulces: Miel de colmena, jarabes, almíbar, bombones, dulces de caramelo

Miscelánea: Sal, especias, condimentos, limón, lima, vinagre, pepinillos, esquite.

No debe comer: Pan de maíz, panes calientes como bizcochos, quesos de crema, requesones, pasteles comerciales, mantequilla, manteca

GRAMMAR AND STRUCTURES DRILLED IN LESSON 18

verbs

deber + infinitive -- should, ought to + verb

¿Debo seguir la dieta?   Should I follow the diet?
Usted debe seguir la dieta. You should follow the diet.

perder, present perfect tense, first and third persons

He perdido peso.   I have lost weight.
Ha perdido peso.   You have lost weight.

Lesson 19
Care of the Patient: Physical Needs

Hospital	Patient
°What's the matter?	I'm hungry.
	thirsty.
	cold.
	hot.
	in pain.
	afraid.
	sleepy.
	I feel like sleeping.
	leaving.
	eating.

°I have to prepare the prescription. Oh, you have to prepare the prescription?

       clean the room.

       clean the bathroom.

       change the bed.

       change the sheets.

       change the pillow cases.

°You have to walk. Do I have to walk?

       take the medicine.

       drink the milk.

       take the treatment.

       go to the bathroom.

       go to the laboratory.

       go to the room.

       rest.

       bend your knee.

       bend your leg.

       speak to the doctor.

Lección 19
Cuidado del paciente: Necesidades físicas

<u>MATERIA NUEVA</u>

Hospital	Paciente
º¿Qué tiene usted?	Tengo hambre.
	sed.
	frío.
	calor.
	dolor.
	miedo.
	sueño.
	Tengo ganas de dormir.
	salir.
	comer.

ºTengo que preparar la receta.
         limpiar el cuarto.
         limpiar el baño.
         cambiar la cama.
         cambiar las sábanas.
         cambiar las fundas.

Ah, ¿tiene que preparar la receta?

ºUsted tiene que caminar.
         tomar la medicina.
         tomar la leche.
         tomar el tratamiento.
         ir al baño.
         ir al laboratorio.
         ir al cuarto.
         descansar.
         doblar la rodilla.
         doblar la pierna.
         hablar al médico.

¿Tengo que caminar?

Hospital	Patient
^o<u>You have to</u> go to bed.	<u>Do I have to</u> go to bed?
get up.	get up?
wash.	wash?
brush your teeth.	brush my teeth?
take a bath.	take a bath?
comb your hair.	comb my hair?
sit up during the day.	sit up during the day?
stay in bed.	stay in bed?
change your clothes.	change my clothes?
change your position.	
change to the left.	
change to the right.	
wrap up.	wrap up?
take care of yourself.	take care of myself?
turn on your side.	turn on my side?
turn over?	turn over?
turn over on the left side.	
(to the left)	
turn over to the right.	
(on the right side)	
get weighed.	get weighed?
shave.	shave?
put on your makeup.	put on my makeup?
^o<u>I have to</u> take <u>your</u> vital signs.	Take <u>my</u> vital signs?
take <u>your</u> blood pressure.	
take <u>your</u> temperature.	
take <u>your</u> pulse.	
raise <u>your</u> bed.	Raise <u>my</u> bed?
lower <u>your</u> bed.	

Hospital	Paciente
°Usted tiene que acostarse.	¿Tengo que acostarme?
levantarse.	levantarme?
lavarse.	lavarme?
lavarse los dientes.	lavarme los dientes?
bañarse.	bañarme?
peinarse.	peinarme?
sentarse durante el día.	sentarme durante el día?
quedarse en la cama.	quedarme en la cama?
cambiarse la ropa.	cambiarme la ropa?
cambiarse de posición.	
cambiarse a la izquierda.	
cambiarse a la derecha.	
abrigarse.	abrigarme?
cuidarse.	cuidarme?
ponerse de lado.	ponerme de lado?
voltearse.	voltearme?
voltearse sobre el lado izquierdo. (a la izquierda)	
voltearse a la derecha. (sobre el lado derecho)	
pesarse.	pesarme?
afeitarse.	afeitarme?
maquillarse.	maquillarme?
°Tengo que tomarle los signos vitales.	¿Tomarme los signos vitales?
tomarle la presión.	
tomarle la temperatura.	
tomarle el pulso.	
levantarle la cama.	¿Levantarme la cama?
bajarle la cama.	

Hospital	Patient
°I have to change your robe.	Change my robe?
change your bandage.	
change your sheets.	
change your clothes.	
give you a bath.	Give me a bath?
give you a bed bath.	
give you a laxative.	
feed you.	
give you an injection.	Give me an injection?
give you an enema.	
put the bedpan under you.	Put the bedpan under me?
take the bedpan (from you).	Take the bedpan (from me)?
take out the thermometer (from you).	
take out the instrument (from you).	
shave your beard.	Shave my beard?
shave your body hair.	Shave my body hair?
shave your pubic hair.	
cut your hair.	Cut my hair?
fix your hair.	Fix my hair?
°You have to tell me	
if you don't eliminate well.	If I don't eliminate well?
if you don't urinate well.	If I don't urinate well?
if you don't defecate well.	If I don't defecate well?
if you don't evacuate well.	If I don't evacuate well?
if you need something.	If I need something?
if you don't sleep well.	If I don't sleep well?

Hospital	Paciente
^o<u>Tengo que</u> cambiar<u>le</u> la bata.	¿Cambiar<u>me</u> la bata?
cambiar<u>le</u> la venda.	
cambiar<u>le</u> las sábanas.	
cambiar<u>le</u> la ropa.	
dar<u>le</u> un baño.	¿Dar<u>me</u> un baño?
dar<u>le</u> un baño de cama.	
dar<u>le</u> un purgante.	
dar<u>le</u> de comer.	
poner<u>le</u> una inyección.	¿Poner<u>me</u> una inyección?
poner<u>le</u> una enema. (lavativa)	
poner<u>le</u> el bacín.	¿Poner<u>me</u> el bacín?
quitar<u>le</u> el bacín.	¿Quitar<u>me</u> el bacín?
quitar<u>le</u> el termómetro.	
quitar<u>le</u> el aparato.	
afeitar<u>le</u> la barba.	¿Afeitar<u>me</u> la barba?
rasurar<u>le</u> el vello.	¿Rasurar<u>me</u> el vello?
rasurar<u>le</u> el pelo púbico.	
cortar<u>le</u> el pelo.	¿Cortar<u>me</u> el pelo?
arreglar<u>le</u> el pelo.	¿Arreglar<u>me</u> el pelo?
^o<u>Usted tiene que decirme</u>	
si no elimin<u>a</u> bien.	¿Si no elimin<u>o</u> bien?
si no orin<u>a</u> bien.	¿Si no orin<u>o</u> bien?
si no defec<u>a</u> bien.	¿Si no defec<u>o</u> bien?
si no evacú<u>a</u> bien.	¿Si no evacú<u>o</u> bien?
si necesit<u>a</u> algo.	¿Si necesit<u>o</u> algo?
si no duerm<u>e</u> bien.	¿Si no duerm<u>o</u> bien?

Nurse: Good morning, ma'am.

Patient: Good morning, nurse.

Nurse: I'm going to give you a bath.

Patient: Do I need a bath now?

Nurse: Yes, ma'am, you need a bath every day. You'll be more comfortable, and you'll get well sooner.

Patient: But it's so early. What time is it?

Nurse: It's 6:00 A.M. You need to have your bath before breakfast.

Patient: What time is breakfast?

Nurse: They'll bring breakfast at 7:00.

Patient: I have to take a bath now, then.

Nurse: Yes, ma'am. You also need to brush your teeth, comb your hair, and change clothes. If you wish, you can put on makeup.

IDENTIFICATION

Read aloud or listen to the conversation below. Jot down or underline key words. Go over the conversation a second time, even a third time if necessary. Check your understanding by answering the three questions that follow the conversation before checking the English.

La enfermera: Buenos días, señora.

Paciente: Buenos días, señorita.

La enfermera: Voy a darle un baño.

Paciente: ¿Necesito un baño ahora?

La enfermera: Sí, señora, usted necesita un baño todos los días. Se sentirá
              más cómoda y sanará más pronto.

Paciente: Pero es tan temprano. ¿Qué hora es?

La enfermera: Son las seis de la mañana. Es necesario que tome su baño antes
              del desayuno.

Paciente: ¿A qué hora es el desayuno?

La enfermera: El desayuno lo traen a las siete.

Paciente: Tengo que bañarme ahora, entonces.

La enfermera: Sí, señora. También necesita limpiarse los dientes, peinarse,
              y cambiarse la ropa. Si quiere, puede maquillarse.

1. Name three things the patient should do before breakfast.

2. When is breakfast?

3. What does the nurse say about bathing? When and why is it necessary?

NOTES

As used in this lesson, both <u>poner</u> and <u>dar</u> may mean "to give" in English.
However, <u>poner</u> implies "to give" in the sense of putting something into a person,
under a person, or on a specific part of the person. <u>Dar</u> conveys the idea "to
give" something externally or for the person himself to take. Compare:

<u>Tengo que darle el laxante</u>. I have to give you the laxative.
(give it to you for you to take)

<u>Tengo que ponerle la inyección</u>. I have to give you the injection.
(place it inside of you)

GRAMMAR AND STRUCTURES DRILLED IN LESSON 19

verbs

regular verbs, present tense, first and third person

<u>tener</u> expressions

<u>Tengo frío</u>.   I'm cold.

<u>tener que</u> + infinitive -- to have to + verb

<u>Tengo que cambiar la cama</u>.   I have to change the bed.

object pronouns

infinitive + indirect object pronouns <u>me</u>, <u>le</u>

<u>Tengo que cambiarle la bata</u>. I have to change your robe.

infinitive + reflexive pronouns <u>me</u>, <u>se</u>

<u>Usted tiene que cambiarse la ropa</u>. You have to change your clothes.

Lesson 20
Care of the Patient: Emotional Needs

<u>NEW MATERIAL</u>

Hospital

Patient

°<u>Are you</u> comfortable (m.)?
          comfortable (f.)?

<u>Yes, I'm</u> comfortable (m.), <u>thanks</u>.
          comfortable (f.)

<u>Why are you</u> worried (m.)?
          worried (f.)?

<u>Because I'm</u> afraid of the operation.

<u>I have</u> pain.

<u>I'm</u> afraid of the pain.

<u>I have</u> problems.

<u>Because I don't have</u> money.

                    work.

                    family here.

°<u>Why are you</u> upset (m.)?
          upset (f.)?

<u>Because I have</u> problems.

                    family problems.

                    problems at work.

<u>Because</u> my son takes drugs.

          my son is in jail.

          my husband has left me.

          my husband is an alcoholic.

°<u>Why are you</u> angry (m.)?
          angry (f.)?

<u>Because I don't like</u> this room.

                    that man.

                    that woman.

                    the food.

                    to be in the
                    hospital.

°<u>Why are you</u> angry (m.)?
          angry (f.)?

<u>Because</u> the doctor hasn't come.

          the nurse hasn't come.

          he hasn't told me why he's going
          to operate.

          he hasn't told me when he's going
          to operate.

Lección 20
Cuidado del paciente: Necesidades emocionales

Hospital	Paciente
°¿Está usted cómodo? 　　　　　　cómoda?	Sí, estoy cómodo, gracias. 　　　　　cómoda
¿Por qué está usted preocupado? 　　　　　　　　　preocupada?	Porque tengo miedo de la operación. 　　　　　　　dolor. 　　　　　　　miedo del dolor. 　　　　　　　problemas.
	Porque no tengo dinero. 　　　　　　　　trabajo. 　　　　　　　　familia aquí.
°¿Por qué está usted mortificado? 　　　　　　　　　mortificada?	Porque tengo problemas. 　　　　　　　problemas en la familia. 　　　　　　　problemas en el trabajo.
	Porque mi hijo toma drogas. 　　　　mi hijo está en la cárcel. 　　　　mi esposo me ha abandonado. 　　　　mi esposo es alcohólico.
°¿Por qué está usted enojado? 　　　　　　　　　enojada?	Porque no me gusta este cuarto. 　　　　　　　　ese señor. 　　　　　　　　　(hombre) 　　　　　　　　esa señora. 　　　　　　　　　(mujer) 　　　　　　　　la comida. 　　　　　　　　estar en el hospital.
°¿Por qué está usted enojado? 　　　　　　　　　enojada?	Porque no ha venido el médico. 　　　　no ha venido la enfermera. 　　　　no me ha dicho por qué me opera. 　　　　no me ha dicho cuándo me opera.

Hospital	Patient
^oWhy are you tired (m.)?	Because I can't sleep.
tired (f.)?	rest.
	walk.
	get up.

^oWhy are you happy (m.)?
            happy (f.)?

Because I don't have pain.
I feel good.
I feel better.
I'm going to leave.
I'm going home.
I can eat.
I can have visits.
the doctor is dismissing me.
everything's going well.

^oWhy are you sad?

Because my husband isn't here.
my family isn't here.
my son is alone.
I don't understand English.
I want to see my family.
I want to see my husband.
I want to go home.
I want to die.
I don't want to die.
I don't want to be in the hospital.
I don't want to be sick.

^oWhy are you laughing?
            crying?
            sleeping?
            walking?

Because I feel like laughing.
                crying.
                sleeping.
                walking.

Hoapital	Paciente
°¿Por qué está usted cansado? cansada?	Porque no puedo dormir. descansar. caminar. levantarme.
°¿Por qué está usted contento? contenta?	Porque no tengo dolor. me siento bien. me siento mejor. voy a salir. voy a casa. puedo comer. puedo tener visitas. el doctor me da de alta. todo va bien.
°¿Por qué está usted triste?	Porque mi esposo no está aquí. mi familia no está aquí. mi hijo está solo. no comprendo inglés. quiero ver a mi familia. quiero ver a mi esposo. quiero ir a casa. quiero morir. no quiero morir. no quiero estar en el hospital. no quiero estar enfermo.
°¿Por qué se ríe? llora? duerme? camina?	Porque tengo ganas de reír. llorar. dormir. caminar.

Mental depression is a very common illness in today's society. There are patients who have headaches, chronic fatigue, neuralgia, constipation, itching, or loss of libido. They visit the doctor often, not because they are physically ill, but because they suffer from mental depression.

1. What symptoms do some patients have?
2. Why do they visit the doctor often?

Many times family and friends don't recognize these symptoms as depression. Doctors are baffled because they find no physical illness in these patients. It is important to discover the problem, because at times depression can lead to suicide. There are drugs that reduce anxiety and help the patient to recover his emotional normalcy.

1. Why are doctors baffled?
2. What can lead to suicide?
3. How do drugs help?

So many people have depression crises that in various cities there are Crisis Hot Lines. One can call a certain telephone number, and someone else listens to him sympathetically. In New York alone, more than 50,000 people use this service each year. More women than men call, and 50 percent of those who call are under 30 years of age. Thirty-five percent have mental depression and 16 percent have marital problems, but the main reason for calling is that they want to talk with someone because they feel lonely.

1. Who listens sympathetically?
2. What age are 50 percent of those who call?

IDENTIFICATION

Read each paragraph aloud two or three times, and then answer the questions orally ih Spanish with as few words as possible.

La depresión mental es una enfermedad muy común en la sociedad de hoy. Hay pacientes que tienen dolores de cabeza, fatiga crónica, neuralgia, constipación, picazón o pérdida del líbido. Visitan al médico con frecuencia pero no porque estén enfermos físicamente, es que sufren de depresión mental.

   1. ¿Qué síntomas tienen unos pacientes?

   2. ¿Por qué visitan al médico con frecuencia?

Muchas veces la familia y los amigos no reconocen esos síntomas como depresión. Los médicos están confusos porque no encuentran males físicos en estos pacientes. Es importante descubrir el problema porque a veces la depresión puede conducir al suicidio. Hay drogas que reducen la ansiedad y ayudan al paciente a recobrar la normalidad emocional.

   1. ¿Por qué están confusos los médicos?

   2. ¿Qué puede conducir al suicidio?

   3. ¿Cómo ayudan las drogas?

Tantas personas tienen crisis depresivas que en varias ciudades hay Centros de Ayuda por Teléfono. Se puede llamar a un número de teléfono, y otra persona le escucha con simpatía. En Nueva York, solamente, más de 50,000 personas usan este servicio al año. LLaman más mujeres que hombres, y el 50 por ciento de los que llaman son personas de menos de 30 años. El 35 por ciento tienen depresión mental, el 16 por ciento tienen problemas maritales, pero la razón principal es que desean hablar con alguien porque se sienten solos.

   1. ¿Quién escucha con simpatía?

   2. ¿Qué edad tienen el 50 por ciento de los que llaman?

GRAMMAR AND STRUCTURES DRILLED IN LESSON 20

verbs

    present tense verbs, first and third person

    estar, first and third person

    tener ganas de + infinitive -- to feel like + -ing form

        Tengo ganas de dormir.   I feel like sleeping.

adjectives

    estar + adjectivo

        ¿Por qué está usted enojado? Why are you angry?

Lesson 21
Care of the Patient: Medicines

<u>NEW MATERIAL</u>

Hospital	Patient

^o<u>Does your</u> head   <u>hurt</u>?   Yes, <u>my</u> head <u>hurts</u>.

        stomach

        throat

        incision

        back

        waist

        arm

        leg

        eye

^o<u>Do your</u> eyes   <u>hurt</u>?   Yes, <u>my</u> eyes <u>hurt</u>.

      feet

      ears

      legs

      shoulders

<u>You have to take</u> aspirin.   ^o<u>My head aches</u>.

        the tablets.

        the pills.

        the pills.
         (the lozenges)

        the capsules.

<u>You have to take</u> the capsule.   ^o<u>I have a sore throat</u>.

        cough syrup.

        medicine.

        a pill.

<u>You have to</u> gargle.

Lección 21
Cuidado del paciente: Las medicinas

Hospital   Paciente

°¿Le duele la cabeza?   Sí, me duele la cabeza.

el estómago?

la garganta?

la herida?

la espalda?

la cintura?

el brazo?

la pierna?

el ojo?

°¿Le duelen los ojos?   Sí, me duelen los ojos.

los pies?

los oídos?

las piernas?

los hombros?

Tiene que tomar aspirina.   °Me duele la cabeza.

las tabletas.

las píldoras.

las pastillas.

las cápsulas.

Tiene que tomar la cápsula.   °Me duele la garganta.

jarabe para la tos.

la medicina.

una pastilla.

Tiene que hacer gárgaras.

Hospital	Patient
You shouldn't scratch it.	^oIt itches.
You have to use germicidal powder.	
a disinfectant powder.	
ointment.	
salve.	My back hurts.
You have to use liniment.	
You have to take a laxative.	I'm constipated (m.).
	constipated (f.).
milk of magnesia.	

You have to take the red liquid.   ^oWhat medicine do I have to take?
    the yellow liquid.
    the white liquid.
    the black liquid.
    (the dark-colored liquid)
    the purple liquid.
    the blue liquid.
    the green liquid.
    the brown liquid.
    the gray liquid.
    the orange liquid.
    the pink liquid.

You should take the red tablet.   ^oMy incision hurts.
    the yellow tablet.
    the white tablet.
    the black tablet.
    the purple tablet.
    the blue tablet.
    the green tablet.
    the brown tablet.
    the gray tablet.
    the orange tablet.
    the pink tablet.

Hospital	Paciente

Hospital

Paciente

No debe rascarse.   °Me pica.

Tiene que usar polvo germicida.

                polvo desinfectante.

                ungüento.

                pomada.

Tiene que usar linimento.   Me duele la espalda.

Tiene que tomar un purgante.   Estoy constipado.
              (un laxante)   constipada.

              leche de magnesia.

Tiene que tomar el líquido rojo.   °¿Qué medicina tengo que tomar?

              el líquido amarillo.

              el líquido blanco.

              el líquido negro.

              el líquido morado.

              el líquido azul.

              el líquido verde.

              el líquido café.

              el líquido gris.

              el líquido color de naranja.

              el líquido color de rosa.

Debe tomar la tableta roja.   °Me duele la herida.

           la tableta amarilla.

           la tableta blanca.

           la tableta negra.

           la tableta morada.

           la tableta azul.

           la tableta verde.

           la tableta café.

           la tableta gris.

           la tableta color de naranja.

           la tableta color de rosa.

Hospital	Patient

<table>
<tr><td>Hospital</td><td>Patient</td></tr>
</table>

Hospital	Patient
Every hour.	^oWhen do I have to take the medicine?
Every 2 hours.	
Every 3 hours.	
According to the label.	
According to the prescription.	
According to the doctor.	
According to the symptoms.	
According to the pain.	
1 tablespoonful.	How much do I have to take?
2 teaspoonfuls.	
2 tablets.	

Hospital	Paciente
Cada hora.	°¿Cuándo tengo que tomar la medicina?
Cada dos horas.	
Cada tres horas.	
Según la etiqueta.	
Según la receta.	
Según el médico.	
Según los síntomas.	
Según el dolor.	
Una cucharada.	¿Cuánto tengo que tomar?
Dos cucharaditas.	
Dos pastillas.	

CONVERSATION 1

Patient: Excuse me, nurse, but I have an awfully bad headache.

Nurse: How long have you had a headache?

Patient: I've had a headache all day, but since I've eaten it's been worse.

Nurse: It could be something you ate. I'm going to call the doctor to ask him what you should have.

CONVERSATION 2

Nurse: May I speak to Dr. Jiménez?

Doctor: This is Dr. Jiménez. What can I do for you?

Nurse: Dr. Jiménez, I'm Miss Rodríguez, the nurse on duty at the General Hospital. Mrs. López Ríos in Room 312 has a headache and fever.

Doctor: Please give her the red tablets every three hours as the label says, and a lot of liquids. If she doesn't feel better, call me again.

Nurse: Thank you, doctor. Good-bye.

Doctor: Good-bye, nurse.

IDENTIFICATION

Extracting from the Context of a Situation

In understanding language, try to go from the general to the specific. First consider the setting, who is speaking, and the order of events. These should give you some general clues. Then listen for specific vocabulary related to the situation. In the following two conversations, a nurse speaks with the patient and then telephones the doctor.

CONVERSACIÓN 1

Paciente: Perdone, señorita, pero me duele mucho la cabeza.

Enfermera: ¿Desde cuándo le duele la cabeza?

Paciente: Me ha dolido la cabeza todo el día, pero después de la comida
            me duele más.

Enfermera: Puede ser algo que comió. Voy a llamar al médico para preguntarle
            qué debe tomar.

CONVERSACIÓN 2

Enfermera: ¿Me permite hablar con el Dr. Jiménez?

Doctor: **Habla el Dr. Jiménez. ¿En qué puedo servirle?**

Enfermera: Dr. Jiménez, le habla la señorita Rodríguez, la enfermera de turno
            del Hospital General. La señora López Ríos, del cuarto 312 tiene
            dolor de cabeza y fiebre.

Doctor: Favor de darle las pastillas rojas cada tres horas como indica
            la receta y líquidos con frecuencia. Si no se siente mejor,
            llame otra vez.

Enfermera: Gracias, doctor. Hasta luego.

Doctor: Adiós, señorita.

Two key words that recur in Conversation 1 give you a general idea about the problem: <u>duele</u> and <u>cabeza</u>. Then, consider: (1) Why would the nurse telephone the doctor? (2) What is his specific advice? (3) What if the patient doesn't feel better? With these three items you have sorted out the important details of the conversation between the nurse and the doctor.

GRAMMAR AND STRUCTURES DRILLED IN LESSON 21

verbs

    tener que + infinitive -- to have to + verb

    doler -- to ache, have pain

        third person singular -- duele

    deber -- should, ought to

indirect object pronoun + duele

Me duele la cabeza.	My head hurts.
Me duelen los ojos.	My eyes hurt.
¿Le duele la herida?	Does the incision hurt?
¿Le duelen los pies?	Do your feet hurt?

Lesson 22
Care of the Patient: Treatments

NEW MATERIAL

Hospital	Patient

°It's necessary to give you a bath.   Is it necessary to give me a bath?
(We have to give you)   (Do you have to give me)

   a warm bath.

   a hot bath.

   a cold bath.

   a partial bath.

   a medicinal bath.

   a cleansing bath.

   a sponge bath.

   a sitz bath.

   a steam bath.

   an alcohol bath.

   a tub bath.

   a shower.

°It's necessary to give you an enema.   Is it necessary to give me an enema?
(We have to give you)   (Do you have to give me)

   an ice pack.

   a hot water bottle.

   a shot.
(an injection)

   an intravenous injection.

   a shot of penicillin.

   an injection of antibiotics.

   an intravenous injection.

Lección 22
Cuidado del paciente: Tratamientos

<u>MATERIA NUEVA</u>

Hospital	Paciente

°<u>Es necesario darle</u> un baño.   ¿<u>Es necesario darme</u> un baño?

    un baño tibio.

    un baño caliente.

    un baño frío.

    un baño parcial.

    un baño medicinal.

    un baño de aseo.

    un baño de esponja.

    un baño de asiento.

    un baño de vapor.

    un baño de alcohol.

    un baño de tina.
            (inmersión)

    un baño de ducha.
            (regadera)

°<u>Es necesario ponerle</u> una enema.   ¿<u>Es necesario ponerme</u> una enema?
                (una ayuda)
                (una lavativa)
                (un lavado)

    una bolsa de hielo.

    una bolsa de agua caliente.

    una inyección.

    una inyección intravenosa.

    una inyección de penicilina.

    una inyección de antibiótico.

    una inyección de suero intravenoso.

Hospital	Patient
°It's necessary to exercise. (You need to)	Yes? Do I need to exercise?

    move your leg.

    move your arm.

    move your hand.

    move your fingers.

    move your leg to the right.

    move your leg to the left.

    lower your leg.

    raise your leg.

    bend your leg.

    walk.

    put you (m.) in traction.
    put you (f.)

Because the doctor says it's necessary. °Why is it necessary?

        the doctor on duty

        the nurse

        the nurse on duty

        the surgeon

        the assistant

        the therapist

°You need a laxative.   Do I? Is it necessary?
                                     Is a laxative necessary?

      a liter of glucose.

      a cobalt treatment.

      an inhalation treatment.

°You need an intravenous injection.   Do I? Is it necessary?
                                      Is an intravenous injection necessary?

    an injection of antitetanus serum.

    an injection of penicillin.

    an injection against infection.

Hospital	Paciente
°Es necesario hacer ejercicios.	¿Sí? ¿Necesito hacer ejercicios?

mover la pierna.

mover el brazo.

mover la mano.

mover los dedos.

mover la pierna a la derecha.

mover la pierna a la izquierda.

bajar la pierna.

levantar la pierna.

doblar la pierna.

caminar.

ponerlo en tracción.
ponerla

Porque el médico dice que es necesario.　°¿Por qué es necesario?

el médico de turno

la enfermera

la enfermera de turno

el cirujano

el ayudante

el terapista

°Necesita un purgante.　　　　　　¿Sí? ¿Es necesario?
　　　　　　　　　　　　　　　　　　¿Es necesario un purgante?

un litro de glucosa.

un tratamiento de cobalto.

un tratamiento de inhalación.

°Necesita una inyección intravenosa.　¿Sí? ¿Es necesaria?
　　　　　　　　　　　　　　　　　　¿Es necesaria una inyección intravenosa

una inyección de suero antitetánico.

una inyección de penicilina.

una inyección contra la infección.

Hospital	Patient
^o<u>You need</u> heat therapy.	<u>Do I</u>? Is it necessary? Is heat therapy necessary?
diathermy.	
hydrotherapy.	
physiotherapy.	
x-ray therapy. (radium)	
^o<u>You need</u> cold compresses.	<u>Do I</u>? Are they necessary? Are cold compresses necessary?
hot compresses.	
Every 2 hours.	^oWhen are they necessary?
Every 15 minutes.	
3 times a day.	
Before bedtime.	
On the affected area.	^oWhere are they necessary?
On the incision.	
^o<u>You need</u> cobalt treatments.	<u>Do I</u>? Are they necessary? Are treatments necessary?
diathermy treatments.	
physical therapy treatments.	

Hospital   Paciente

ᵒNecesita termoterapia.   ¿Sí? ¿Es necesaria?
                                                      ¿Es necesaria la termoterapia?

        diatermia.
        hidroterapia.
        fisioterapia.
        radioterapia.

ᵒNecesita compresas frías.   ¿ Sí? ¿Son necesarias?
                                                       ¿Son necesarias las compresas frías?

        compresas calientes.

Cada dos horas.   ᵒ¿Cuándo son necesarias?
Cada quince minutos.
Tres veces al día.
Antes de dormir.
En la parte afectada.   ᵒ¿Dónde son necesarias?
En la herida.

ᵒNecesita tratamientos de cobalto.   ¿Sí? ¿Son necesarios?
                                                      ¿Son necesarios los tratamientos?

        tratamientos de diatermia.
        tratamientos de fisioterapia.

1. The doctor says that the patient needs an intravenous injection.
2. The man says that he needs an ice pack.
3. The nurse says to give you a bath.
4. The doctor won't permit you to eat too much.
5. The assistant says the compresses shouldn't be too cold.
6. **The anesthetist has ordered me to give you a shot that's a sedative.**
7. The nurse says to use hot compresses three times a day.
8. The nurse on duty says to give you a hot water bottle.

9. The therapist says to move your leg to the left.
10. The nurse says that the woman can't move the joints in her arm.

IDENTIFICATION

In the following sentences someone orders something done or says that a certain condition exists. Try to determine who is saying what in each sentence.

1. El doctor dice que el paciente necesita una inyección intravenosa.

2. El señor dice que necesita una bolsa de hielo.

3. La enfermera dice que le dé un baño.

4. **El médico no le permite que coma demasiado.**

5. El ayudante dice que las compresas no deben ser demasiado frías.

6. El anestesista manda que le ponga una inyección sedante.

7. La enfermera dice que le ponga compresas calientes tres veces al día.

8. La enfermera de turno dice que es necesario ponerle una bolsa de agua caliente.

9. El terapista dice que mueva la pierna a la izquierda.

10. La enfermera dice que la señora no puede mover las articulaciones del brazo.

GRAMMAR AND STRUCTURES DRILLED IN LESSON 22

verbs

necesitar + infinitive -- to need to + verb

es necesario + infinitive -- it is necessary to + verb

adjectives

necesario, -a, -os, -as -- agreement with noun.

pronouns

infinitive + indirect object pronoun me, le

Lesson 23
Communicable Diseases

<u>NEW MATERIAL</u>

Hospital

°<u>We must give you</u> an injection.
<u>(One must)</u>

                a booster shot.

<u>We must give you a vaccination</u>
<u>(One must)</u>

   for colds.

   for influenza.
     (flu)

   for measles.

   for German measles.

   for smallpox.

   for chickenpox.

   for diphtheria.

   for whooping cough.

   for scarlet fever.

°<u>We must give you a vaccination</u>
<u>(One must)</u>

   for tetanus.

   for polio.
     (poliomyelitis)

   for mumps.

   for typhus.

   for malaria.

   for cholera.

   for yellow fever.

   for typhoid fever.

Patient

<u>Oh, an injection</u>?

<u>Oh, a vaccination</u> for colds?

<u>Do you have to give me a vaccination</u>

   for tetanus?

Lección 23
Enfermedades transmisibles

Hospital	Paciente
°Hay que ponerle una inyección.	Ah, ¿una inyección?

una inyección secundaria.

Hay que ponerle vacuna	Ah, ¿vacuna para el resfriado?
	(el catarro)

    para el resfriado.
      (el catarro)

    para la influenza.
      (la gripe)

    para el sarampión.

    para la rubéola.

    para la viruela.

    para las viruelas locas.
      (la varicela)

    para la diftoria.

    para la tos ferina.

    para la escarlatina.

°Hay que ponerle una vacuna	¿Tiene que ponerme una vacuna

    para el tétano.   para el tétano?
    para la poliomielitis.

    para las paperas.
      (la parotiditis)
      (las parótidas)

    para el tifo.

    para el paludismo.
      (la malaria)

    para el cólera.

    para la fiebre amarilla.

    para la fiebre tifoidea.

Hospital	Patient
	°What does the vaccine do?
The vaccine protects you against infection.	
°Did your vaccination take?	Yes, my vaccination took.
	No, it did not take.
It's from 10 to 21 days.	°How long is the incubation period?
Yes, they're very contagious.	°Are measles very contagious?
Yes, it's very contagious. Yes, very. No, it's not very contagious. No, not very.	°Is anthrax <u>very contagious</u>?

malaria

typhus

tetanus

impetigo

Hospital	Patient
Yes, it's very contagious. Yes, very. No, it's not very contagious. No, not very.	°Is rabies <u>very contagious</u>?

plague

meningitis

dysentery

brucellosis

hepatitis

smallpox

whooping cough

typhoid

malaria

tuberculosis (TB)

pneumonia

pleurisy

yellow fever

Hospital	Paciente
La vacuna protege contra la infección.	°¿Qué hace la vacuna?
°¿Le prendió la vacuna?	Sí, me prendió la vacuna.
	No, no me prendió.
Dura de diez a veintiún días.	°¿Cuánto dura el período de incubación?
Sí, es muy contagioso.	°¿Es muy contagioso el sarampión?
<u>Sí, es muy contagioso.</u> <u>Sí, mucho.</u>	°¿Es muy <u>contagioso</u> el ántrax?
<u>No, no es muy contagioso.</u> <u>No, no mucho.</u>	
	el paludismo?
	el tifo?
	el tétano?
	el impétigo?
<u>Sí, es muy contagiosa.</u> <u>Sí, mucho.</u>	°¿Es muy <u>contagiosa</u> la rabia?
<u>No, no es muy contagiosa.</u> <u>No, no mucho.</u>	
	la peste bubónica?
	la meningitis?
	la disentería?
	la brucelosis?
	la hepatitis?
	la viruela?
	la tos ferina?
	la tifoidea?
	la malaria?
	la tuberculosis?
	la pulmonía?
	la pleuresía?
	la fiebre amarilla?

Hospital	Patient

Hospital

Yes, there are many (m.).
Yes, there are many (f.).

Patient

^oAre there many doctors?

many vaccinations?

many contagious diseases?

many patients?

many nurses?

many surgeons?

many immunizations?

many injections?

Yes, when you disinfect the dishes.

when you wash the clothes.

when you see the patient.

when you wash your hands.

^oMust I be careful?
(Must one)

You must immunize the patient.
(One must)

immunize the family.

take care of the patient.

call the doctor.

isolate the patient.

separate the patient.

^oWhat must I do?
(What must be done?)

You must avoid contagion.
(One must)

use a private room.

use a hospital gown.

use a protective apron.

use a mask.

keep the door closed.

not have visitors.

be careful for a long time.

wash the bed linens separately.
(linens)
(sheets and pillowcases)

wash your hands.

protect yourself from the infection.

put on a robe.

^oWhen you get the disease, what must you do?
(one gets)   (one)

Hospital	Paciente
Sí, hay muchos.	°¿Hay muchos médicos?
Sí, hay muchas.	muchas vacunas?

                    Hospital   Paciente

Sí, hay muchos.   °¿Hay muchos médicos?
Sí, hay muchas.   muchas vacunas?
                                                   muchas enfermedades contagiosas?
                                                   muchos pacientes?
                                                   muchas enfermeras?
                                                   muchos cirujanos?
                                                   muchas inmunizaciones?
                                                   muchas inyecciones?

Sí, al desinfectar los utensilios.   °¿Hay que tener cuidado?

    al lavar la ropa.
    al ver al paciente.
    al lavarse las manos.
Hay que inmunizar al paciente.   °¿Qué hay que hacer?

        inmunizar a la familia.
        cuidar al paciente.
        llamar al médico.
        aislar al paciente.
        separar al paciente.

Hay que evitar el contagio.   °Al contraer la enfermedad, ¿qué hay que
                                               hacer?

    usar un cuarto privado.
    usar una bata de hospital.
    usar un delantal protector.
    usar una mascarilla.
    tener la puerta cerrada.
    no tener visitas.
    tener cuidado por mucho tiempo.
    lavar las ropas de cama separadas.

    lavarse las manos.
    protegerse de la infección.
    ponerse una bata.

Conversation

Doctor: Come in, ma'am, and tell me how you feel.

Woman: I'm very upset because a friend of my son's has TB. I'm afraid my son may have caught it. They're always together at my house.

Doctor: Don't worry. Although tuberculosis is a very contagious illness, and one must be careful, it is possible to do something.

Woman: What can we do?

Doctor: We'll do an x-ray of your son immediately and also several tests to see if there are any signs of infection.

Woman: What should I do at home with my family?

Doctor: Clean and disinfect your house well, and always wash your hands before preparing food. Let the boy follow his normal life, have him rest and exercise moderately outdoors. Bring the boy again next week. If you have any questions, call me.

IDENTIFICATION

Conversación

Doctor: <u>Pase</u>, señora, y <u>dígame</u> cómo se siente.

Señora: Estoy muy nerviosa porque un amigo de mi hijo tiene tuberculosis.
Temo que mi hijo se contagie. Siempre están juntos en mi casa.

Doctor: <u>No se preocupe</u>. Aunque la tuberculosis es una enfermedad muy
contagiosa y hay que tener cuidado, es posible hacer algo.

Señora: ¿Qué podemos hacer?

Doctor: Vamos a hacerle una radiografía a su hijo inmediatamente y también
varios análisis para ver si se ha contagiado.

Señora: ¿Qué debo hacer en casa con la familia?

Doctor: <u>Limpie</u> y <u>desinfecte</u> bien la casa y siempre <u>lávese</u> las manos antes
de preparar la comida. Que el niño <u>siga</u> una vida normal, <u>descanse</u>
y <u>haga</u> ejercicio moderado al aire libre. <u>Tráigame</u> al niño otra
vez la semana que viene. Si tiene preguntas <u>llámeme</u>.

The underlined forms in the above conversation are commands. They tell someone
to do (or, if negative, not to do) something. You have learned an easy way around
these forms: <u>favor de</u> + infinitive. Change the following commands to this simple
way to say <u>please</u>.

Command	Infinitive (+ pronoun)		Please
pase	pasar	to come in	<u>favor de</u> pasar
dígame	decir(me)	to tell me	
no se preocupe	preocupar(se)	to worry (oneself)	
limpie	limpiar	to clean	
desinfecte	desinfectar	to disinfect	
lávese	lavar(se)	to wash (oneself)	
siga	seguir	to follow	
descanse	descansar	to rest	
haga	hacer	to do	
tráigame	traer(me)	to bring (me)	
llámeme	llamar(me)	to call (me)	

Now, can you pick out the key words to answer the following questions?

1. What is the mother worried about?

2. What is the doctor going to do?

3. What are some of the things the doctor tells the mother to do?

GRAMMAR AND STRUCTURES DRILLED IN LESSON 23

verbs

<u>hay</u> -- there is, there are

<u>hay que</u> + infinitive -- one must (we must, you must) + verb

idioms

<u>al</u> + infinitive -- when + verb

<u>al desinfectar</u> -- when you disinfect

adjective

agreement with noun

<u>¿Es contagioso el tifo?</u> Is typhus contagious?
<u>¿Es contagiosa la varicela?</u> Is chickenpox contagious?

<u>mucho</u> -- very

<u>¿Es contagiosa la viruela?</u> <u>Sí, mucho.</u> Is smallpox contagious? Yes, very.

personal <u>a</u>

<u>Hay que inmunizar a la familia.</u> One must immunize the family.

Lesson 24
Antiseptics

Hospital	Patient

○ <u>I have to</u> wash the wound.

<u>Oh, do you have to</u> wash <u>it</u> (f.)?

   clean the wound.

   sterilize the wound.

   dry the wound.

   cure the wound.

   change the bandage.

   change the gauze.

   change the bed.

   use boiled water.

   use sodium peroxide.

   use medicine.

   use an antiseptic solution.

   use adhesive tape.

○ <u>I have to</u> wash the wounds.

<u>Oh, do you have to</u> wash <u>them</u> (f.)?

   clean the wounds.

   sterilize the wounds.

   dry the wounds.

   cure the wounds.

   change the bandages.

   use antiseptic solutions.

○ <u>I have to</u> use bleach.

<u>Oh, do you have to</u> use <u>it</u> (m.)?

   use disinfectant.

   use soap.

   use ointment.

   use ammonia.

   use iodine.

   use alcohol.

   change the bandage.

Lección 24
Antisépticos

Hospital   Paciente

°<u>Tengo que</u> lavar la herida.   <u>Ah, ¿tiene que</u> lavar<u>la</u>?

limpiar la herida.

esterilizar la herida.

secar la herida.

curar la herida.

cambiar la venda.

cambiar la gasa.

cambiar la cama.

usar agua hervida.

usar agua oxigenada.

usar medicina.

usar solución antiséptica.

usar tela adhesiva.

°<u>Tengo que</u> lavar las heridas.   <u>Ah, ¿tiene que</u> lavar<u>las</u>?

limpiar las heridas.

esterilizar las heridas.

secar las heridas.

curar las heridas.

cambiar las vendas.

usar soluciones antisépticas.

°<u>Tengo que</u> usar cloro.   <u>Ah, ¿tiene que</u> usar<u>lo</u>?

usar desinfectante.

usar jabón.

usar ungüento.

usar amoníaco.

usar yodo.

usar alcohol.

cambiar el vendaje.

Hospital	Patient

^o<u>You have to</u> use disinfectants.

<u>Oh, do I have to</u> use <u>them</u> (m.)?

         use germicides.
         avoid germs.
         use bandages.
         use water and soap.
         wash the equipment.
         sterilize the equipment.
         dry the equipment.
         clean the equipment.

<u>Yes</u>, you should change <u>it</u> (f.).

^oShould I change the bandage?

    one must

Must one change the bandage?

    you can

Can I change the bandage?

    you need to

Do I need to change the bandage?

    it is necessary to

Is it necessary to change the bandage?

<u>Yes</u>, you should <u>clean it</u> (m.).

Should I clean the instrument?
Must one clean the instrument?
Can I clean the instrument?
Do I need to clean the instrument?

^o<u>It's necessary to clean</u> the instrument.

<u>I understand</u>. <u>It's necessary</u>
      <u>to clean it</u> (m.).

        the wound.

          <u>it</u> (f.).

        the equipment.

          <u>them</u> (m.).

        the wounds.

          <u>them</u> (f.).

<u>It's necessary to expose</u> the wound to
    the air.

    to expose <u>it</u> (f.) to the air.

Hospital	Paciente
°<u>Usted tiene que</u> usar desinfectantes.	Ah, <u>¿tengo que</u> usar<u>los</u>?
usar germicidas.	
evitar microbios.	
usar vendajes.	
usar agua y jabón.	
lavar los aparatos.	
esterilizar los aparatos.	
secar los aparatos.	
limpiar los aparatos.	
<u>Sí</u>, debe cambiar<u>la</u>.	°¿Debo cambiar la venda?
hay que	¿Hay que cambiar la venda?
puede	¿Puedo cambiar la venda?
necesita	¿Necesito cambiar la venda?
es necesario	¿Es necesario cambiar la venda?
<u>Sí</u>, debe <u>limpiarlo</u>.	¿Debo limpiar el aparato?
	¿Hay que limpiar el aparato?
	¿Puedo limpiar el aparato?
	¿Necesito limpiar el aparato?
°<u>Es necesario limpiar</u> el aparato.	Comprendo. Es necesario <u>limpiarlo</u>.
la herida.	<u>la</u>
los aparatos.	<u>los</u>
las heridas.	<u>las</u>
Es necesario exponer la herida al aire.	exponerla al aire.

Disinfectants

1. The proper use of a disinfectant in the laundry can prevent or reduce the spread of bacteriological infections.

2. Some disinfectants that are effective in reducing the number of bacteria in clothing are bleach, pine oil, and the quaternary disinfectants, such as benzalkonium. The quaternary disinfectants, used especially in hospitals, should be put only in the final rinse of the laundry.

3. These disinfectants can be bought in supermarkets, drugstores, or in stores that sell cleaning products.

4. Warning: Disinfectants should be kept out of the reach of children.

IDENTIFICATION

Read through the following paragraphs. Try to get a general idea of what is being said through cognate words.

Desinfectantes

1. El uso apropriado de un desinfectante en el lavado de ropa puede prevenir o reducir la propagación de infecciones bacteriológicas.

2. Algunos desinfectantes efectivos en reducir el número de bacterias en la ropa son cloro, aceite de pino y los cuaternarios, como Benzylkonyum. Los desinfectantes cuaternarios, usados especialmente en los hospitales, deben ponerse solamente en el enjuague final del lavado.

3. Estos desinfectantes pueden comprarse en los supermercados, en las farmacias o en los establecimientos que venden materiales de limpieza.

4. Advertencia: Los desinfectantes deben estar fuera de alcance de los niños.

Underline these key words in the foregoing paragraphs.

1.	uso	2.	desinfectantes	3.	desinfectantes	4.	advertencia
	desinfectante(s)		efectivos		comprarse		desinfectantes
	lavado de ropa		cloro		supermercados		fuera
	prevenir		aceite de pino		farmacias		alcance
	reducir		cuaternarios				niños
	infecciones		enjuague final				
			lavado				

Notice that most of these key words are cognates. Others are related to words that you have studied, such as lavado from lavar. Can you guess the ones you don't know from the context of each paragraph?

GRAMMAR AND STRUCTURES DRILLED IN LESSON 24

verbs

    tener que + infinitive -- to have to + verb

pronouns

    direct object pronoun attached to the infinitive

        lo, la -- it   los, las -- them

        Tengo que usar cloro.   I have to use bleach.
        Tengo que usarlo.   I have to use it (m.).

        Tengo que usar medicina. I have to use medicine.
        Tengo que usarla.   I have to use it (f.).

Lesson 25
Maternity: Prenatal Care

NEW MATERIAL

Hospital	Patient
°Why are you coming to see the doctor?	I think I'm pregnant.
Why do you think so?	Because I haven't had my period for 7 weeks.
You haven't had menstruation?	No, I haven't had menstruation.
What symptoms do you have?	I'm nauseated.
Are you nauseated?	Yes, I'm nauseated. No, I'm not nauseated.

Do you vomit?

Do you have acidity in your stomach?

        heartburn?

        cramps in your legs?

        swollen legs?

        piles?
(hemorrhoids)

        pain at the waist?

        discharge of blood?

        change in your breasts?

You should rest more.	°What should I do?
rest every day.	
keep your body clean.	
keep your normal weight.	
stay in a good frame of mind. (stay in a good mood)	
exercise moderately.	
walk every day.	
Yes, ma'am, you should visit the doctor often.	°Should I visit the doctor often?
	use comfortable clothing?
	use loose-fitting clothes?
	keep on working?

Lección 25
Maternidad: Cuidado prenatal

<u>MATERIA NUEVA</u>

Hospital	Paciente
°¿Por qué viene usted al médico?	Creo que estoy embarazada.
¿Por qué lo cree?	Porque hace siete semanas que no tengo mi regla.
¿No tiene usted menstruación?	No, no tengo menstruación.
¿Qué tiene usted?	Tengo náuseas.
¿<u>Tiene usted</u> náuseas?	<u>Sí, tengo</u> náuseas.
	<u>No, no tengo</u> náuseas.
vómitos?	
acidez en el estómago?	
hervor?	
calambres en las piernas?	
las piernas hinchadas?	
almorranas? (hemorroides)	
dolor de cintura?	
flujo de sangre?	
cambio en los senos? (cambio en los pechos)	
<u>Debe</u> descansar más.	°¿<u>Qué debo hacer</u>?
descansar todos los días.	
conservar su cuerpo limpio.	
conservar su peso normal.	
conservar su buen humor.	
hacer ejercicio moderado.	
caminar todos los días.	
<u>Sí, señora, usted debe</u> visitar al médico con frecuencia.	°¿<u>Debo</u> visitar al médico con frecuencia?
	usar ropa cómoda?
	usar ropa amplia?
	seguir trabajando?

259

Hospital	Patient

Hospital

It lasts 9 months.
     10 lunar months.
     40 weeks.
     from 273 to 280 days after your
     last menstrual period.

Patient

°How long does the pregnancy last?

Hospital

°Have you had problems?

     miscarriages or abortions?
     rapid weight gain?
     headaches?
     vision difficulties?

Do you see black spots?
Yes, ma'am, you have toxemia.
No, ma'am, you don't have

Yes, there is danger.
No, there is no danger.

If you have a discharge of blood.

     strong pains.
     frequent contractions.
If your bag of waters breaks.
You should take a suitcase.
Yes, you should take it (f.).
             it (m.).
             them (m.).
             them (f.).

Patient

Yes, doctor, I've had problems.
No, doctor, I haven't had

No, I don't see black spots.
°Do I have toxemia?
        high blood pressure?

Is there danger of eclampsia?

°When should I call the doctor?
        go to the hospital?

What should I take to the hospital?
Should I take a suitcase?
        my robe?
        my slippers?
        personal articles?
        articles for the baby?
        my toothbrush?
        my hairbrush?

Hospital	Paciente

<u>Dura</u> nueve meses.

    diez meses lunares.

    cuarenta semanas.

    de doscientos setenta y tres a
    doscientos ochenta días después
    del último período.

°¿<u>Ha tenido</u> problemas?

      abortos?

      aumento rápido de peso?

      dolores de cabeza?

      trastornos en la visión?

¿Ve puntos negros?

<u>Sí, señora, usted tiene</u> toxemia.
<u>No, señora, usted no tiene</u>

Sí, hay peligro.
No, no hay peligro.

<u>Si tiene</u> flujo de sangre.

      dolores fuertes.

      contracciones frecuentes.

Si se le rompe la fuente.

Debe llevar una maleta.

<u>Sí, debe llevarla.</u>
        lo.
        los.
        las.

°¿<u>Cuánto dura el período de gestación</u>?

<u>Sí, doctor, he tenido</u> problemas.
<u>No, doctor, no he tenido</u>

No, no veo puntos negros.
°¿<u>Tengo</u> toxemia?
      la presión alta?

¿Hay peligro de eclampsia?

°¿<u>Cuándo debo</u> llamar al médico?
      ir al hospital?

¿Qué debo <u>llevar al hospital</u>?
¿<u>Debo llevar</u> una maleta?
      la bata?
      las zapatillas?
      artículos personales?
      artículos para el bebé?
      el cepillo de dientes?
      el cepillo de cabeza?

1. I should go to the doctor because I think I'm pregnant. I haven't men-struated for six weeks, and in the morning I feel bad. Besides, my breasts ache.

2. You know I'm working, and I don't have easy pregnancies. I was pregnant before, and I had a miscarriage at four months. This will be my second pregnancy, and I don't know if the doctor will let me keep on working.

IDENTIFICATION

In Paragraph 1, underline these key words.

ir	embarazada	menstruación	mañanas	me duelen
médico	no	seis semanas	mal	pechos

Then read the paragraph aloud and summarize what you think the speaker is saying.

1. Debo ir al médico porque creo que estoy embarazada. No he tenido menstruación desde hace seis semanas, y por las mañanas me siento mal. Además me duelen los pechos.

Read Paragraph 2 aloud for a general idea of what is being said. Then read it again, underlining what you think are the key words.
If you can answer the questions that follow the paragraph, you understand most of what the native speaker said.

2. Usted sabe que estoy trabajando fuera de casa y yo no tengo embarazos fáciles. Antes estuve embarazada y a los cuatro meses tuve un aborto. Este va a ser mi segundo embarazo y no sé si el médico me va a permitir seguir trabajando.

1. What does the woman wonder if the doctor will let her do?

2. What problem does she have and what has happened before?

3. Is this her first pregnancy?

GRAMMAR AND STRUCTURES DRILLED IN LESSON 25

verbs

tener, first and third person, present and present perfect tense

deber, first and third person, + infinitive

pronouns

infinitive + direct object pronoun

Lesson 26
Maternity: Labor and Delivery

<u>NEW MATERIAL</u>

Hospital	Patient
^oWho is your doctor?	It's Dr. Sánchez.
Do you want to go to the bathroom?	<u>No, I don't need to</u> go to the bathroom.
Do you need to urinate?	urinate.
Has your bag of waters broken?	No, my bag of waters hasn't broken.
<u>Take off</u> your clothes, <u>please</u>.	<u>All right</u>.
	<u>Of course</u>!
your coat	
your dress	
your blouse	
your hose	
all your clothes	
your panties	
^o<u>Sit down</u> here, <u>please</u>.	<u>Here? Thanks</u>.
on the bed	
on the chair	
The baby's about to be born.	
<u>We're going</u> to the maternity floor.	<u>Well, let's go</u> to the maternity floor.
to the predelivery room.	
to the labor room.	
to the delivery room.	
^o<u>We're going to</u> prepare <u>you</u>.	<u>Are you (pl.) going to</u> prepare <u>me</u>?
shave <u>you</u>.	
observe <u>you</u>.	
take <u>your</u> blood pressure.	take <u>my</u> blood pressure?
take <u>your</u> temperature.	
take <u>your</u> pulse.	
do a rectal exam (on <u>you</u>).	
give <u>you</u> an enema.	

Lección 26
Maternidad: Labor y parto

Hospital	Paciente
°¿Quién es su médico?	Es el doctor Sánchez.
¿Quiere ir al baño?	No, no necesito ir al baño.
¿Necesita orinar?	orinar.
¿Ha perdido agua?	No, no he perdido agua.
Quítese la ropa, por favor.	Muy bien.
el abrigo	¡Cómo no!
el vestido	
la blusa	
las medias	
toda la ropa	
los calzones	
°Siéntese aquí, por favor.	¿Aquí? Gracias.
en la cama	
en la silla	
Ya el niño va a nacer.	
Vamos al piso de maternidad.	Bueno, vamos al piso de maternidad.
a la sala prenatal.	
a la sala de labor.	
a la sala de partos.	
°Vamos a prepararla.	¿Van a prepararme?
afeitarla. (rasurarla)	
observarla.	
tomarle la presión.	tomarme la presión?
tomarle la temperatura.	
tomarle el pulso.	
hacerle un tacto rectal.	
ponerle una enema. (ponerle una ayuda) (ponerle una lavativa)	

Hospital	Patient

^oDo you have frequent pains?   Yes, I have pains.

    frequent contractions?

    frequent expulsive contractions?

Very strong?   Yes, very strong.

How often?   Every 20 minutes.

                                  Every 12 minutes.

                                  Every 7 minutes.

                                  Every 3 minutes.

You must breathe deeply.   But it hurts so much.

       be calm.

Not yet. You're just beginning.   ^oI want medicine.

He's coming soon.   to see the doctor.

^oWhat kind of anesthesia do you want?   I want a local anesthetic.

                                  a spinal.

                                  natural childbirth.

                                  what the doctor recommends.

I think so.   ^oAm I going to have a normal birth?

I don't think so.

I hope so.   a difficult birth?

I hope not.

                       Are they going to do a caesarean section?

                       Are they going to use forceps?

                                     tongs?

                                     pincers?

^oIf you lose water, you have to stay in   All right.

    bed.

(If your bag of waters breaks)

Hospital	Paciente
°¿<u>Tiene</u> dolores frecuentes?	Sí, tengo dolores.
dolores de parto frecuentes?	
pujos seguidos?	
¿Muy fuertes?	Sí, muy fuertes.
¿<u>Con qué frecuencia</u>?	Cada veinte minutos.
	Cada doce minutos.
	Cada siete minutos.
	Cada tres minutos.
<u>Hay que</u> respirar profundo.	Pero me duele mucho.
estar tranquila.	
Todavía no. Apenas empieza.	°<u>Quiero</u> medicina.
Viene pronto.	ver al médico.
°¿<u>Qué clase de anestesia quiere</u>?	Quiero anestesia local.
	raquídea.
	un parto natural.
	la que recomiende el doctor.
<u>Creo que sí.</u>	°¿<u>Voy a tener</u> un parto normal?
<u>Creo que no.</u>	un parto difícil?
<u>Ojalá que sí.</u>	
<u>Ojalá que no.</u>	
	¿Van a hacerme una operación cesárea?
	¿<u>Van a usar</u> forceps?
	tenazas?
	pinzas?
°Si pierde agua, <u>tiene que quedarse en cama</u>.	Muy bien.
(Si se le rompe la fuente)	

Hospital	Patient

<u>If</u> you need to urinate, <u>we'll</u> bring you <u>All right</u>.
a bedpan.

<u>If</u> you have fever, <u>we'll</u> take your
temperature <u>again</u>.

<u>If</u> you have high blood pressure, <u>we'll</u>
take your blood pressure.

^oPlease wake up.   Yes? So early?

Wake up.

<u>It's a boy</u>.   Great!
     <u>a girl</u>.

                                 Wonderful! Great!

Yes, he's normal.   ^oIs he normal?
   (she's)   (she)

Yes, just fine.   Is he all right?
                                (she)

<u>He weighs</u> 8 pounds.   <u>How much does he weigh</u>?
(<u>She</u>)   (<u>she</u>)
       8 pounds 3 ounces.
       6 pounds 12 ounces.
       7 1/2 pounds.
       6 pounds 2 ounces.

<u>He's very</u> handsome (m.)!   <u>Yes, very</u> pretty.
(<u>She's</u>)   pretty (f.)!

Hospital	Paciente
Si necesita orinar, <u>vamos a</u> ponerle el bacín.	Muy bien.
Si tiene fiebre, <u>vamos a</u> tomarle la temperatura <u>otra vez</u>.	
Si tiene alta presión, <u>vamos a</u> tomarle la presión.	
°Favor de despertarse.	¿Sí? ¿Tan temprano?
Despiértese.	
<u>Es un niño.</u> una niña.	¡Qué bueno!
	¡Excelente! ¡Qué bueno!
Sí, es normal.	°¿Es normal?
Sí, está bien.	¿Está bien?
<u>Pesa</u> ocho libras.	¿<u>Cuánto pesa</u>?
ocho libras y tres onzas. seis libras y doce onzas. siete libras y media. seis libras y dos onzas.	
¡<u>Es muy</u> bonito! bonita!	<u>Sí, muy</u> bonito. bonita.

What is your husband's full name?

Where was your husband born?

What is the date of his birth?

Where does your husband work?

With what company?

What is your home address?

What is your full maiden name?

Where were you born?

What is the date of your birth?

What date did the doctor give you for this birth?

Is this your first pregnancy?

How many children have you had?

Have you had any miscarriages or abortions?

What is your religion?

What kind of anesthesia do you want?

Are you going to breastfeed the child?

IDENTIFICATION

The following questions might be asked of the mother before the child is born to obtain information for the birth certificate and other information concerning the child. Compare the questions with those in Lesson 7 (En el hospital: Admisión y formas). All the important vocabulary should be either in that lesson or in this one. Imagine asking an imaginary mother these questions and record her answers.

¿Cuál es el nombre completo de su esposo? _____

¿Dónde nació su esposo? _____

¿Cuál es la fecha de su nacimiento? _____

¿Dónde trabaja su esposo? _____

¿En qué compañía? _____

¿Cuál es la dirección de su casa? _____

¿Cuál es su nombre completo de soltera? _____

¿Dónde nació usted? _____

¿Cuál es la fecha de su nacimiento? _____

¿Qué fecha le dio el médico para este parto? _____

¿Es su primer embarazo? _____

¿Cuántos niños ha tenido? _____

¿Ha tenido abortos? _____

¿Cuál es su religión? _____

¿Qué tipo de anestesia desea? _____

¿Va a darle el pecho al niño? _____

GRAMMAR AND STRUCTURES DRILLED IN LESSON 26

verbs

  ir a + infinitive -- to be going to + verb

idioms

  Creo que sí.   I think so.
  Creo que no.   I think not.

  Ojalá que no.   I hope not.
  Ojalá que sí.   I hope so.

pronouns

  indirect object pronoun attached to infinitive

  direct object pronoun attached to infinitive

Lesson 27
Maternity: Postnatal Care of the Mother

<u>NEW MATERIAL</u>

Hospital	Patient
It's necessary to take pills.	^oWhat is necessary?
take pills six times.	Is it necessary to take pills?
take pills every 4 hours.	
take a sedative at bedtime.	
take a laxative every night.	
contract your uterus.	
give you shots.	
give you an enema.	
use cream.	
use a lamp.	
use a lamp for 20 minutes.	
On the perineum.	^oWhere?
the incision.	
the stitches.	
To dry up the incision.	What for?
^oIt's necessary to	Is it necessary to watch for it (m.)?
watch for excessive flow.	it (f.)?
prepare the formula.	them (f.)?
prepare the milk.	
sterilize the bottles.	
wash the bottles.	
boil the bottles.	
rinse the bottles.	
dry the bottles.	
give medicines.	

Lección 27
Maternidad: Cuidado posnatal de la madre

MATERIA NUEVA

Hospital	Paciente

Es necesario tomar píldoras.

    tomar píldoras seis veces.

    tomar píldoras cada cuatro horas.

    tomar un calmante al acostarse.

    tomar un laxante todas las noches.

    contraer el útero.

    ponerle inyecciones.

    ponerle una enema.

    ponerle crema.

    ponerle una lámpara.

    ponerle una lámpara veinte minutos.

En el perineo.

  la herida.

  (la incisión)

    las puntadas.

Para secarle la herida.

°Es necesario

    observar el exceso de flujo.

    preparar la formula.

    preparar la leche.

    esterilizar las botellas.

    lavar las botellas.

    hervir las botellas.

    enjuagar las botellas.

    secar las botellas.

    dar medicinas.

Paciente column:

°¿Qué es necesario?

¿Es necesario tomar píldoras?

°¿Dónde?

¿Para qué?

¿Es necesario observarlo?

                la?

                las?

Hospital	Patient

Hospital

°<u>It's necessary to</u>
  take care of the baby (m.).
  change the baby.
  go to see the baby.
  keep the baby clean.

°<u>It's necessary to</u>
  take care of the baby (f.).
  change the baby.
  go to see the baby.
  keep the baby clean.

<u>It's necessary to</u> **give him water.**
                    (her)

                 nurse   him.
              (breastfeed) (her)
                 change his diaper.
                       (her)
If the baby (m.) is wet.
  the baby (f.) is wet.
If the baby (m.) is dirty.
  the baby (f.) is dirty.

<u>You should</u> drink a lot of liquids.
              drink a lot of water.
              rest enough.

<u>You can</u> eat a **regular diet.**
  let your legs dangle.
  sit up.
  sit in a chair.
  get up.
  walk.
  take a shower.

Patient

<u>It's necessary to</u> take care of <u>him</u>.
              change <u>him</u>.
              go to see <u>him</u>.
              keep <u>him</u> clean.

<u>It's necessary to</u> take care of <u>her</u>.
              change <u>her</u>.
              go to see <u>her</u>.
              keep <u>her</u> clean.

°<u>Is it necessary to</u>
  give the baby (m.) water?
       the baby (f.)
  nurse   the baby (m.)?
  (breastfeed) the baby (f.)?
  change the baby's (m.) diaper?
         the baby's (f.)
When should I change his diaper?
                     (her)

°<u>What should I do</u>?

°<u>What can I do</u>?   The first day?
                    From the first day?
                    The second day?
                    From the second day?

Hospital   Paciente

°Es necesario
   cuidar al bebé.   Es necesario cuidar<u>lo</u>.

   cambiar al bebé.   cambiar<u>lo</u>.

   ir a ver al niño.   ir a ver<u>lo</u>.

   mantener al niño limpio.   mantener<u>lo</u> limpio.

°Es necesario
   cuidar a la niña.   Es necesario cuidar<u>la</u>.

   cambiar a la niña.   cambiar<u>la</u>.

   ir a ver a la niña.   ir a ver<u>la</u>.

   mantener a la niña limpia.   mantener<u>la</u> limpia.

Es necesario darle agua.   °¿**Es necesario**
                            dar agua al niño?
                                    a la niña?

        darle de mamar.   dar de mamar al niño?
        (darle el pecho)   (dar el pecho) a la niña?

        cambiarle el pañal.   **cambiarle el pañal al niño?**
                                  a la niña?

Si el niño está mojado.   ¿Cuándo hay que cambiarle el pañal?
  la niña está mojada.

Si el niño está sucio.
  la niña **está sucia.**

<u>Usted debe</u> tomar muchos líquidos.   °¿<u>Qué debo</u> hacer?

        tomar mucha agua.

        descansar bastante.

<u>Usted puede</u> comer una **dieta general.**   °¿<u>Qué puedo hacer?</u>   ¿El primer día?
                                         ¿Desde el primer día?
   colgar las piernas.   ¿El segundo día?
   sentarse.   ¿Desde el segundo día?

   sentarse en una silla.

   levantarse.

   andar.

   darse un baño   de regadera.
      (una ducha)

Hospital	Patient
Yes, you can see the baby.	^oCan I see the baby?
No, you can't	nurse the baby?
	go to the bathroom?
	eat everything?
	smoke?
Every 4 hours.	When can I nurse the baby?
After 6 weeks.	can I have intercourse with my husband?
The doctor will tell you.	can I go home?
Right away.	When are they going to bring the baby?
Very soon.	should I see the doctor again?
	are they going to discharge me?
It's necessary to dry up your milk.	^oWhat is necessary
	if I'm not going to nurse the baby?
put cream on your breasts.	if I'm going to nurse the baby?
give you an injection.	if I have nausea?
give you the bedpan.	if I want to urinate?
put in a catheter.	if I can't urinate?

Hospital	Paciente
	°¿Puedo ver al niño?
Sí, usted puede ver al niño.	dar el pecho al bebé?
No, usted no puede	ir al baño?
	comer de todo?
	fumar?

Hospital	Paciente
Cada cuatro horas.	¿Cuándo puedo dar de mamar al bebé?
Después de seis semanas.	puedo tener relaciones con mi esposo?
El médico va a decirle.	puedo ir a casa?
En seguida.	¿Cuándo va a traer al bebé?
Muy pronto.	debo volver al médico?
	van a darme de alta?

Hospital	Paciente
Es necesario secarle la leche.	°¿Qué es necesario
	si no voy a darle el pecho?
ponerle crema en los pechos.	si voy a darle el pecho?
ponerle una inyección.	si tengo náuseas?
ponerle el bacín.	si quiero orinar?
ponerle una sonda. (un catéter)	si no puedo orinar?

Conversation

Mrs. Pérez: Here's a gift for your baby. I brought him diapers and
plastic pants. The little fellow looks like his father.
He has blue eyes and blond hair.

Mrs. Sánchez: He's a very good boy. He almost never cries. He sleeps a
lot. He's not excitable.

Mrs. Pérez: When are you going home?

Mrs. Sánchez: The doctor's going to discharge me Monday or Tuesday if
everything goes well.

Mrs. Pérez: Do you have milk already?

Mrs. Sánchez: Yes, I have enough milk.

Mrs. Pérez: Do your breasts hurt?

Mrs. Sánchez: Yes, they hurt. I need to nurse the baby frequently.

IDENTIFICATION

Conversación

Señora Pérez: Aquí tengo un regalo para su niño. Le traigo pañales y
pantalones de plástico. El bebito se parece a su papá.
Tiene los ojos azules y el pelo rubio.

Señora Sánchez: Es un niño muy bueno. Casi nunca llora. Duerme mucho.
No es nervioso.

Señora Pérez: ¿Cuándo vuelve a casa?

Señora Sánchez: **El médico va a darme de alta el lunes o el martes si todo
va bien.**

Señora Pérez: ¿Ya le bajó la leche?

Señora Sánchez: Sí, tengo bastante leche.

Señora Pérez: ¿Le duelen los pechos?

Señora Sánchez: Sí, me duelen. Necesito dar de mamar al niño con frecuencia.

Underline the following key words in this conversation.

regalo	martes
pañales	si
papá	bien
ojos azules	ya
pelo rubio	leche
niño	tengo
bueno	leche
no llora	duelen
duerme	pechos
¿Cuándo?	sí
médico	duelen
darme de alta	mamar
lunes	con frecuencia

Write the English beside each word you know in the above list. For each of the
words you do not know, guess, look it up in the vocabulary, or ask your instructor,
"¿Qué quiere decir . . . ?" ("What does . . . mean?") Summarize the conversation
in English before checking the translation.

GRAMMAR AND STRUCTURES DRILLED IN LESSON 27

verbs

    es necesario + infinitive -- it is necessary + infinitive

    deber + infinitive -- should, ought to + verb

    poder + infinitive -- can + verb

personal a

    Es necesario ver a la niña.   It's necessary to see the baby.

pronouns

    indirect object pronoun attached to infinitive

    direct object pronoun attached to infinitive

Lesson 28
Maternity: Care of the Newborn

<u>NEW MATERIAL</u>

<table>
<tr><td style="text-align:center">Hospital</td><td style="text-align:center">Patient</td></tr>
</table>

Yes, <u>you must bathe</u> him <u>every day.</u>   ^o<u>Must I</u>   bathe the baby <u>every day</u>?
    (<u>one must</u>)   (her)   (<u>Must one</u>)   the baby (m.)
                                        the baby (f.)

                                 <u>Must I</u>   bathe the baby (f.) <u>in warm water</u>?
                                 (<u>Must one</u>)   the baby (m.)

Every day.   .   When <u>must I</u>   bathe him ?
                                    (<u>must one</u>)   (her)

In warm water.   How <u>must I bathe</u> him ?
                                      (her)

With your elbow.   How <u>must I</u>   test the water?
                              (<u>must one</u>)

<u>After</u> the umbilical cord falls off.   When can I put him into the water?
                                      (her)

    the navel heals.

^o<u>You must</u> avoid drafts.   Avoid them?
(<u>One must</u>)

    dry him well.   Dry him well?
      (her)   (her)

    feed him every 3 or 4 hours.
      (her)

    feed him according to the doctor's
      (her)

      recommendations.

Lección 28
Maternidad: Cuidado del recién nacido

MATERIA NUEVA

Hospital	Paciente
Sí, hay que bañarlo todos los días. bañarla	°¿Hay que bañar al bebé todos los días? al niño a la niña
	¿Hay que bañar a la niña en agua tibia? al niño
Todos los días.	¿Cuándo hay que bañarlo? la
En agua tibia.	¿Cómo hay que bañarlo? la
Con el codo.	¿Cómo hay que probar el agua?
Después de caérse el ombligo. (cordón umbilical) secársele el ombligo.	¿Cuándo puedo sumergilo en agua? la
°Hay que evitar las corrientes de aire.	¿Evitarlas?
secarlo bien. la	¿Secarlo bien? la
alimentarlo cada tres o cuatro horas. la	
alimentarlo según diga el médico. la	

Hospital	Patient

^o<u>You must</u> prepare the formula.   Prepare <u>it</u> (f.)?
(<u>One must</u>)   <u>it</u> (m.)?

    use a measuring cup.   <u>them</u> (m.)?

    use a sterilizer.   <u>them</u> (f.)?

    have 8 or 10 baby bottles.

    have 8 or 10 bottles.

    wash the baby bottles <u>in hot water</u>.

    wash the bottles.

    wash the utensils.

    put the bottle in the sterilizer.   Put <u>it</u> (f.)?

    put the baby bottle in the sterilizer.   <u>it</u> (m.)?

    sterilize the utensils.   <u>them</u> (m.)?

    sterilize the bottles.   <u>them</u> (f.)?

    sterilize the baby bottles.

    sterilize the nipples.

    test the milk.

    test the milk on the inner part of
        your arm.

^o<u>You must</u> give the baby a bath.   Give <u>him</u> a bath?
(<u>One must</u>)

      give him a sponge bath.

      nurse him every 3 hours.

      put talcum powder on him.

      change his diaper.

^o<u>You must</u> burp the baby.   Burp?
(<u>One must</u>)

<u>The baby has to</u> burp.

    eliminate well.   Eliminate well?

    eliminate regularly.

<u>You have to</u>

    put cream on <u>your</u> breasts.   Put cream on (<u>me</u>)?

    put cream on <u>your</u> nipples.

    wash <u>your</u> breasts.

    wash each breast before nursing
        the baby.

Hospital	Paciente
ᵒ<u>Hay que</u> preparar la fórmula.	¿Preparar<u>la</u>?
	<u>lo</u>?
usar una taza de medir.	<u>los</u>?
usar un esterilizador.	<u>las</u>?
tener ocho o diez biberones.	
tener ocho o diez botellas.	
lavar los biberones <u>en agua caliente</u>.	
lavar las botellas.	
lavar los utensilios.	
poner la botella en el esterilizador.	¿Poner<u>la</u>?
poner el biberón en el esterilizador.	<u>lo</u>?
esterilizar los utensilios.	<u>los</u>?
esterilizar las botellas.	<u>las</u>?
esterilizar los biberones.	
esterilizar las teteras.	
(los tetos)	
probar la leche.	
probar la leche en la parte interior del brazo.	
ᵒ<u>Hay que</u> darle un baño al niño.	¿Dar<u>le</u> un baño?
darle un baño de esponja.	
darle el pecho cada tres horas.	
ponerle talco.	
cambiarle el pañal.	
ᵒ<u>Hay que</u> hacer eructar el niño.	¿Eructar?
<u>El niño tiene que</u> eructar.	
eliminar bien.	¿Eliminar bien?
eliminar con regularidad.	
<u>Usted tiene que</u> poner<u>se</u> crema en los pechos.	¿Poner<u>me</u> crema?
poner<u>se</u> crema en los pezones.	
lavar<u>se</u> los pechos.	
lavar<u>se</u> cada pecho antes de dar de mamar al bebé.	

Formula for Your Baby

BOILING

Put a clean rack in a clean pan. Put the empty bottles in the pan. Add several inches of water. Put the pan without a cover on the stove. When it begins to boil, put on the lid and let it boil 25 minutes.

KEEPING

Turn off the stove. Take the pan off the burner, put it aside without removing the cover, and let it cool from 1 1/2 to 2 hours. Take the cover off, take out the bottles, and tighten the tops. Open milk cans should be kept covered in the refrigerator with the bottles.

WARNINGS ABOUT THE FORMULA

The baby's formula is very special. Try to follow directions exactly. Don't make any change without consulting your doctor. Always sterilize the milk -- this kills germs and aids the baby's digestion. Don't change the formula to homogenized milk without first checking with your doctor.

There are two methods for sterilizing the formula. (1) The bottles can be sterilized before filling them with the formula. (2) The formula can be put in the clean bottles, and then the formula and the bottles can be sterilized at the same time.

IDENTIFICATION

Fórmula para su bebé

HERVIR

Ponga una parrilla en una cacerola limpia. Ponga las botellas vacías en la cacerola. Añada unas pulgadas de agua. Ponga la cacerola sin tapa en la estufa. Cuando empiece a hervir, ponga la tapa y déjela hervir 25 minutos.

GUARDAR

Apague la lumbre. Quite la olla de la lumbre, póngala al lado sin quitarle la tapa y déjela enfriar de una y media a dos horas. Quítele la tapa, saque las botellas y apriétele las tapas. Latas de leche abiertas deben mantenerse cubiertas y guardarse con las botellas en el refrigerador.

ADVERTENCIAS PARA LA FÓRMULA

La fórmula del bebé es muy especial. Procure seguir las instrucciones exactamente. No haga ningún cambio sin antes consultar con el médico. Siempre esterilice la leche -- esto mata los microbios y facilita la digestión del bebé. No cambie de fórmula a leche homogenizada sin antes consultar con el médico.

Hay dos métodos de esterilizar la fórmula. (1) Se pueden esterilizar las botellas antes de llenarlas con la fórmula. (2) Se puede poner la fórmula en las botellas limpias y esterilizar la fórmula y las botellas a la vez.

The three main headings of this section about preparing the baby's formula are: Boiling, Keeping, and Warnings About the Formula. Combine your knowledge of cognates and of the subject at hand to finish each of the following statements in English.

BOILING

Put a clean rack in a clean pan. Put_____.

Add_____. Put the pan on the stove. Don't _____

_____. When the water begins to boil, cover the pan and_____

_____.

KEEPING

Turn off the stove. Put the pan to one side and _____. Take
the cover off _____. Open milk cans should

_____.

WARNING ABOUT THE FORMULA

The baby's formula is very special. Try to follow_____.

Always sterilize the milk to_____.

Don't change the formula to homogenized milk without_____.

GRAMMAR AND STRUCTURES DRILLED IN LESSON 28

verbs

hay que + infinitive -- one must + verb

tener que + infinitive -- to have to + verb

pronouns

infinitive + direct object pronoun

infinitive + indirect object pronoun

preposition + infinitive

Después de caérsele el ombligo.   After the umbilical cord falls off.

Lesson 29
Contraception

NEW MATERIAL

Hospital	Patient

Hospital

Some women use the pill.

    the diaphragm.

    the intrauterine device (IUD).

    the spiral.

    the loop.

    the bow.

    the ring.

    the shield.

    the cervical cap.

°Some use creams.

    gelatins.

    vaginal spermicides.

Some use the rhythm method.

    suppositories.

    oral contraceptives.

    douches.

Some have an abortion.

Some men use prophylactics.

    condoms.

    rubbers.

    coitus interruptus.
(withdrawal)

    sterilization.

Some have a vasectomy.

Patient

°What are some methods for birth control?

Yes? Do they use it (f.)?
      Do they use it (m.)?

Yes? Do they use them (f.)?

Yes? Do they use it (m.)?
            it (f.)?
          them (m.)?
          them (f.)?

Yes? Do they have one?

°What can men use?

Yes? Do they use it (m.)?
            it (f.)?

Yes? A vasectomy?

Lección 29
Contracepción

Hospital	Paciente
Algunas mujeres usan la píldora.	ᵒ¿Cuáles son algunos métodos de contracepción?
el diafragma.	¿Sí? ¿La usan?
el aparato intrauterino.	¿Lo usan?
(el dispositivo intrauterino)	
el espiral.	
el lazo.	
el nudo.	
el anillo.	
el escudo.	
el gorro cervical.	
ᵒAlgunas usan cremas.	¿Sí? ¿Las usan?
jaleas.	
espermicidas vaginales.	
Unas usan el método de ritmo.	¿Sí? ¿Lo usan?
supositorios.	¿La
anticonceptivos orales.	¿Los
	¿Las
ducha vaginal.	
(lavado vaginal)	
Algunas tienen un aborto.	¿Sí? ¿Lo tienen?
Algunos hombres usan un profiláctico.	ᵒ¿Qué pueden usar los hombres?
un condón.	¿Sí? ¿Lo usan?
una goma.	¿La
interrupción de coito.	
(la "retirada")	
esterilización.	
Algunos se hacen una vasectomía.	¿Sí? ¿Una vasectomía?

Hospital	Patient

Hospital

Some <u>methods</u> are effective.

   are very effective.

   aren't very effective.

   <u>have</u> advantages.

      disadvantages.

      advantages and disadvantages.

Some <u>are not effective.</u>
Others
All

^oWhat do you use?

<u>You should</u> consult your doctor.

You and your husband should decide.

<u>Some women have</u> cramps.

   sore breasts.

   discharge of blood.

   headache.

   negative results.

   positive results.

<u>Some</u> gain weight.

   lose hair.

   get pregnant.

   have multiple births.

They prevent the joining of **sperm** and
                      (semen)

   ovum.

<u>You should</u> go to the doctor for an
   examination.

      have a laboratory test.

<u>If you don't have</u> menstruation.
        (your period)

Patient

^o<u>Are they effective?</u>

<u>Really? Aren't they effective?</u>

I don't use anything.
^o<u>What method is best for me?</u>

<u>Can there be complications with the pill?</u>

^o<u>What effects can it have on women?</u>

<u>What happens if one stops taking the
   pill?</u>

^o<u>What do contraceptives do?</u>

<u>How do I know if I'm pregnant?</u>

Hospital	Paciente

Algunos métodos son eficaces.

   son muy eficaces.

   no son muy eficaces.

   tienen ventajas.

      desventajas.

      ventajas y desventajas.

°¿Son eficaces?

Unos no son eficaces.
Otros
Todos

¿De veras? ¿No son eficaces?

¿Qué usa usted?

No uso nada.

Debe consultar con su médico.

   decidirlo con su esposo.

°¿Qué método es mejor para mí?

Algunas mujeres tienen calambres.

   dolor en los senos.

   flujo de sangre.

   jaqueca.

   resultados negativos.

   resultados positivos.

¿Puede haber complicaciones con la píldora?

Unas aumentan de peso.

   pierden el pelo.

   quedan embarazadas.

   tienen partos múltiples.

°¿Qué efecto puede tener en la mujer?

¿Qué pasa si se deja de tomar la píldora?

Evitan el encuentro de la esperma y
         (del semen)
         (de la semilla)
   el óvulo.

°¿Qué hacen los anticonceptivos?

Debe ir al médico para hacerse un examen.

   hacerse un examen de laboratorio.

¿Cómo voy a saber si estoy embarazada?

Si no tiene menstruación.
      (el período)
      (la regla)

Conversation

Mrs. M.: Doctor, I have just had a little girl, and I don't want to get pregnant again. We already have a 3-year-old boy and don't want any more children right now. What can I do?

Doctor R.: I have here a booklet explaining different contraceptive methods used today.

Mrs. M.: How do I know which one is best?

Doctor R.: All methods have advantages and disadvantages. Read the booklet and discuss with your husband the possibilities of each method. Contraceptives are useful to many people. There are young couples who are not ready for the responsibilities of parenthood. There are other cases, like yours, where the parents have all the children they want or can raise properly. Other times, for health reasons, the mother or father doesn't want to have children because of some hereditary trait that may run in the family. In other cases, the mother's life may be endangered during pregnancy or at delivery, and it is advisable to avoid having children.

Mrs. M.: Thank you, doctor. I can see that the use of contraceptives is more common than I thought.

Doctor R.: Yes, Mrs. Martínez. Besides, it is not unusual for single adults to be sexually active, and few unmarried women would want to get pregnant.

Mrs. M.: You're right. It's better to be protected in those cases. After discussing contraceptive methods with my husband I will come back to see you.

Doctor R.: All right. Good-bye, Mrs. Martínez.

Mrs. M.: Good-bye, Dr. Ramírez.

IDENTIFICATION

Conversación

Señora M.: Doctor, acabo de tener una bebita y no deseo salir embarazada otra vez. Ya tenemos un niño de tres años y no queremos más ahora. ¿Qué puedo hacer?

Doctor R.: Aquí tengo un folleto que explica distintos métodos anticonceptivos que se usan hoy en día.

Señora M.: ¿Cuál es el mejor método?

Doctor R.: Todos tienen sus ventajas y sus desventajas. Lea el librito y discuta con su esposo las posibilidades de cada método. Los anticonceptivos son útiles a muchas personas. Hay recién casados que no están listos para las responsabilidades de la paternidad. Hay otros casos, como el suyo, en que los padres tienen todos los niños que desean o que pueden criar bien. Otras veces, por razones de salud, la madre o el padre no desea tener hijos para evitar algún defecto que exista en la familia. En otros casos la vida de la madre puede estar en peligro durante el embarazo o el parto, y es preferible evitar los hijos.

Señora M.: Gracias, doctor. Ya veo que el uso de los anticonceptivos es más común de lo que yo pensaba.

Doctor R.: Sí, Señora Martínez. Además, no es raro que los solteros sean sexualmente activos y pocas mujeres desean salir embarazadas si no están casadas.

Señora M.: Usted tiene razón. Es mejor usar alguna precaución en esos casos. Después de leer el librito volveré a verlo y discutiremos lo que decidamos mi esposo y yo.

Doctor R.: Está bien. Hasta pronto, señora Martínez.

Señora M.: Adiós, doctor Ramírez.

Check to see if you have understood the main points of this conversation by answering the questions.

1. After reading the booklet, what should Mrs. Martínez do?
2. Name, in order, the five cases the doctor mentions in which people use contraceptives.
3. When will Mrs. Martínez come to see the doctor again?

GRAMMAR AND STRUCTURES DRILLED IN LESSON 29

verbs

present tense, third person plural

indefinite adjectives and pronouns

algunos, algunas -- some
unos, unas -- some

pronouns

direct object pronoun preceding verb

Lesson 30
Surgery: Preparation and Anesthesia

Hospital	Patient

°You have to sign the permission to operate.

    All right.

You can't eat anything.

          eat anything after 12.

          have anything but liquids.

Yes, we're going to prepare you (m.).
                  you (f.).

    Are you going to prepare me?

        shave me?

        disinfect me?

        take me to the operating room?

Yes, we're going to prepare you (m.).
                  you (f.).

    Are you going to prepare me?

        shave me?

        disinfect me?

        take me to the operating room?

We're going to give you an injection.

    °Are you going to give me an injection?
                    an enema?

We're going to give you a sedative.
                    an analgesic.

    Are you going to give me a sedative?

    °What anesthetic are you going to give me?

We're going to give you
    a general anesthetic.

    Are you going to give me a general anesthetic?

    a local anesthetic.

    a partial anesthetic.

    a spinal.

    sodium pentothal.

    gas.

Lección 30
Cirugía: Preparación y anestesia

MATERIA NUEVA

Hospital	Paciente

Tiene que firmar el permiso para operar.   Muy bien.

No puede comer nada.

        comer nada después de las doce.

        tomar sino líquidos.

Sí, lo vamos a preparar.
     la

                                ¿Van a prepararme?

                                    afeitarme?

                                    desinfectarme?

                                    llevarme a la sala de operaciones?

Sí, vamos a prepararlo.   ¿Me van a preparar?

            prepararla.   afeitar?

                                    desinfectar?

                                    llevar a la sala de operaciones?

Vamos a ponerle una inyección.   ¿Me van a poner una inyección?

                                    una enema?
                                    (un lavado)

Vamos a darle un calmante.   ¿Me van a dar un calmante?

            un analgésico.

                                ¿Qué anestesia me van a dar?

Le vamos a dar   ¿Me van a dar anestesia general?

  anestesia general.

  anestesia local.

  anestesia parcial.

  raquídea.

  pentotal de sodio.

  gas.

Hospital	Patient

°<u>The anesthesiologist</u> wants to
   see you (m.).
      you (f.).

Very well.

What medicines do you take, sir?

I don't take medicines.

<u>Do you suffer from</u>
   heart disease, ma'am?

<u>No, doctor, I don't suffer from</u>
   <u>heart disease.</u>

   kidney trouble?

   lung problems?

Do you smoke much, miss?

I don't smoke at all.

°<u>Do you have</u> any allergies, sir?

<u>No, I don't.</u>
<u>Yes, I do.</u>

        gallstones

        kidney stones

        a cough

        dentures
        (bridgework)

        high blood pressure

        low blood pressure

        a scar

        stitches

°<u>Do you have</u> the permit?

Yes, I have it.
No, I don't have it.

        the authorization?

<u>Take out</u>
(<u>Take off</u>)

   your bridge, please.

Okay, if it's necessary.

   your wig

   your rings

<u>You must</u> tape your rings.
(<u>One</u>)   (one's)

Tape my rings?

      examine the patient.

      give him oxygen.
         (her)

      give him drugs.

      give him a transfusion.

      give him intravenous serum.

Hospital	Paciente
°El anestesiólogo quiere verlo.	Muy bien.
quiere verla.	
lo quiere ver.	
la quiere ver.	
¿Qué medicinas toma, señor?	No tomo medicinas.
¿Padece	No, doctor, no padezco
del corazón, señora?	del corazón.
de los riñones?	
de los pulmones?	
¿Fuma mucho, señorita?	No fumo nada.
°¿Tiene alergias, señor?	No, no tengo.
cálculos biliares	Sí, sí tengo.
cálculos renales	
tos	
dientes postizos	
la presión alta	
la presión baja	
una cicatriz	
puntos	
(puntadas)	
°¿Tiene el permiso?	Sí, lo tengo.
la autorización?	Sí, la tengo.
Quítese	
los dientes postizos, por favor.	Bien, si es necesario.
la peluca	
los anillos	
Hay que asegurar los anillos con	¿Asegurar los anillos?
tela adhesiva.	
examinar al paciente.	
darle oxígeno.	
darle drogas.	
ponerle una transfusión.	
ponerle suero intravenoso.	

Doctor: Nurse, do you have the authorization signed for the operation?

Nurse: Yes, doctor. Here it is with the clinical record.

Doctor: Remember that I prefer to use local anesthetic in these cases.

Nurse: I'll put it on the sheet. I have shaved the patient. I only need to sterilize the area of the operation.

Doctor: You can give her a sedative tonight so that she'll sleep well.

Nurse: Shall I give her an enema in the morning too?

Doctor: Yes. It's better for her to be completely clean to avoid any gastrointestinal problems.

Nurse: How much serum are you going to need?

Doctor: Have three bottles ready just in case. Also oxygen and blood.

Nurse: At what time is the anesthesiologist coming?

Doctor: At 6:00 A.M.

IDENTIFICATION

Doctor: Señorita, ¿tiene la autorización firmada para la operación?

Enfermera: Sí, doctor, aquí está con la hoja clínica.

Doctor: Recuerde que yo prefiero usar anestesia local en estos casos.

Enfermera: Lo anotaré en la hoja. Ya he rasurado a la paciente. Sólo necesito esterilizar la región de la operación.

Doctor: Puede darle un sedante esta noche para que duerma bien.

Enfermera: ¿Debo ponerle un lavado por la mañana también?

Doctor: Sí, señorita. Es preferible que esté bien limpia para evitar trastornos gastrointestinales.

Enfermera: ¿Cuánto suero va a necesitar?

Doctor: Tenga tres botellas preparadas en caso de necesidad. También oxígeno y sangre.

Enfermera: ¿A qué hora viene el anestesiólogo?

Doctor: A las seis de la mañana.

Answer each question in Spanish with as few words as possible.

1. ¿Para qué es la autorización?
2. ¿Qué anestesia prefiere el doctor?
3. ¿Ha rasurado a la paciente?
4. ¿Debe ponerle un lavado?
5. ¿Qué hay que evitar?
6. ¿Cuánto suero va a necesitar?
7. ¿Va a necesitar algo más?
8. ¿A qué hora viene el anestesiólogo?

GRAMMAR AND STRUCTURES DRILLED IN LESSON 30

verbs

ir a + infinitive -- to be going to + verb

tener que + infinitive -- to have to + verb

hay que + infinitive -- one must + verb

pronouns

direct or indirect object pronouns attached to infinitive or preceding conjugated verb

Vamos a prepararlo. We're going to prepare you (m.).
Lo vamos a preparar.

Lesson 31
Surgery: Operations and Results

<u>NEW MATERIAL</u>

Hospital	Patient
^o<u>What operation are they going to do</u>?	<u>They're going to do an</u> exploratory operation.
<u>Yes</u>? <u>You're going to have</u> a biopsy?	^o<u>They're going to do</u> a biopsy (on me).
	a trepanation of the cranium
	plastic surgery
	a hysterectomy
	a laparoscopy
	a vasectomy
	a mastectomy
^o<u>What are they going to do to you</u>?	<u>They're going to take out</u> my tonsils.
	my ovaries.
	my appendix.
	a tumor.
	a fibroma.
	a cyst.
	a blood cyst.
	a fatty cyst.
	a sebaceous cyst.
	a kidney.
	my uterus.
^o<u>What are they going to do to you</u>?	<u>They're going to</u> dilate the urethra.
	tie my tubes. (Fallopian tubes)
	set a fracture (on me).
	repair tissues (on me).
	repair my nose.
	repair my jaw.

Lección 31
Cirugía: Operaciones y resultados

MATERIA NUEVA

<table>
<tr><th>Hospital</th><th>Paciente</th></tr>
<tr><td>°¿Qué operación le van a hacer?</td><td>Me van a hacer una operación exploratoria.
(de exploración)</td></tr>
<tr><td>¿Sí? ¿Le van a hacer una biopsia?</td><td>°Me van a hacer una biopsia.</td></tr>
<tr><td></td><td>una trepanación del cráneo.</td></tr>
<tr><td></td><td>cirugía plástica.</td></tr>
<tr><td></td><td>una histerectomía.</td></tr>
<tr><td></td><td>una laparoscopía.</td></tr>
<tr><td></td><td>una vasectomía.</td></tr>
<tr><td></td><td>una mastectomía.</td></tr>
<tr><td>°¿Qué le van a hacer?</td><td>Me van a sacar las amígdalas.</td></tr>
<tr><td></td><td>los ovarios.</td></tr>
<tr><td></td><td>el apendice.</td></tr>
<tr><td></td><td>un tumor.</td></tr>
<tr><td></td><td>un fibroma.</td></tr>
<tr><td></td><td>un quiste.</td></tr>
<tr><td></td><td>un quiste de sangre.</td></tr>
<tr><td></td><td>un quiste de sebo.</td></tr>
<tr><td></td><td>un quiste sebáceo.</td></tr>
<tr><td></td><td>un riñón.</td></tr>
<tr><td></td><td>el útero.</td></tr>
<tr><td>°¿Qué le van a hacer?</td><td>Me van a dilatar la uretra.</td></tr>
<tr><td></td><td>ligar los tubos uterinos.
(los tubos de Falopio)
(las trompas)</td></tr>
<tr><td></td><td>componer una fractura.</td></tr>
<tr><td></td><td>reparar los tejidos.</td></tr>
<tr><td></td><td>reparar la nariz.</td></tr>
<tr><td></td><td>reparar la mandíbula.</td></tr>
</table>

Hospital	Patient

Hospital

We're going to operate on your finger.

    your appendix.

    your throat.

    your foot.

    your tonsils.

    your gallbladder.

    your pancreas.

    an ulcer.

    a hernia.

    a slipped disc.

    a calcified disc.

    cataracts.

    a cancer.

Patient

°What are you going to operate on?

Yes, are you going to operate on it (m.)?
                  it (f.)?
                them (m.)?
                them (f.)?

Hospital

°What operation are they going to do?

Patient

They're going to operate on my heart.

    my brain.

    my ear.

    my ovaries.

    my prostate.

    my thyroid.

    my eyes.

Hospital

°We're going to do
    an exploratory operation.

    a heart operation.

    a hysterectomy.

    a biopsy.

Patient

Yes? You're going to do it (f.) to me?

Hospital

°We're going to take out your appendix.

    your tonsils.

    a cyst.

    a tumor.

    2 cysts.

    your ovaries.

    a kidney.

    the stitch.

    the stitches.

Patient

You're going to take it (m.) out?
             it (f.)
           them (m.)
           them (f.)

Hospital	Paciente
Le vamos a operar el dedo.	°¿Qué me van a operar?
el apéndice.	
la garganta.	<u>Sí</u>, ¿me lo van a operar?
el pie.	<u>me la</u>
las amígdalas.	<u>me los</u>
la vesícula.	<u>me las</u>
el páncreas.	
una úlcera.	
una hernia.	
un disco desplazado.	
un disco calcificado.	
las cataratas.	
un cáncer.	
°¿Qué operación le van a hacer?	**Me van a operar** del corazón.
	del cerebro.
	del oído.
	de los ovarios.
	de la próstata.
	del tiroides.
	de los ojos.
°Le vamos a hacer	Sí? ¿Me la van a hacer?
una operación exploratoria.	
una operación del corazón.	
una histerectomía.	
una biopsia.	
°**Le vamos a sacar** el apéndice.	¿Me lo van a sacar?
las amígdalas.	<u>Me la</u>
un quiste.	<u>Me los</u>
un tumor.	<u>Me las</u>
dos quistes.	
los ovarios.	
un riñón.	
Le vamos a quitar los puntos.	
las puntadas.	

Hospital	Patient

                    Hospital   Patient

It came out well.   °How did the operation come out?

He came out well.   How did he come out?
She   she
      didn't come out well.

The patient is all right.   How is the patient?

          is delirious.

          is very ill.

          is not rational.

          has pain.

          has no pain.

          doesn't understand.

          is going to live.

          is not going to live.

          is going to die.

          died.

We don't know if the patient   °Is he going to live?
   is going to live.

   is going to die.

There is nothing else we can do.   What can be done?

°Should I call a priest?   Please call a priest.

          a minister?

          his family?
          her

          his relatives?
          her

Hospital	Paciente
Resultó bien.	°¿Cómo resultó la operación?
Salió bien.	¿Cómo salió?
No salió bien.	
El paciente está bien.	¿Cómo está el paciente?
está delirando.	
está muy grave.	
no está racional.	
tiene dolor.	
no tiene dolor.	
no comprende.	
va a vivir.	
no va a vivir.	
va a morir.	
murió.	
No sabemos si el paciente va a vivir.	°¿Va a vivir?
va a morir.	
No podemos hacer nada más.	¿Qué se puede hacer?
°¿Debo llamar a un cura?	Favor de llamar a un cura.
un ministro?	
su familia?	
sus parientes?	

Case 1: Mrs. Cantú

The woman in 411 is suffering from rheumatoid arthritis. She says that a chiropractor has been treating her, but she needs more intensive treatment. It's a typical case. She needs therapy.

Case 2: Mr. Gutiérrez

The man in 418 has a spasm in the lower part of his esophagus. He has a phobia about the thermometer. It's believed this is a psychiatric case.

Case 3: Miss Ramos

There is a young girl in 422. By the symptoms, the doctor suspects that she has difficulties in the lymphatic system or perhaps with the thyroid. She hopes to leave the hospital as soon as they finish doing the diagnostic tests.

Case 4: Mrs. Vela

The woman in 315 is hemorrhaging. They are giving blood transfusions. If they can't control the hemorrhaging, they're going to do a hysterectomy.

IDENTIFICATION

The following cases contain several cognate words. Remembering the spelling equivalents below will make many Spanish words easier to recognize.

English ph = Spanish f   English initial s + consonant =
        y =   i   Spanish initial es + consonant
        th =   t

Answer with as few Spanish words as possible the questions that follow each case.

Caso 1: Sra. Cantú

La señora ingresada en el 411 padece de artritis reumatoide. Dice que la ha atendido un quiropráctico pero necesita un tratamiento más intenso. Es un caso típico. Hay que darle terapia.

¿Quién la ha atendido?

¿Qué necesita?

Caso 2: Sr. Gutiérrez

El señor del 418 tiene espasmo en la parte inferior del esófago. Le tiene fobia al termómetro. Se cree que es un caso psiquiátrico.

¿Dónde tiene espasmo?

¿Qué se cree?

Caso 3: Srita. Ramos

Hay una jovencita en el 422. Por los síntomas el médico sospecha que tiene dificultades en el sistema linfático o tal vez en la tiroides. Ella espera salir del hospital en cuanto termine los análisis de diagnóstico.

¿Qué tiene la jovencita?

¿Qué análisis van a hacerle?

Caso 4: Sra. Vela

La señora del 315 tiene hemorragia. Le están dando transfusiones de sangre. Si no se le contiene la hemorragia van a hacerle una histerectomía.

¿Qué van a hacerle si no se le contiene la hemorragia?

GRAMMAR AND STRUCTURES DRILLED IN LESSON 31

verbs

ir -- first and third person plural, present tense

<u>vamos</u> -- we're going   <u>van</u> -- they're going, you (pl.) are going

<u>ir a</u> + infinitive -- to be going to + infinitive

pronouns

indirect and direct object pronouns preceding conjugated verb

<u>Me van a sacar las amígdalas</u>. They're going to take my tonsils out (of me).

<u>Sí, me las van a sacar</u>. They're going to take them out (of me).

definite article used to show possession with parts of the body (see above example)

Lesson 32
Medicine in the Home

Nurse	Patient

Nurse

He   has normal temperature.
(She)

   98.6 degrees Fahrenheit.

   100 degrees.

   37 degrees Centigrade.

   38.5 degrees Centigrade.

What a shame!
What a pity!
How awful!
What a problem!

Does he have it?   What a shame!

What a shame! Does she have it (m.)?
                    it (f.)?

Patient

°What temperature does   he   have?
                        (she)

The boy has a burn.
(The girl)

      has sunstroke.

      is frostbitten (m.).
      is frostbitten (f.).

      is sunburned (m.).
      is sunburned (f.).

°**The child has** an allergy.

   a nosebleed.

   a snakebite.

   diarrhea.

   general malaise.

   indisposition.

   an ingrown nail.

   an infected nail.

   a scab.

   a speck in his eye.

   a rash.

°**The child has** a foreign body in her eye.

   a callus.

   a sty.

   a wart.

   a tick in her ear.

   a splinter in her finger.

   a blister.

Lección 32
Medicinas en el hogar

MATERIA NUEVA

Enfermera	Paciente
Tiene temperatura normal.	°¿Qué temperatura tiene?

   noventa y ocho seis grados Fahrenheit.

   cien grados.

   treinta y siete grados centígrados.

   treinta y ocho cinco grados
      centígrados.

Enfermera	Paciente
¡Qué lástima! ¡Qué pena! ¡Qué malo! ¡Qué problema!	El niño tiene una quemadura. La niña

      tiene insolación.

      está congelado.
         congelada.

      está quemado del sol.
         quemada

Enfermera	Paciente
¿La tiene? ¡Qué lástima!	°El niño tiene alergia.

   hemorragia nasal.

   una mordida de serpiente.

   diarrea.

   destemplanza.

   indisposición.

   una uña enterrada.

   una uña infectada.

   postilla.

   una paja en el ojo.

   salpullido.

Enfermera	Paciente
¡Qué lástima! ¿Lo tiene? La	°La niña tiene un cuerpo extraño en el ojo.

   un callo.

   un orzuelo.

   una verruga.

   una garrapata en el oído.

   una astilla en el dedo.

   una ampolla.

Nurse	Patient
<u>Poor thing</u>! <u>Does he have them</u> (f.)?	^o<u>He has</u> insect bites.
	worms.
	nits.
	fleas.
	crab lice.
<u>Poor thing</u>! <u>Does she have them</u> (m.)?	<u>She has</u> lice.
	parasites.
<u>You can buy it</u> (m.) <u>in the pharmacy</u>.	^o<u>I need</u> alcohol.
	Merthiolate.
	a bottle of Merthiolate.
	iodine.
	cotton.
	ointment.
	liniment.
	cough syrup.
	bicarbonate.
	a laxative.
<u>You can buy it</u> (f.) <u>in the pharmacy</u>.	^o<u>Where can I buy</u> adhesive tape?
	aspirin?
	gauze?
	milk of magnesia?
	salve?
	antibiotic ointment?

Enfermera	Paciente

<table>
<tr><td>Enfermera</td><td>Paciente</td></tr>
</table>

¡<u>Pobrecito</u>! ¿<u>Las tiene</u>?
              ^o<u>El tiene</u> picaduras.
                     (picadas)
                  lombrices.
                  liendres.
                  pulgas.
                  ladillas.

¡<u>Pobrecita</u>! ¿<u>Los tiene</u>?
              <u>Ella tiene</u> piojos.
                      parásitos.

<u>Lo puede comprar</u> en la farmacia.
(<u>Puede comprarlo</u>)
              ^o<u>Necesito</u> alcohol.
                  mertiolato.
                  un frasco de mertiolato.
                  yodo.
                  algodón.
                  ungüento.
                  linimento.
                  jarabe para la tos.
                  bicarbonato.
                  un laxante.

<u>La puede comprar en la farmacia</u>.
(<u>Puede comprarla</u>)
              ^o¿<u>Dónde puedo comprar</u> tela adhesiva?
                  aspirina?
                  gasa?
                  leche de magnesia?
                  pomada?
                  crema antibiótica?

Nurse	Patient

You can buy them (m.) in the pharmacy.   °Where can I buy bandages?
                                                            (dressings)

                                                            dressings?

                                                            poultices?

                                                            medicine plasters?

                                                            mustard plaster?

You can buy them (f.) in the supermarket. °I need Band-Aids.

                                                    pills.

                                                    drops.

                                                    bandages.

                                                    children's aspirin.

It's in the medicine cabinet.   °I need medicine.
You should get a prescription.   What should I do?
          read the label.
          give him an antidote.
               (her)
°Do you need tissue?   Yes, he has to blow his nose.
                                              (she)   (her)

                                                    sneeze.

Enfermera	Paciente
<u>Los puede comprar</u> en la farmacia. (<u>Puede comprarlos</u>)	°¿<u>Dónde puedo comprar</u> vendajes?
	parches?
	apósitos?
	emplastos?
	sinapismo?
<u>Las puede comprar</u> en el supermercado. (<u>Puede comprarlas</u>)	°<u>Necesito</u> curitas.
	píldoras.
	gotas.
	vendas.
	aspirinas para niños.
Está en el botiquín.	°Necesito medicina.
<u>Debe</u> obtener una receta.	¿<u>Qué debo hacer</u>?
leer la etiqueta.	
darle el antídoto.	
°¿Necesita kleenex?	Sí, <u>tiene que</u> soplarse la nariz.
	sonarse
	estornudar.

Daughter: We need to clean out the medicine cabinet. There are so many bottles of medicine, there isn't any more space.

Mother: Let's see. What things don't we need so we can throw them out?

Daughter: This jar of acne cream is almost empty. Put it in the trash.

Mother: We don't need these empty bottles of iodine or Mercurochrome, or this dry sponge.

Daughter: These eye drops are quite old, and the boric acid isn't any good now.

Mother: We should keep these antispasm drops. And let's put the date on them, because we're going to clean out the medicine chest every three months.

Daughter: That's a good idea! Now we can have the things we need: sterile cotton, aspirin for adults and for children, peroxide, **germicidal soap, cough syrup, and of course Band-Aids.**

IDENTIFICATION

Hija: Tenemos que limpiar el botiquín. Hay tantos frascos de medicina
         que no hay más espacio.

Madre: A ver, ¿qué cosas no necesitamos para disponer de ellas?

Hija: Este pote de crema para el acné está casi vacío. Ponlo en la
         basura.

Madre: Tampoco necesitamos estos frascos vacíos de yodo y de mercurocromo,
         ni esta esponja seca.

Hija: Estas gotas para los ojos están muy viejas y el ácido bórico ya
         no sirve.

Madre: Debemos guardar estas gotas antiespasmódicas. Y vamos a poner
         la fecha porque debemos limpiar el botiquín cada tres meses.

Hija: ¡Es una buena idea! Ahora podemos tener las cosas que necesitamos:
         algodón estéril, aspirina para adultos y para niños, agua
         oxigenada, **jabón germicida,** jarabe para la tos y por supuesto,
         curitas.

1. ¿Qué cosas no van a guardar? Favor de hacer una lista.

2. ¿Qué cosas necesitan?

GRAMMAR AND STRUCTURES DRILLED IN LESSON 32

verbs

necesitar + infinitive -- to need to + verb

poder + infinitive -- can + verb

pronouns

direct object pronouns, attached to infinitive or before conjugated verb or
    verb phrase

subject pronouns él, ella -- he, she

Lesson 33
Emergencies: First Aid

<u>NEW MATERIAL</u>

Hospital

<u>One must</u> ask for help.
(<u>You</u>)

   not move the patient.

   put a tourniquet on him.
                       (her)

   give him artificial respiration.
     (her)

   give mouth-to-mouth rescuscitation.

   give oxygen.

<u>It's</u> a minor <u>injury</u>.
   serious

<u>It's</u> a heart attack.

   a minor injury.

   a rash from a plant.
              a poisonous plant.

   poison ivy.

<u>He has</u> convulsions.
(<u>She</u>)

   fits.

   tremors.

   fainting spells.

   allergy.

   hemorrhaging.

   sunstroke.

   heatstroke.

   fatigue.

   burns.

   a fracture.

   acidosis.

Patient

°<u>What must one do</u>?
         (<u>I</u>)

<u>He almost</u> drowned.
(<u>She</u>)

           died.

°<u>How serious is the injury</u>?

<u>What's the matter with him</u>?
               (her)

°<u>What's wrong with</u> the patient (m.)?
                 the patient (f.)?
                 the sick man?
                 the sick woman?

Lección 33
Emergencias: Primeros auxilios

MATERIA NUEVA

Hospital	Paciente
Hay que pedir socorro.	°¿Qué hay que hacer?
no mover al paciente.	
ponerle un torniquete.	
darle respiración artificial.	Por poco se ahoga.
darle respiración boca a boca.	
darle oxígeno.	se muere.
La herida es leve.	°¿Cómo es la herida?
es grave.	
Es un ataque cardíaco.	¿Qué le pasa?
una lesión menor.	
una erupción de una planta.	
una planta venenosa.	
hiedra venenosa.	
Tiene convulsiones.	°¿Qué tiene el paciente?
	la paciente?
	el enfermo?
	la enferma?
ataques.	
temblores.	
desmayos.	
alergia.	
hemorragia.	
insolación.	
postración del calor.	
fatiga.	
quemaduras.	
fractura.	
acidosis.	

Hospital	Patient

What a shame! Has he had an accident?   °He had an accident.

He tried to commit suicide.

He had a fall.

He cut himself.

He hurt himself.

He had contusions.

He got burned.

He twisted a muscle.

He broke his leg.

        his hip.

He fractured a bone.
  (broke)

He got frostbitten.

Yes, I'm going to give it (m.)
  to you.   °The treatment? Are you going to give it
    (m.) to me?

The alcohol?

The antidote?

Yes, I'm going to give them (m.)
  to you.   The bandages? Are you going to give
    them (m.) to me?

The treatments?

Yes, I'm going to give it (f.)
  to you.   °The medicine? Are you going to give
    it (f.) to me?

The prescription?

The label?

Yes, I'm going to give them (f.)
  to you.   The bandages? Are you going to give
    them (f.) to me?

The medicines?

The pills?

Hospital	Paciente

;Qué lástima! ¿Ha tenido un accidente?   °Ha tenido un accidente.

Ha tratado de suicidarse.

Se ha caído.

Se ha cortado.

Se ha herido.

Se ha dado golpes.

Se ha quemado.

Se ha torcido un músculo.

Se ha fracturado la pierna.

la cadera.

Se ha fracturado un hueso.
   (quebrado)
   (roto)

Se ha congelado.

Sí, se lo voy a dar.   °¿El tratamiento? ¿Me lo va a dar?

¿El alcohol?

¿El antídoto?

Sí, se los voy a dar.   ¿Los vendajes? ¿Me los va a dar?

¿Los tratamientos?

Sí, se la voy a dar.   °¿La medicina? ¿Me la va a dar?

¿La receta?

¿La etiqueta?

Sí, se las voy a dar.   ¿Las vendas? ¿Me las va a dar?

¿Las medicinas?

¿Las píldoras?

<table>
<tr><td>Hospital</td><td>Patient</td></tr>
</table>

Hospital   Patient

°It's the treatment.
   I'm going to give <u>it</u> (m.) to you.   <u>You're going to give it to me</u>?

It's the tourniquet. I'm going to
   give it to you.

It's the medicine. I'm going to give
   it to you.

It's the bandage. I'm going to give
   it to you.

They're the medicines. I'm going to
   give them to you.

They're the tourniquets. I'm going
   to give them to you.

They're the bandages. I'm going to
   give them to you.

They're the prescriptions. I'm going
   to give them to you.

They're the bottles. I'm going to
   give them to you.

Hospital   Paciente

⁰Es el tratamiento.   ¿<u>Me lo va a dar</u>?
     Se lo voy a dar.   <u>Me la</u>
                                                      <u>Me los</u>
                                                      <u>Me las</u>

Es el torniquete. Se lo voy a dar.

Es la medicina. Se la voy a dar.

Es el vendaje. Se lo voy a dar.

Son las medicinas. Se las voy a dar.

Son los torniquetes. Se los voy a dar.

Son las vendas. Se las voy a dar.

Son las recetas. Se las voy a dar.

Son los frascos. Se los voy a dar.

Juan:	Listen, Ernesto, call the pool lifeguard. Your brother's drowning.
Ernesto:	Hey, mister, come here, my brother's drowning.
Lifeguard:	What's the matter? We've got to help the boy.
Ernesto:	It was an accident. He was playing and he fell. He doesn't know how to swim.
Juan:	Here he is.
Lifeguard:	It's not serious. He appears to be breathing. Yes, he's breathing. Let's see his pulse. I feel a pulse, but slow. . . . Now his pulse is regular, and his breathing is rhythmical.
Ernesto:	What a scare! We've got to be more careful. Should I take him to the doctor?
Lifeguard:	Watch him awhile, and if you don't see anything wrong you won't need to go to the doctor.
Ernesto:	Thanks for your help.

IDENTIFICATION

Two key phrases will help you understand the conversation that follows.

<u>Llama al salvavidas de la piscina</u>. Call the pool lifeguard.
<u>No sabe nadar</u>. He doesn't know how to swim.

Juan: Oye, Ernesto, llama al salvavidas de la piscina, que tu hermano
            se está ahogando.

Ernesto: Venga acá, señor, mi hermano se ahoga.

Salvavidas: ¿Qué pasa? Hay que ayudar al muchacho.

Ernesto: Fue un accidente. Estaba jugando y se cayó. No sabe nadar.

Juan: Aquí está.

Salvavidas: No es nada serio. Parece que respira. Sí, está respirando.
            A ver el pulso. Siento pulso, pero lento. . . . Ahora tiene
            el pulso regular y la respiración rítmica.

Ernesto: ¡Qué susto! Tenemos que tener más cuidado. ¿Lo llevo al médico?

Salvavidas: Obsérvelo un rato y si no nota nada anormal no será necesario
            ir al médico.

Ernesto: Gracias por su ayuda.

1. ¿A quién hay que llamar?
2. ¿Qué pasa?
3. ¿Sabe nadar el hermano de Ernesto?
4. ¿Siente pulso?
5. ¿Está bien el muchacho?

GRAMMAR AND STRUCTURES DRILLED IN LESSON 33

verbs

    ir a + infinitive -- to be going to + verb

    hay que + infinitive -- one must + verb

pronouns

    two object pronouns preceding verb

    se as third person, indirect object pronoun

        Se lo voy a dar. I'm going to give it to you.
        ¿Me lo va a dar? Are you going to give it to me?

idioms

    Por poco + present tense verb

        Por poco se ahoga. He almost drowned.

Lesson 34
Emergencies: The Emergency Room

NEW MATERIAL

Hospital	Patient
One must call an ambulance. (We)	°What are we going to do?
take him to the hospital. (her)	
take him to the emergency room.	
take him to the emergency center.	
take him on a stretcher.	
He has a minor fracture.	°What's the matter?
a bad fracture. (serious)	
a compound fracture.	
a complete fracture.	
a multiple fracture.	
One must put a cast on his leg. (We)	°What must be done?
What's the matter with him?	He has a bean in his nose.
What's wrong?	He's hurt. She's hurt.
	dehydrated (m.). dehydrated (f.).
	drunk.
	in a coma.
°What's wrong?	He's been stabbed. (She's)
	She's been raped. attacked.
	He's bleeding profusely. (She's)
	bleeding.

334

Lección 34
Emergencias: La sala de emergencia

MATERIA NUEVA

Hospital	Paciente

Hospital

Hay que llamar la ambulancia.

    llevarlo al hospital.
    (llevarla)

    llevarlo a la sala de emergencia.
                   (urgencia)

    llevarlo al centro de emergencias.

    llevarlo en camilla.

Tiene una fractura menor.
    una fractura mayor.

    una fractura compuesta.
    una fractura total.
    una fractura múltiple.

Hay que enyesar la pierna.

º¿Qué tiene?
 ¿Qué pasa?

º¿Qué pasa?

Paciente

º¿Qué vamos a hacer?

º¿Qué tiene?

º¿Qué hay que hacer?

Tiene un frijol en la nariz.

Está lastimado (m.).
     lastimada (f.).

     deshidratado (m.).
     deshidratada (f.).

     borracho (m.).
     borracha (f.).

     en estado de coma.

Le dieron una puñalada.

La violaron.
   atacaron.

Se desangra.

Está sangrando.

Hospital   Patient

There are victims.   °What's the matter?
         dead persons.
         badly hurt persons.

It was a disaster.   °What happened?
        a shot.
        a gunshot wound.
        a reaction against medicine.
        an automobile accident.

°What happened?   He tried to commit suicide.
                                                  shoot himself.
                                                  get up.
                                                  kill himself.
                                                  take drugs.
                                                  walk.

How frightening! Did he take it (m.)? °He took poison.
                             it (f.)?   drugs.
                             them (m.)?   sleeping pills.
                             them (f.)?   bleach.
                                               lye.
                                               carbon tetrachloride.
                                               insecticide.
                                               medicines.
                                               tranquilizers.
                                               turpentine.

How frightening! Did he   °He swallowed a pin.
    swallow it (m.)?   a coin.
            it (f.)?   a marble.

                                                    a button.

Hospital   Paciente

Hay víctimas.   º¿Qué pasa?
    muertos.
    heridos.

Fue un desastre.   º¿Qué pasó?
    un tiro.
    una herida de bala.
    una reacción contra la medicina.
    un accidente de automóvil.

º¿Qué pasó?   Trató de suicidarse.
                                                   darse un tiro.
                                                   levantarse.
                                                   matarse.
                                                   tomar drogas.
                                                   caminar.

¡Qué susto! ¿Lo tomó?   ºTomó veneno.
             ¿La   drogas.
             ¿Los   píldoras para dormir.
             ¿Las   cloro.
                                                lejía.
                                                tetracloruro de carbón.
                                                insecticida (m.).
                                                medicinas.
                                                tranquilizantes (m.).
                                                trementina.

¡Qué susto! ¿Se lo tragó?   ºSe tragó un alfiler.
             la   una moneda.
                                                   un mármol.
                                                   una canica.
                                                   un botón.

Memorial Medical Testing Center

Hello, and welcome to Memorial Medical Testing Center. Please be seated and make yourself comfortable. If you will give me your history, I will go over it to make sure you answered each question.

While I am checking your history and preparing your chart, I will give you a summary of the testing you will be receiving.

The first thing we will do is take a urine sample. We will test you for your vital signs, and take your height and weight. Then you will be given a hearing test and a vision screening test. Then we will give you an electrocardiogram, or a heart tracing test, and your eyes will be tested for glaucoma. After that, you will have a chest x-ray and a lung screening test.

There will be little physical discomfort from these tests. After I have finished preparing your chart, I will ask you to sign a consent form. This form is just to give us permission to administer the testing and to release the results to your doctor.

Then I will ask you for the fee, make out your receipts, and give them to you. Afterward, I will call the technician, and she will start the testing.

Reprinted by permission of Memorial
Hospital System, Houston, Texas

IDENTIFICATION

Centro de Exámenes Médicos Memorial

Bienvenido al Centro de Exámenes Médicos Memorial. Siéntese, por favor, y póngase cómodo. Ahora yo tomaré sus datos personales y usted me ayudará para estar segura de que hemos contestado todas las preguntas.

Mientras reviso su historia clínica y preparo su hoja de registro, yo le explicaré los exámenes que le van a hacer.

El primero es el análisis de orina para el cual usted nos da una muestra. Después le tomaremos sus signos vitales (el pulso, la presión, etc.) y lo mediremos y lo pesaremos. Entonces le haremos el examen para medir su capacidad de oír y su visión. Luego le haremos el electrocardio-grama o un trazado del funcionamiento del corazón y le haremos una prueba para ver si tiene síntomas de glaucoma. Después le haremos una radiografía del pecho y una prueba para medir su capacidad vital, o sea el aire que puede contener en sus pulmones.

Estos exámenes le causan muy poca molestia física. Después de haber preparado su historia clínica, le pediré que firme una autorización. Esta forma es para darnos el permiso para someterse a los exámenes y enviarle los resultados a su médico.

Entonces le pediremos su pago y le daremos los recibos. Después de haber hecho los recibos llamaré a la persona que le va a hacer los exámenes y ella comenzará a examinarlo.

Reprinted by permission of Memorial
Hospital System, Houston, Texas

Answer each question in Spanish in as few words as possible.

1. ¿Qué datos va a tomar?
2. ¿Qué le va a explicar?
3. ¿Qué análisis van a hacer primero?
4. ¿Qué más van a examinar?
5. ¿Qué es un electrocardiograma?
6. ¿Qué radiografía le van a hacer?
7. ¿Qué tiene que firmar?
8. ¿Quién va a recibir los resultados?

GRAMMAR AND STRUCTURES DRILLED IN LESSON 34

verbs

   preterit tense -- third person, regular -ar verbs

   ser -- to be

   fue -- it was

pronouns

   reflexive pronoun se

   se + direct object pronoun preceding conjugated verb

Lesson 35
Heart Disease

Hospital	Patient
	ᵒWhat's the matter?

He has bad color.
(She)

He's pale.
She's pale.

      bluish (m.).
      bluish (f.).

ᵒHe needs to go to
(She)

    the intensive care unit.

    the room for patients with heart
      disease.

    the postoperative room.

ᵒHe needs intensive care.
(She)

      oxygen.

      better circulation.

      prolonged rest.

      a blood transfusion.

      an electrocardiogram.

      a special nurse.

Patient column:

Does he need it (m.)?
   (she)   it (f.)?

Does he need it (m.)?
   (she)   it (f.)?

Lección 35
Enfermedades del corazón

Hospital	Paciente
Tiene mal color.	○¿Qué tiene?

Está pálido.
    pálida.

    azuloso.
    azulosa.

○Necesita ir a

    la sala de cuidado intensivo.   ¿Lo necesita?
    (la unidad de cuidado intensivo)

    la sala de los enfermos del corazón.

    la sala de observación postoperatoria.

○Necesita cuidado intensivo.   ¿Lo necesita?
                                La

    oxígeno.

    mejor circulación.

    descanso prolongado.

    una transfusión de sangre.

    un electrocardiograma.

    una enfermera especial.

Hospital	Patient

Hospital

^oHe has high blood pressure.
(She)

      low blood pressure.

      normal blood pressure.

      hypertension.

      hypotension.

      a rapid heartbeat.
      (tachycardia)

      a slow heartbeat.

      a rhythmical heartbeat.

      an irregular beat.

      aortic insufficiency.

      atrial fibrillation.

      coronary thrombosis.

      arteriosclerosis.

      a heart murmur.

      irregular pulse.

      irregular heartbeats.

      varicose veins.

^oHe had a heart attack.
(She)

      a stroke.

      a coronary attack.

      a cardiac arrest.

      an embolism.

      an infarct.

He's going to take his blood pressure.
           (her)

^oHe's going to take his temperature.
           (her)

    take blood.

    measure the arterial tension.

Patient

Oh, does he have it (f.)?
   (she)   it (m.)?
          them (m.)?
          them (f.)?

Oh, did he have it (m.)?
   (she)   it (f.)?

^oWhat is the doctor going to do?
       the surgeon
       the technician
       the nurse

Yes? Is he going to take it (f.) for him?
                    (her)

Hospital	Paciente
°<u>Tiene</u> la presión alta.	Ah, ¿ <u>la tiene</u>?
	<u>lo</u>
la presión baja.	<u>los</u>
la presión normal.	<u>las</u>
hipertensión.	
hipotensión.	
palpitación rápida. (taquicardia)	
palpitación lenta.	
palpitación rítmica.	
palpitación irregular.	
insuficiencia aórtica.	
fibrilación auricular.	
trombosis coronaria.	
arterioesclerosis.	
un murmullo. (un soplo)	
el pulso irregular.	
latidos irregulares.	
venas varicosas. (várices)	
°<u>Tuvo</u> un ataque al corazón.	Ah, ¿ <u>lo tuvo</u>?
	<u>la</u>
un ataque al cerebro.	
un ataque coronario.	
un paro cardíaco. (un fallo cardíaco)	
una embolia.	
un infarto cardíaco.	
<u>Le va a tomar la presión</u>.	°¿<u>Qué va a hacer</u> el médico?
	el cirujano?
	el técnico?
	la enfermera?
°<u>Le va a</u> tomar la temperatura.	<u>Sí</u>? ¿<u>Se la va a</u> tomar?
sacar sangre.	
medir la tensión arterial.	

Hospital	Patient
^oHe's going to take his pulse. (her)	Yes? Is he going to take it (m.) for him? (her)
do an electrocardiogram.	
do an arterial graft.	
^oDo you smoke a lot?	Yes, doctor, I smoke a lot. No, doctor, I don't smoke much.
Do you walk	
Do you work	
Do you drive	
^oDo you drink a lot of coffee?	I drink some, but not a lot.
Do you drink many alcoholic beverages?	I drink some, but not a lot.
Do you smoke many cigarettes?	I smoke some, but not a lot.
Do you need to rest?	Yes, I need to rest.
Do you use medicine?	
Do you need medicine?	
Do you try to exercise?	
Do you speak English?	

Hospital   Paciente

°Le va a tomar el pulso.   ¿Sí? ¿Se lo va a tomar?

   hacer un electrocardiograma.

   hacer un injerto en una arteria.

°¿Fuma usted mucho?   Sí, doctor, fumo mucho.
                                          No, doctor, no fumo mucho.

¿Camina

¿Trabaja

¿Maneja

°¿Toma usted mucho café?   Tomo, pero no mucho.

¿Toma usted muchas bebidas alcohólicas? Tomo, pero no muchas.

¿Fuma usted muchos cigarillos?   Fumo, pero no muchos.

¿Necesita descanso?   Sí, necesito descanso.

¿Usa medicina?

¿Necesita medicina?

¿Trata de hacer ejercicio?

¿Habla inglés?

Telephone Conversation

Luisa: Hi! How's everything?

María: Fine, thanks, and you?

Luisa: Fine, too, thanks. What's new?

María: You know, I went to see the doctor because I wasn't feeling well.

Luisa: Yes, that's why I called you, to find out what the doctor said.

María: He gave me a complete examination, with an electrocardiogram and everything.

Luisa: And you're okay?

María: Yes, he told me I have tachycardia, but it's because of nerves.

Luisa: Tachy . . . what?

María: TACHYCARDIA. That means I have a rapid heartbeat, but not always, you know. Only sometimes.

Luisa: Is it serious?

María: He says it isn't, that it's a symptom to be watched, like high blood pressure. I should take tranquilizers, and relax and have more fun.

Luisa: I especially like the part about having more fun.

María: Me, too. We'll have to get together soon. Thanks for your interest in my health.

Luisa: See you soon. Remember me to Pedro.

María: Good-bye. Say hello to Juan.

IDENTIFICATION

The following conversation is typical in that the main information is contained in the middle part; the beginning and the end are greetings and small talk. The familiar form of address is used in conversation between friends. You have not learned to use this form, but see if you can recognize it in the conversation.

Conversación por teléfono

Luisa: Hola, ¿qué tal?

María: Bien, gracias, ¿y tú?

Luisa: Bien también, gracias. ¿Qué se cuenta?

María: Sabes, que fui a ver al médico porque no me sentía bien.

Luisa: Sí, por eso te llamé, para saber qué te dijo el médico.

María: Me hizo un examen completo con electrocardiograma y todo.

Luisa: ¿Y estás bien?

María: Sí, me dijo que tengo taquicardia pero es de los nervios.

Luisa: Taqui . . . ¿qué?

María: TAQUICARDIA. Eso quiere decir que tengo palpitación rápida, pero no siempre, ¿sabes? Algunas veces solamente.

Luisa: ¿Eso es serio?

María: El dice que no, que es un síntoma que hay que vigilar, como la presión alta. Debo tomar tranquilizadores y distraerme.

Luisa: Me gusta sobre todo la parte de la distracción.

María: A mí también. Tenemos que reunirnos pronto. Gracias por tu interés en mi salud.

Luisa: Hasta pronto. Recuerdos a Pedro.

María: Adiós. Saluda a Juan.

Answer each question in Spanish as briefly as possible.

1. ¿Qué examen le hizo el médico?
2. ¿Qué tiene?
3. ¿Qué es taquicardia?
4. ¿Qué debe tomar?

GRAMMAR AND STRUCTURES DRILLED IN LESSON 35

verbs

   ir a + infinitive -- to be going to + verb

   tener -- third person present and third person preterit

      tiene -- he has   tuvo -- he had

   present tense, regular -ar verbs, first and third person

pronouns

   direct object pronoun preceding conjugated verb

   indirect object pronoun preceding conjugated verb

   se as indirect object pronoun

   two object pronouns preceding conjugated verb

   lo as neuter (n.) direct object to refer to whole concept

Lesson 36
Disabilities and Major Illnesses

<u>NEW MATERIAL</u>

Hospital	Patient

Hospital

<u>He has</u> heart trouble.
(<u>She</u>)

     kidney trouble.

     tuberculosis.

     diabetes.

     muscular dystrophy.

     multiple sclerosis.

     epilepsy.

     leukemia.

     insanity.

     hemophilia.

     anemia.

     cystic fibrosis.

<u>He has</u> poliomyelitis.
(<u>She</u>) (polio)

°<u>He has</u> infantile paralysis.
(<u>She</u>)

     tuberculosis.
     (TB)

     diabetes.

     epilepsy.

     arthritis.

     leukemia.

     arteriosclerosis.

     a congenital disease.

     a genetic disease.

     cancer.

     a birth defect.

     a hereditary defect.

Patient

°<u>What does he   suffer from?</u>
     (<u>she</u>)(<u>have</u>)

°<u>What disease does he have?</u>
                 (<u>she</u>)

<u>Does he have it</u> (f.)?
    (<u>she</u>)   <u>it</u> (m.)?

Lección 36
Incapacidades y enfermedades mayores

	Hospital	Paciente
	Padece del corazón.	°¿De qué padece?
	de los riñones.	
	de tuberculosis.	
	de diabetes.	
	de distrofia muscular.	
	de esclerosis múltiple.	
	de epilepsia.	
	de leucemia.	
	de locura.	
	de hemofilia.	
	de anemia.	
	de fibrosis quística.	
	Tiene poliomielitis.	°¿Qué enfermedad tiene?
	°Tiene parálisis infantil.	¿La tiene?
		Lo
	tuberculosis.	
	diabetes.	
	epilepsia.	
	artritis.	
	leucemia.	
	arterioesclerosis.	
	una enfermedad congénita.	
	una enfermedad genética.	
	cáncer.	
	un defecto congénito.	
	un defecto hereditario.	

Hospital	Patient
°He's mongoloid. (She's)	Does he have it (m.)? (she)
He has gangrene. (She)	Does he have it (f.)? (she)
He suffered a trauma. (She)	Did he suffer it (m.)? (she)
a nervous breakdown.	
a heart attack.	
°He had a serious accident. (She)	Can he walk? (she)

He has to use a brace.
(She)
	Does he have to use it (m.)?
	(she) it (f.)
	                           them (m.)
	                           them (f.)

a crutch.	
a wheelchair.	
a walker.	
crutches.	
braces.	
He should (She)	Should he hold them (f.) out? (she)
hold the crutches out from his body. (her)	
follow a program of rehabilitation.	follow it (m.)?
follow a program of exercise.	
have therapy.	have it (f.)?
Yes, they're going to amputate it (m.).	°Are they going to amputate a finger from him ? (her)
amputate it (f.).	a leg from him ? (her)
amputate it (m.).	an arm from him ? (her)
Yes, they're going to amputate it (m.).	Are they going to amputate a finger from him ? (her)
amputate it (f.).	a leg from him ? (her)
amputate it (m.).	an arm from him ? (her)

Hospital	Paciente
⁰Tiene mongolismo.	¿Lo tiene?
Tiene gangrena.	¿La tiene?
Sufrió un trauma.	¿Lo sufrió?
un colapso nervioso.	
un ataque al corazón.	
⁰Tuvo un accidente serio.	¿Puede andar?
Tiene que usar un soporte.	¿Tiene que usarlo?
	usarla
	usarlos
	usarlas
una muleta.	
una silla de ruedas.	
un andador.	
muletas.	
soportes.	
Debe	¿Debe separarlas?
separar las muletas del cuerpo.	
seguir un programa de rehabilitación.	seguirlo?
seguir un programa de ejercicios.	
tomar terapia.	tomarla?
Sí, van a amputárselo.	⁰¿Van a amputarle un dedo?
amputársela.	una pierna?
amputárselo.	un brazo?
Sí, se lo van a amputar.	¿Le van a amputar un dedo?
se la van a amputar.	una pierna?
se lo van a amputar.	un brazo?

Hospital	Patient
He's lame. (She's)	°What disability does he have? (she)

    blind (m.).
    blind (f.).

    deaf (m.).
    deaf (f.).

    a stutterer (m.).
    a stutterer (f.).

| Yes, he has a crippled hand (m.).
 (she) (maimed) | Is he crippled?
 (she) (maimed) |

      (is) crippled (m.).
      (is) crippled (f.).

      (is) hunchbacked (m.).
      (is) hunchbacked (f.).

| Yes, he's lame now, but he's
 (she's) (she's) | °Is he lame?
 (she) |

    going to get better.

                                 deaf (m.)?
                                 deaf (f.)?

                                 anemic (m.)?
                                 anemic (f.)?

Hospital	Paciente

Hospital

Es cojo.
   coja.

   ciego.
   ciega.

   sordo.
   sorda.

   tartamudo.
   tartamuda.

Sí, es manco.
      manca.

    tullido.
    tullida.

    jorobado.
    jorobada.

Sí, está cojo ahora, pero va a
       coja

mejorarse.

Paciente

°¿Qué incapacidad tiene?

¿Es lisiado?
   lisiada?

°¿Está cojo?
      coja?

      sordo?
      sorda?

      anémico?
      anémica?

Patient: The nurse must be busy because I keep ringing the bell and she doesn't come.

Nurse: May I help you, sir?

Patient: I want to get up, and I can't without my crutches.

Nurse: Here they are. Let me help you. The therapist will be here soon. You need to learn to use your crutches.

Patient: Yes, it's very difficult to walk with crutches.

Nurse: There's a correct way to hold crutches and an incorrect way. You should hold the crutches out from your body and lean them carefully on the floor.

Patient: Evidently, it's more difficult than it seems.

Nurse: After you go home, you should continue your program of rehabilitatation. Little by little, you'll get used to them.

Patient: Thank you, nurse.

IDENTIFICATION

Two key words that are new should make the main points of the conversation below easy for you to understand: <u>sin</u> -- without; <u>aprender</u> -- to learn. Answer the questions that follow as briefly as possible in Spanish.

Paciente: La enfermera debe estar ocupada porque toco el timbre y no viene.

Enfermera: ¿En qué puedo servirle, señor?

Paciente: Quiero levantarme y no puedo sin las muletas.

Enfermera: Aquí las tiene. Permítame ayudarlo. El terapista viene pronto. Usted necesita aprender a usar las muletas.

Paciente: Sí, es muy difícil andar con muletas.

Enfermera: Hay un modo correcto de sujetar las muletas y otro incorrecto. Debe separar las muletas del cuerpo y apoyarlas con cuidado en el suelo.

Paciente: Evidentemente, es más difícil de lo que parece.

Enfermera: Después de ir a casa usted debe continuar con su programa de rehabilitación. Poco a poco se acostumbra.

Paciente: Gracias, señorita.

1. ¿Qué necesita para levantarse?
2. ¿Quién va a venir?
3. ¿Qué necesita aprender?
4. ¿Cómo debe usar las muletas?
5. ¿Qué debe continuar?

GRAMMAR AND STRUCTURES DRILLED IN LESSON 36

verbs

<u>tener</u> –– to have

<u>tener que</u> + infinitive –– to have to + verb

<u>padecer de</u> –– to have, to suffer from (disease)

<u>sufrir</u> –– to suffer

<u>sufrió</u> –– he (she, you) suffered

adjectives

<u>ser</u> + adjectives indicating characteristics

<u>Es ciego.</u>   He's blind.

<u>estar</u> + adjectives indicating conditions

<u>Ahora está enfermo.</u>   He's sick now.

pronouns

position of two object pronouns, either attached to infinitive or preceding
conjugated verb

<u>Van a amputárselo.</u>   They're going to amputate it from him.
<u>Se lo van a amputar.</u>

Lesson 37
Venereal Diseases

Hospital	Patient
What symptoms do you have?	°Do I have a venereal disease?
	I have a chancre on the genitals.
	a sore that doesn't heal.
	a sore.
	a rash.
Do you have inflammation on the groin?	No, I don't.
inflammation on the membranes?	
a sore on the mucous membranes?	
a chancre?	
a discharge of pus?	
°How long have you been feeling bad?	For several days.
	a week.
	2 weeks.
	a month.
When have you had sexual relations?	A few days ago.
	3 weeks ago.
	Frequently.
°It's necessary to give you a blood test.	A blood test?
Yes, the test is positive.	°Is the test positive?
negative.	negative?
Yes, you have gonorrhea.	Do I have gonorrhea?
No, you don't have	
	a venereal virus?
	syphilis?
It's in the first stage.	In what stage?
secondary	
advanced	

Lección 37
Enfermedades venéreas

<u>MATERIA NUEVA</u>

Hospital	Paciente

Hospital

¿Qué síntomas tiene?

<u>¿Tiene</u> inflamación en la ingle?
   inflamación en las membranas?
   ulceración en las mucosas?
   un chancro?
   flujo purulento?

°<u>¿Desde cuándo se siente mal?</u>

¿<u>Cuándo ha tenido relaciones sexuales?</u>

°Es necesario hacerle un examen de sangre.

<u>Sí, el examen es</u> positivo.
             negativo.

<u>Sí, usted tiene</u> gonorrea.
<u>No, usted no tiene</u>

<u>Está en estado</u> primario.
        secundario.
        avanzado.

Paciente

°¿Tengo una enfermedad venérea?

<u>Tengo</u> un chancro en los genitales.
     un grano que no sana.
     una lesión.
     una erupción.

<u>No, no tengo.</u>

<u>Hace</u> varios días.
     una semana.
     dos semanas.
     un mes.

<u>Hace</u> unos días.
     tres semanas.
Frecuentemente.

¿Un examen de sangre?

°¿<u>Es</u> positivo <u>el examen?</u>
    negativo

¿<u>Tengo</u> gonorrea?

     un virus venéreo?
     sífilis?
¿En qué estado?

Hospital	Patient

Hospital

It's good to take   antibiotics.
It's better to take
It's possible to take
It's necessary to take

        aureomycin.

        sulfa.

        streptomycin.

        penicillin.

It's better to go to the doctor.
It's necessary

    to have preventive treatment.

    to have early treatment.

    to abstain from sexual relations.

    to use a condom.

    not to cover up the symptoms without
       curing them.

    to be clean (m.).
        clean (f.).

Yes, there is one (m.).
          one (f.).

It's possible, but it's not certain.
It's probable, but it's not certain.

Patient

°What should I take?

°What should I do?

°Is there a preventive method?

Is there a rapid cure?

Is there danger of direct infection?

Is there danger of infection through
    sexual contact?

°Can it produce mental deterioration?

            emotional deterioration?

            physical deterioration?

Am I going to have scars?

Am I going to have marks?

Hospital	Paciente

Hospital

Es bueno tomar   antibióticos.
Es mejor tomar
Es posible tomar
Es necesario tomar

       aureomicina.

       sulfa.

       estreptomicina.

       penicilina.

Es mejor ir al médico.
Es necesario

    tener tratamiento preventivo.

    tener tratamiento temprano.

    abstenarse de las relaciones sexuales.

    usar un condón.

    no encubrir los síntomas sin curarse.

    estar limpio.
         limpia.

Sí, lo hay.
    la

Es posible, pero no es seguro.
Es probable, pero no es seguro.

Paciente

°¿Qué debo tomar?

°¿Qué debo hacer?

°¿Hay un método preventivo?

¿Hay una cura rápida?

¿Hay peligro de contagio directo?

¿Hay peligro de contagio por contacto sexual?

°¿Puede producir deterioración mental?

                 deterioración emocional?

                 deterioración física?

¿Voy a tener cicatrices?

¿Voy a tener marcas?

Venereal Diseases

The Department of Health is trying to inform the public concerning the prevention and cure of venereal disease.

The public should be aware that syphilis can cause loss of vision, loss of hearing, heart disorders, insanity, paralysis, and even death.

Gonorrhea can cause, among other things, sterility in men and women, and rheumatism.

Also it is important to know that these diseases are acquired by direct contact with a person who has the disease.

One should go to the doctor as soon as he suspects that he may have syphilis or gonorrhea.

Adequate and early treatment can quickly cure these diseases. Be careful! Be alert! Protect your health!

IDENTIFICATION

Enfermedades venéreas

El Departamento de Sanidad está tratando de divulgar información para la prevención y cura de las enfermedades venéreas.

Es necesario que el público sepa que la sífilis puede causar pérdida de la vista, pérdida del oído, complicaciones en el funcionamiento del **corazón, locura, parálisis y hasta la muerte.**

La gonorrea puede causar, entre otras cosas, esterilidad en hombres y mujeres y reumatismo.

También es importante saber que se adquieren esas enfermedades por contacto directo con una persona enferma.

Uno debe ir al médico tan pronto como sospeche que tiene sífilis o gonorrea.

El tratamiento adecuado y temprano puede curar pronto estas enfermedades. **¡Tenga cuidado! ¡Esté alerta! ¡Proteja su salud!**

Answer the following questions in Spanish in as few words as possible.

1. ¿Quién quiere divulgar información?
2. ¿Para qué es la información?
3. ¿Qué puede causar la sífilis?
4. ¿Qué puede causar la gonorrea?
5. ¿Cómo puede uno contagiarse?
6. **Cuando una persona sospeche que tiene sífilis, ¿qué debe hacer?**

GRAMMAR AND STRUCTURES DRILLED IN LESSON 37

impersonal expression + infinitive

Es bueno tomar antibióticos.	It's good to take antibiotics.
Es mejor	It's better
Es posible	It's possible
Es necesario	It's necessary
Es probable	It's probable
No es seguro	It's not certain

time expressions

¿desde cuándo + present tense verb -- how long + present perfect

hace -- for, ago

pronouns

direct object pronoun before hay

¿Hay un método preventivo?	Is there a preventive method?
Sí, lo hay.	Yes, there is.

Lesson 38
Drugs

NEW MATERIAL

| Hospital | Patient |
| | |

° One must give drugs to the patient.   What drugs?
(We)

        penicillin   Penicillin?
        morphine
        sodium pentothal
        Demerol
        codeine
        barbiturates

° What did he take?   The young man took drugs.
                                          narcotics.
                                          an overdose.
                                          LSD.
                                          STP.
                                          DMT.
                                        amphetamines.
                                          barbiturates.
                                          quads.

° Does the young man take drugs?   I don't know. I think so.
  What does he take?   I think barbiturates.
  For how long?   I think for quite a while.
  When?   I think frequently.
  How much?   I think quite a bit.

Lección 38
Las drogas

Hospital	Paciente
⁰Hay que darle drogas al paciente.	¿Qué drogas?
	¿Penicilina?

      penicilina

      morfina

      pentotal de sodio

      demerol

      codeína

      barbituratos

⁰¿Qué tomó?

El joven tomó drogas.

        narcóticos.

        una dosis excesiva.

        LSD. (ele ese de)

        STP. (ese te pe)

        DMT (de eme te)

        anfetaminas.

        barbituratos.

        cuads.

⁰¿Toma el joven drogas?   No sé. Creo que sí.

 ¿Qué toma?   Creo que barbituratos.

 ¿Desde cuándo?   Creo que hace tiempo.

 ¿Cuándo?   Creo que frecuentemente.

 ¿Cuánto?   Creo que bastante.

Hospital	Patient

Hospital

°Is he addicted to drugs?

        alcohol?

        morphine?

        heroin?

        cocaine?

What does he use?

°What's the matter with him?

What symptoms does he have?

Does he have hallucinations?

        cold hands and feet?

        vomiting?

        poor appetite?

        excessive appetite?

        extreme fatigue?

        dryness of the mouth?

        dilated pupils?

        itching?

        lethargy?

        suicidal tendencies?

Is he alienated?
    (withdrawn)

Patient

Yes, he's addicted.
No, he's not

He uses methadone.
He takes cough syrup.
        cough syrup with codeine.
He sniffs glue.
He smokes marijuana.

He has needle marks.
He has tremors.
Yes, he does.
    (has)

Hospital	Paciente
°¿Es adicto a las drogas?	Sí, es adicto.
	No, no es
al alcohol?	
a la morfina?	
a la heroína?	
a la cocaína?	
¿Qué usa?	Usa metadona.
	Toma jarabe para la tos.
	jarabe con codeína.
	Inhala goma.
	Fuma marihuana.
°¿Qué tiene?	Tiene marcas de aguja.
¿Qué síntomas tiene?	Tiene temblores.
¿Tiene alucinaciones?	Sí, las tiene.
las manos y los pies fríos?	los
vómitos?	la
poco apetito?	lo
apetito excesivo?	
fatiga extrema?	
sequedad en la boca?	
pupilas dilatadas?	
picazón?	
aletargamiento?	
tendencias suicidas?	
alienación?	

Hospital	Patient

^oDoes he cry a lot?

Does he speak incoherently?
Does he laugh a lot?
He has hepatitis.
He has to take some treatments.
         stop using drugs.
You must watch him.

^oWhat do you take?
         use?
         buy?
         eat?
         have?
         write?
         feel?

Yes, he cries a lot.
No, he doesn't cry a lot.

^oWhat's the matter with him?

What does he have to do?

What must I do to help him?

I don't take anything.

Hospital	Paciente
º¿Llora mucho?	<u>Sí</u>, llora mucho.
	<u>No</u>, no llora mucho.
¿Habla incoherentemente?	
¿Se ríe mucho?	
Tiene hepatitis.	º¿Qué tiene?
<u>Tiene que</u> tomar tratamientos.	¿<u>Qué tiene que hacer</u>?
dejar de usar drogas.	
Debe vigilarlo.	¿Qué debo hacer para ayudarlo?
º¿Qué tom<u>a</u> <u>usted</u>?	<u>No</u> tom<u>o</u> <u>nada</u>.
us<u>a</u>	
compr<u>a</u>	
com<u>e</u>	
tien<u>e</u>	
escrib<u>e</u>	
sient<u>e</u>	

Nurse 1:   What a shame about that young man! An ambulance just brought
           him in. He took an overdose of narcotics. He's unconscious.

Nurse 2:   The doctor on duty is trying to help him. Narcotics are very
           dangerous, because drug addicts take more and more to get the
           same effect.

Nurse 1:   The worst thing to cure is the psychological addiction of the addict.

Nurse 2:   Yes, when someone stops taking drugs for 18 hours he gets certain
           symptoms that make him feel miserable.

Nurse 1:   We had another emergency case in the hospital. The ambulance
           brought a woman who took barbiturates and alcohol. Of course
           she died. It was a very sad case.

Nurse 2:   Really, these cases are a shame.

IDENTIFICATION

Enfermera 1: ¡Qué lástima con este pobre joven! Una ambulancia lo acaba de traer. Tomó una dosis excesiva de narcóticos. Está inconsciente.

Enfermera 2: El médico de turno está tratando de ayudarlo. Los narcóticos son muy peligrosos porque los adictos a las drogas toman más cada vez para sentir el mismo efecto.

Enfermera 1: Lo peor de curar es la dependencia psicológica del adicto.

Enfermera 2: Sí, cuando una persona suspende el uso de las drogas por 18 horas aparecen ciertos síntomas que lo hacen sentir miserable.

Enfermera 1: Tuvimos otro caso de emergencia en el hospital. La ambulancia trajo a una señora que tomó barbituratos y bebidas alcohólicas. Por supuesto que murió. Fue un caso muy triste.

Enfermera 2: De veras son una lástima estos casos.

Answer the following questions about the conversation in Spanish in as few words as possible.

1. ¿Por qué está el joven en el hospital?

2. ¿Quién trata de ayudarlo?

3. ¿Qué es un peligro con las drogas?

4. ¿Qué tomó la señora?

5. ¿Qué pasó?

GRAMMAR AND STRUCTURES DRILLED IN LESSON 38

verbs

hay que + infinitive -- one must + verb

tener que + infinitive -- to have to + verb

present tense, first and third person

negatives

nada -- nothing

Lesson 39
The Dentist

NEW MATERIAL

Hospital	Patient
°<u>Please</u> sit down in the chair.	Thank you.
take off your lipstick.	All right.
open your mouth.	Open it?
close your mouth.	Close it?
raise your head.	Raise it?
lower your head.	Lower it?
rinse your mouth.	Rinse it?
<u>brush your teeth</u>	Brush them?
before going to bed.	
after eating.	
spit in the bowl.	Okay.

Hospital	Patient
°<u>I'm going to</u> extract your tooth.	<u>You're going to</u> extract <u>it</u> (m.)?
extract your molar.	<u>it</u> (f.)?
deaden the nerve.	<u>them</u> (m.)?
block the nerve.	
straighten your teeth.	
<u>You have</u> good teeth.	I have? I'm glad.
a cavity in one tooth.	What a shame! I have?
a cavity in a molar.	
°<u>You have</u> a loose tooth.	<u>What a shame!</u> <u>Do I</u> (have it) (m.)?
an abscessed tooth.	<u>I'm glad!</u> (have it) (f.)?
an impacted molar.	(have them) (m.)?
a loose eyetooth.	(have them) (f.)?
healthy gums.	
inflamed gums.	
stained teeth.	
white teeth.	
even teeth.	
pretty teeth.	
pyorrhea.	
gingivitis.	

Lección 39
El dentista

Hospital	Paciente
°Favor de sentarse en la silla.	Gracias.
quitarse la pintura de labios.	Muy bien.
abrir la boca.	¿Abrirla?
cerrar la boca.	¿Cerrarla?
levantar la cabeza.	¿Levantarla?
bajar la cabeza.	¿Bajarla?
enjuagarse la boca.	¿Enjuagármela?
cepillarse los dientes.	¿Cepillármelos?
antes de dormir.	
después de comer.	
escupir en la taza.	Bien.
°Le voy a extraer el diente.	¿Me lo va a extraer?
extraer la muela.	la
adormecer el nervio.	los
obstruir el nervio.	
enderezar los dientes.	
Usted tiene una dentadura buena.	¿La tengo? Me alegro.
una carie en un diente.	¡Qué lástima! ¿La tengo?
una carie en una muela.	
°Usted tiene un diente flojo.	¡Qué lástima! ¿Lo tengo?
un absceso en un diente.	¡Me alegro! La
un molar impactado.	Los
un colmillo flojo.	Las
las encías sanas.	
las encías inflamadas.	
los dientes manchados.	
los dientes blancos.	
los dientes parejos.	
los dientes bonitos.	
piorrea.	
gingivitis.	

Hospital	Patient
°You need to go to the orthodontist.	Really? Do I need to? it?

to visit the dentist every 6 months.

to return next week.

an x-ray.

to massage your gums.

a denture.

a partial plate.

a filling.

a crown.

°You need a bridge in front.	Really? Do I need it?

in the upper jaw.

in the lower jaw.

on the upper right side.

on the lower right side.

on the upper left side.

on the lower left side.

°Does your molar hurt?	Yes, it hurts. No, it doesn't hurt.

       tooth

Does something hot on your teeth bother you?

              cold

              sweet

              sour

Do your teeth hurt?

        molars hurt?

        teeth hurt when you chew?

                when you bite?

Do your gums bleed?

Hospital		Paciente

°<u>Necesita</u> ir al ortopédico dental.   ¿<u>De veras</u>? ¿Lo <u>necesito</u>?
              ortodontista.   La

   visitar al dentista cada seis meses.

   volver la semana que viene.

   una radiografía.

   masaje en la encía.

   una dentadura postiza.

   una dentadura parcial.

   un empaste.

   una corona.

°<u>Necesita un puente</u> en el frente.   ¿<u>De veras</u>? ¿<u>Lo necesito</u>?

   en la mandíbula superior.

   en la mandíbula inferior.

   en el lado derecho superior.

   en el lado derecho inferior.

   en el lado izquierdo superior.

   en el lado izquierdo inferior.

°¿<u>Le duele</u> la muela?   <u>Sí, me duele.</u>
                                     <u>No, no me duele.</u>

       el diente?

¿<u>Le molesta</u> lo caliente <u>en los dientes</u>?

         lo frío

         lo dulce

         lo agrio

¿<u>Le duelen</u> los dientes?

       las muelas?

       <u>los dientes</u> al mascar?

              al morder?

¿Le sangran las encías?

Mental Alertness and Body Image

YES   NO

____ ____	Knows name, first and last
____ ____	Knows age
____ ____	Knows name of school
____ ____	Can count to 20
____ ____	Counts to 50 by 10
____ ____	Can identify coins
____ ____	Knows value of coins
____ ____	Knows days of the week
____ ____	Knows days of the month
____ ____	Knows the months of the year
____ ____	Tells what time it is
____ ____	Knows left from right
____ ____	Identifies four colors
____ ____	Knows morning from night
____ ____	Knows parts of body, knee, ankle, neck, elbow
____ ____	Can move part of body pointed to
____ ____	Can repeat short sentences
____ ____	Can repeat essence of a story
____ ____	Knows alphabet
____ ____	Can spell
____ ____	Can read Level_____

IDENTIFICATION

The following form is part of an "Intellectual and Social Appraisal" used by a school health service. The key word is <u>sabe</u> -- "he knows," or "he knows how to." Try to guess as many of the skills as you can before checking the English. The six questions at the end, dealing with body image, use structures you have not studied. However, look for key words with which you are familiar, and if necessary consult the English, and then try to answer the questions for an imaginary child.

Disposición mental e imagen corporal

SI   NO

____ ____ Sabe su nombre, primer nombre y apellido
____ ____ Sabe su edad
____ ____ Sabe el nombre de la escuela
____ ____ Sabe contar hasta veinte
____ ____ Sabe contar hasta 50 de diez en diez
____ ____ Sabe identificar las monedas
____ ____ Sabe el valor de las monedas
____ ____ Sabe los días de la semana
____ ____ Sabe los días del mes
____ ____ Sabe los meses del año
____ ____ Sabe decir la hora
____ ____ Puede distinguir entre derecha e izquierda
____ ____ Identifica cuatro colores
____ ____ Puede distinguir entre mañana y noche
____ ____ Conoce las partes del cuerpo, rodilla, tobillo, cuello, codo
____ ____ Puede mover la parte del cuerpo que se le indique
____ ____ Puede repetir oraciones cortas
____ ____ Puede resumir un cuento
____ ____ Sabe el alfabeto
____ ____ Sabe deletrear
____ ____ Sabe leer   Nivel_____

1. What animal would you like to be? Why?

2. If you had three wishes what would you wish for?

3. If you were going away on a deserted island, with whom would you like to go? Why?

4. Do you like school? Why?

5. Do people like you? Why?

6. What games do you like to play? Why?

-- Reprinted by permission from "Developmental, Intellectual, Physical and Social Indepth Health Appraisal," School Health Services, Houston Independent School District, Houston, Texas

1. ¿Qué animal te gustaría ser? ¿Por qué?

2. Si pudieras tener tres cosas, ¿qué cosas desearías?

3. Si estuvieras en un desierto, ¿con quién quisieras estar? ¿Por qué?

4. ¿Te gusta la escuela? ¿Por qué?

5. ¿Tú le gustas a la gente? ¿Por qué?

6. ¿Qué juegos te gusta jugar? ¿Por qué?

-- Translated from "Developmental, Intellectual, Physical and Social Indepth Health Appraisal," School Health Services, Houston Independent School District, Houston, Texas

GRAMMAR AND STRUCTURES DRILLED IN LESSON 39

verbs

    ir a + infinitive -- to be going to + verb

pronouns

    indirect object pronoun with doler, molestar, sangrar

    direct object pronoun + verb

idioms

    favor de + infinitive -- please + verb

Lesson 40
The Sick Child

NEW MATERIAL

Hospital		Patient

°<u>Listen</u>, love.

What?
What is it?
Leave me alone!

    little one.

<u>Look</u>, dear.

    darling.

    sweetheart.

<u>Come on</u>, precious.

    baby.

°<u>That's good</u>! Give me a hug.   <u>I love you</u>.
<u>How pretty</u>! Give me a kiss.   <u>But I don't want to</u>.
<u>How cute</u>!
<u>How darling</u>!

    Open your mouth.

    Close your eyes.

    Sleep well.

    Stay nice and quiet.

°<u>Darling</u>, be good.

<u>I don't want to</u>.
<u>Leave me alone</u>.

    say "ah."

    tell me what's the matter.

    go to sleep.

°<u>Darling</u>, be quiet.

<u>I don't want to</u>.
<u>Leave me alone</u>.

    wake up.

    sit down.

    stand up.

    get up.

Lección 40
El niño enfermo

<u>MATERIA NUEVA</u>

                    Hospital   Paciente

^o<u>Oye</u>, amorcito.   ¿Qué?
                                                  ¿Qué cosa?
                                                  Déjame.

        mi hijito.
        mi hijita.

    <u>Mira</u>, muchachito.
          muchachita.

        nene.
        nena.

        nenito.
        nenita.

    <u>Ven</u>, precioso.
         preciosa.

        chiquitín.
        chiquitina.

^o¡<u>Qué bueno</u>!   Hazme un cariñito.   <u>Te quiero</u>.
 ¡<u>Qué chulo</u>!   Dame un besito.   <u>Si no quiero</u>.
 ¡<u>Qué mono</u>!
 ¡<u>Qué precioso</u>!

              Abre la boquita.

              Cierra los ojitos.

              Duerme tranquilito.

              Estáte tranquilito.

^o<u>Mi hijito</u>, sé bueno.   <u>No tengo ganas</u>.
 <u>Mi hijita</u>,   Déjame.

            di "ah."

            dime qué te pasa.

            duérmete.

^o<u>Mi hijito</u>, cállate.   <u>No tengo ganas</u>.
 <u>Mi hijita</u>,   Déjame.

            despiértate.

            siéntate.

            levántate.

            párate.

Hospital	Patient
°<u>Sweetheart</u>, don't talk now.	I'm not talking.
don't cry now.	I'm not crying.
don't be bad.	I'm not being bad.
don't be afraid.	I'm never afraid.
it's not going to hurt.	I'm strong.
don't take that.	I'm not taking anything.
°<u>Dear</u>, did you take your medicine?	No, I forgot.
did you sleep well?	Yes, of course.
how do you feel?	Okay, thanks.
do you feel better?	Yes, thanks.
°<u>Honey, what do you want</u>?	I don't want anything.
<u>Do you want</u> your toys?	<u>Yes, I want</u> my toys.
your storybook?	
your doll?	
°<u>Honey, do you want to come with me</u>?	<u>Yes, I want to.</u> <u>No, I don't want to.</u> <u>Not now.</u>
do you want to rest?	<u>Later.</u>
do you want to make water?	
do you want to go to the bathroom?	
do you want to have a bowel movement?	
do you want to play?	
do you want to have something?	
°<u>Do you want to</u> breathe deeply?	<u>I don't feel like it.</u> <u>I can't.</u>
bend your arm?	<u>Help me.</u>
turn on your side?	
turn on this side?	
get up a little bit?	

Hospital	Paciente
°<u>Precioso</u>, no hables ahora. <u>Preciosa</u>,	Yo no hablo.
no llores ahora.	Yo no lloro.
no seas malo.	Yo no soy malo.
no tengas miedo.	Yo nunca tengo miedo.
no te va a doler.	Yo soy fuerte. (valiente)
no tomes esto.	Yo no tomo nada.
°<u>Chiquito</u>, ¿tomaste la medicina? <u>Chiquita</u>,	No, se me olvidó.
¿dormiste bien?	Sí, cómo no.
¿cómo te sientes?	Bien, gracias.
¿te sientes mejor?	Sí, gracias.
°<u>Nenito</u>, ¿qué quieres? <u>Nenita</u>,	No quiero nada.
¿<u>quieres</u> tus juguetes?	Sí, <u>quiero</u> mis juguetes.
tu librito de cuentos?	
tu muñeca?	
°<u>Chiquitín</u>, ¿<u>quieres venir conmigo</u>? <u>Chiquitina</u>,	Sí, <u>quiero</u>. <u>No, no quiero</u>. <u>No ahora</u>. <u>Luego</u>.
¿quieres descansar?	
¿quieres orinar?	
¿quieres ir al baño?	
¿quieres ensuciar?	
¿quieres jugar?	
¿quieres tomar algo?	
°¿<u>Quieres</u> respirar profundamente?	<u>No tengo ganas</u>. <u>No puedo</u>. <u>Ayúdame</u>.
doblar el brazo?	
ponerte de lado?	
ponerte en este lado?	
levantarte un ratito?	

Hospital	Patient
^OLet me comb your hair, honey.	Wait a minute.
	a little bit.

    change your clothes
    change your bed
    put on your shoes
    fasten your shoes
    fasten your shirt
    fasten your pants
    carry you

Hospital	Patient
I hope so!	^OWhen's mom coming? Soon?
	mommy Today?
	Now?
	Right now?
	dad Tomorrow?
	daddy
	poppy

Hospital	Patient
Do you like the doctor?	Yes, I like the doctor.
the nurse?	
the ice cream?	
the milk?	
Does it hurt?	Yes, it hurts.
Does it itch?	

Hospital   Paciente

°Déjame peinarte, nene.   Espérate un momentito.
                nena.   un momentico.

        cambiarte la ropa   un ratito.
        cambiarte la cama   un ratico.
        ponerte los zapatos
        abrocharte los zapatos
        abrocharte la camisa
        abrocharte el pantalón
        llevarte
        cargarte

Ojalá que sí.   °¿Cuándo viene mamá?   ¿Pronto?
                                            mami?   ¿Hoy?
                                            mamita? ¿Ahora?
                                            papá?   ¿Ahorita?
                                            papi?   ¿Mañana?
                                            papito?

°¿Te gusta el médico?   Sí, me gusta el médico.
         la enfermera?
         el helado?
         la leche?
¿Te duele?   Sí, me duele.
¿Te pica?

Child: You're going to take me to the doctor's office, aren't you?

Mother: Yes, my love. We have to go.

Child: But, mommy, I don't want to go to the doctor.

Mother: Why, darling?

Child: Because I don't like what they do to me.

Mother: Don't be afraid. The nurse is very nice, and she'll take care
          of you.

Child: Yes, she's nice, but when she tells me "Give me your finger," she
          pricks me and takes out blood.

Mother: Oh, that doesn't matter. It barely hurts at all. It's like a
          mosquito bite.

Child: Ha, ha, ha! . . . But I'm ashamed to say I wet the bed . . .
          sometimes. . . .

Mother: It's not your fault. You only wet the bed when you have nightmares
          and you wake up afraid. Don't be silly. Give me a hug and a kiss
          and let's go.

Child: But I'm tired! Let me sit on your lap.

Mother: Come here. Do your legs hurt?

Child: No, it's just that I want a little hug.

IDENTIFICATION

Niña: Tú me vas a llevar a la consulta del médico, ¿no?

Madre: Sí, mi amor, tenemos que ir.

Niña: Mamá, no quiero ir al médico.

Madre: ¿Por qué, amorcito?

Niña: Porque no me gusta lo que me hacen.

Madre: No tengas miedo, la señorita es muy simpática y ella te atiende.

Niña: Sí, es muy simpática, pero cuando me dice "dame el dedito" me pincha
y me saca sangre.

Madre: ¡Ah! Eso no importa, no duele mucho. Es como la picada de un
mosquito.

Niña: Ja, ja, ja . . . pero me da vergüenza decir que me orino en la cama
. . . algunas veces . . .

Madre: Tú no tienes la culpa, tú mojas la cama sólo cuando tienes pesadilla
y te despiertas asustada. No seas tontina. Dame un abrazo y un
besito y vamos.

Niña: ¡Si estoy cansada! Déjame sentarme en tus piernas.

Madre: ¡Ven acá! ¿Te duelen las piernas?

Niña: No, es que quiero un cariñito.

Answer the questions in Spanish in as few words as possible.

1. ¿Adónde tienen que ir la madre y la niña?

2. ¿Qué no quiere la niña?

3. ¿Qué no le gusta?

4. ¿Qué va a hacer la señorita al decir "dame el dedito"?

5. ¿Por qué se orina en la cama la niña?

6. ¿Por qué quiere sentarse en las piernas de su mamá?

NOTES

THE FAMILIAR FORM

Throughout this text, you have learned the more formal way to say you (usted) rather than the familiar (tú) because that is the form one would use in most cases in dealing with patients. However, children are addressed in familiar forms, some of which you have practiced in this lesson. In addition to the familiar commands used here, the main differences between these forms and the ones you have practiced throughout the text are as follows:

Formal	Familiar
usted	tú
su	tu
le	te
lo, la	te
se	te

verbs in present tense -- add s

(quiere -- quieres)

ENDEARMENTS

Endearments generally are used more by Spanish-speaking people than they are by most English-speaking people. These affectionate terms so necessary for dealing with children in Spanish cannot be translated well. In this lesson the English translations attempt to show the affection and, if possible, a little of the literal meaning.

DIMINUTIVES

Diminutives are endings added to words to show something little or small, and to give the idea of affection and warmth. The most common ending is -ito or -ita. Diminutives may be added to nouns, and even to adjectives and adverbs. As with terms of endearment, there are no exact equivalents in English.

GRAMMAR AND STRUCTURES DRILLED IN LESSON 40

verbs

    familiar commands

        affirmative   <u>Déjame</u>. Let me.

        negative   <u>No hables ahora</u>. Don't talk now.

    <u>querer</u> + infinitive -- to want to + verb

pronouns

    indirect object pronoun = <u>te</u>

       <u>Déjame ponerte los zapatos</u>. Let me put on your shoes.

    reflexive pronoun = <u>te</u>

       ¿<u>Quieres ponerte de lado</u>? Do you want to turn on your side?

    position of object pronouns

Lesson 41
Physical Characteristics and Personality

<u>NEW MATERIAL</u>

Hospital	Patient

^o<u>What's</u> he   <u>like</u>?   <u>He's</u> short.
        she   <u>She's</u>
        the man
        the woman
        your husband
        your wife

What is John like?   thin.
     Mary
                                  skinny.

                                  fat.

  heavy.

  pleasant.
(nice)

  unpleasant.
(disagreeable)

  ugly.

  good.

  darling.

  handsome.

  beautiful.

  nervous.

  attentive.

^oWhat are John and Mary <u>like</u>?   <u>They're</u> old (m., or m. and f.).
     Mary and Anna   <u>They're</u> old (f.).

  wise.

  studious.

  obese.

Lección 41
Características físicas y personalidad

<u>MATERIA NUEVA</u>

	Hospital	Paciente
°¿Cómo es	él?	<u>Es</u> bajo.
	ella?	baja.
	el hombre?	
	la mujer?	
	su esposo?	
	su esposa?	

¿Cómo es Juan?   delgado.
          María?   flaco.

                                                    gordo.

                                                    grueso.

                                                    simpático.

antipático.
(pesado)
feo.
bueno.
precioso.
guapo.
hermoso.
nervioso.
atento.

°¿Cómo son Juan y María?   <u>Son</u> viejos.
          María y Ana?   viejas.

                                                      sabios.

                                                    estudiosos.

                                                    obesos.

Hospital	Patient
^o<u>What are</u> your children <u>like</u>?	<u>They're</u> funny.
they	impudent.
those people	proud.
those men (and women),	rich.
that couple	simple.
	(plain)
	cute.
^o<u>What is</u> your father <u>like</u>?	<u>He's</u> kind.
your mother	<u>She's</u>
<u>What is</u> your son <u>like</u>?	<u>He's</u> courteous.
your daughter	<u>She's</u>
	large.
	humble.
	sensitive.
	flexible.
	inflexible.
	poor.
	sociable.
	strong.
	interesting.
^o<u>What are</u> your parents <u>like</u>?	<u>They're</u> competent.
<u>What are</u> your children <u>like</u>?	
	incompetent.
	hard-working.
	pleasing.
	unpleasant.
	courteous.
	impatient.
	impertinent.
	important.
	brave.

Hospital	Paciente

°¿__Cómo son__ sus hijos?   __Son__ graciosos.
                ellos?   frescos.
                esas personas?
                esos señores?   orgullosos.

                                       ricos.

                                       sencillos.

                                       monos.

°¿__Cómo es__ su padre?   __Es__ amable.
                su madre?
 ¿__Cómo es__ su hijo?   __Es__ cortés.
                su hija?

                                       amable.

                                       grande.

                                       humilde.

                                       sensible.

                                       flexible.

                                       inflexible.

                                       pobre.

                                       sociable.

                                       fuerte.

                                       interesante.

°¿__Cómo son__ sus padres?   __Son__ competentes.
 ¿__Cómo son__ sus hijos?

                                       incompetentes.

                                       diligentes.

                                       complacientes.

                                       desagradables.

                                       corteses.

                                       impacientes.

                                       impertinentes.

                                       importantes.

                                       valientes.

Hospital	Patient
^o<u>How is</u> the man <u>today</u>? the woman	<u>Today he's</u> ill. <u>she's</u> ill.

Today he's ill.
she's ill.

nervous.

happy.

tired.

upset.

worried.

agitated.

fatter.

thinner.

proud of his (her) stitches.

acting crazy.

well.

sad.

weak.

strong.

very ill.

impatient.

lying down.

sitting up.
    (down)

asleep.

Hospital	Paciente
°¿<u>Cómo está</u> el señor <u>hoy</u>?	<u>Hoy está</u> enfermo.
la señora	enferma.
	nervioso.
	contento.
	cansado.
	turbado.
	preocupado.
	agitado.
	más gordo.
	más flaco.
	orgulloso de sus puntos.
	loco.
	bien.
	triste.
	débil.
	fuerte.
	grave.
	impaciente.
	acostado.
	sentado.
	dormido.

Anthem to Health

Traditional Air
Translated by Julia J. Tabery

Wash us clean with plenty of water and with soap
For our beauty, for our vigor and our health.
Let us play and exercise in the fresh air,
Let us breathe life deeply running in the sun.

For from God are also happiness and laughter
And of all things in life, health is the best.
Be our journey a joyous stroll without fatigue,
Let's forget our anxious strife and our pain.

IDENTIFICATION

Music and poetry are an intrinsic part of Hispanic culture. In a tribute to this and to the subject matter of this text, this anthem to health expresses fundamental, timeless values. It is especially appropriate for those involved in health care in bilingual school situations.

Himno a la salud

Aire tradicional

Viva el agua, viva el baño y el jabón

que nos lavan, embellecen, dan vigor.

Viva el baile, el ejercicio y la alegría,

la carrera respirando a pleno sol.

Justo al cuerpo, a la dicha y a la risa,

de la vida la salud es lo mejor.

Sea la vida movimiento sin fatiga,

rechacemos la violencia y el dolor.

GRAMMAR AND STRUCTURES DRILLED IN LESSON 41

adjectives

ser + adjectives indicating characteristics or inherent qualities

estar + adjectives indicating conditions or things subject to change

Es nervioso. He is nervous (by nature).
Está nervioso. He's nervous (because of unusual excitement).

agreement with implied or stated subject of ser or estar

Himno a la salud

Traditional Air
Arrangement by Julia J. Tabery

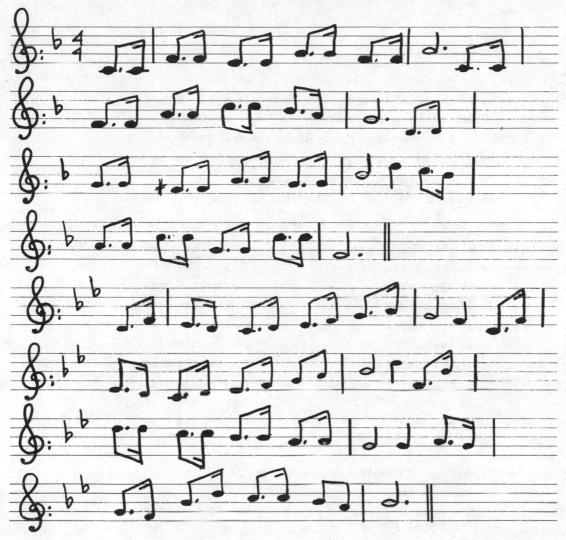

Evaluation

LESSON 1

A. Subraye la parte del cuerpo que no pertenece a este grupo.

1. the ankle, the wrist, the leg, the knee, the foot
2. the head, the eyelid, the eyelash, the eye, the hand
3. the nail, the armpit, the chest, the shoulder, the back
4. the waist, the neck, the buttock, the hip, the crotch
5. the foot, the sole of the foot, the toe, the heel, the ear

B. Cubra la columna de la derecha y conteste cada pregunta en plural.

1.	Is it the arm?	They're the arms.
2.	Is it the ear?	They're the ears.
3.	Is it the eye?	They're the eyes.
4.	Is it the finger?	They're the fingers.
5.	Is it the leg?	They're the legs.
6.	Is it the hip?	They're the hips.
7.	Is it the hand?	They're the hands.
8.	Is it the nail?	They're the nails.
9.	Is it the ankle?	They're the ankles.
10.	Is it the knee?	They're the knees.
11.	Is it the shoulder?	They're the shoulders.

C. Escoja la mejor respuesta a la frase dada.

1. How do you feel today?

    a. I'm sorry.　　　　　b. It's nothing.
    c. See you later.　　　d. Better, thanks.

2. Hi! How's everything?

    a. Not very good.　　　b. You have it.
    c. Pardon.　　　　　　d. Excuse me.

3. I feel bad.

    a. Thank you.　　　　　b. I'm sorry.
    c. Very well.　　　　　d. Gladly.

4. How's it going?

    a. Don't mention it.　　b. Very well, thanks.
    c. Hi!　　　　　　　　d. Good-bye.

Evaluación

LECCION 1

A. Underline the part of the body that does not belong with each group.

1. el tobillo, la muñeca, la pierna, la rodilla, el pie
2. la cabeza, el párpado, la pestaña, el ojo, la mano
3. la uña, la axila, el pecho, el hombro, la espalda
4. la cintura, el cuello, la nalga, la cadera, la entrepierna
5. el pie, la planta del pie, el dedo del pie, el talón, la oreja

B. Cover the right-hand column, and answer each question in the plural.

1. ¿Es el brazo?	Son los brazos.
2. ¿Es la oreja?	Son las orejas.
3. ¿Es el ojo?	Son los ojos.
4. ¿Es el dedo?	Son los dedos.
5. ¿Es la pierna?	Son las piernas.
6. ¿Es la cadera?	Son las caderas.
7. ¿Es la mano	Son las manos.
8. ¿Es la uña?	Son las uñas.
9. ¿Es el tobillo?	Son los tobillos.
10. ¿Es la rodilla?	Son las rodillas.
11. ¿Es el hombro?	Son los hombros.

C. Select the best reply to the phrase given.

1. ¿Cómo se siente usted hoy?

    a. Lo siento.
    c. Hasta la vista.
    b. No es nada.
    d. Mejor, gracias.

2. ¡Hola! ¿Qué tal?

    a. No muy bien.
    c. Perdón.
    b. Usted lo tiene.
    d. Con permiso.

3. Me siento mal.

    a. Gracias.
    c. Muy bien.
    b. Lo siento.
    d. Con mucho gusto.

4. ¿Cómo le va?

    a. No hay de qué.
    c. ¡Hola!
    b. Muy bien, gracias.
    d. Adíos.

LESSON 2

A. Añada por lo menos una palabra que se pueda asociar con las otras dadas.

1. the spleen, the liver,

2. the throat, the lungs,

3. the vagina, the uterus,

4. the penis, the testicles,

5. the intestines, the colon,

B. Relacione cada órgano y parte del cuerpo en la columna A con la parte correspondiente en la columna B. Escriba la letra en el espacio al lado de la palabra.

A				B	
1. wrist	___	eye	___	a.	head
2. spleen	___	gallbladder	___	b.	chest
3. hand	___	knee	___	c.	abdomen
4. bronchial tubes	___	ear	___	d.	arm
5. eyelash	___	thigh	___	e.	leg
6. elbow	___	nostrils	___		
7. ankle	___	foot	___		
8. breast	___	ear (inner)	___		

C. Escoja la mejor respuesta a la frase dada.

1. With your permission.

    a. Good-bye.   b. You have it.
    c. Please.   d. Not very well.

2. Do you understand?

    a. What a shame!   b. No, very little.
    c. Stupendous!   d. Same to you.

3. I feel very good.

    a. Marvelous.   b. Poor thing!
    c. Yes, very little.   d. Good luck.

4. Please speak more slowly.

    a. Fantastic!   b. Thanks a million.
    c. Repeat, please.   d. Yes, sir, gladly.

LECCION 2

A. To each group add at least one more word that might be associated with those given.

1. el esplín, el hígado,

2. la garganta, los pulmones,

3. la vagina, la matriz,

4. el pene, los testículos,

5. los intestinos, el colon,

B. Match each organ or part of the body in Column A with its general location in Column B. Write the corresponding letter in the blank next to the word.

A

				B
1. muñeca ___	ojo ___			a. cabeza
2. bazo ___	vesícula ___			b. pecho
3. mano ___	rodilla ___			c. abdomen
4. bronquios ___	oreja ___			d. brazo
5. pestaña ___	muslo ___			e. pierna
6. codo ___	fosas nasales ___			
7. tobillo ___	pie ___			
8. seno ___	oído ___			

C. Select the best reply to the phrase given.

1. Con su permiso.

    a. Adiós.   b. Usted lo tiene.
    c. Por favor.   d. No muy bien.

2. ¿Comprende?

    a. ¡Qué lástima!   b. No, muy poco.
    c. ¡Estupendo!   d. Igualmente.

3. Me siento muy bien.

    a. Maravilloso.   b. ¡Pobrecito!
    c. Sí, un poco.   d. Buena suerte.

4. Favor de hablar más despacio.

    a. ¡Fantástico!   b. ¡Un millón de gracias!
    c. Repita, por favor.   d. Sí, señor, con mucho gusto.

LESSON 3

A. Escoja la mejor respuesta a cada pregunta.

1. Do you have a cough?

   a. Yes, I have a cold.
   b. Yes, I have hives.
   c. Yes, I have burning when I urinate.

2. Do you have sweating?

   a. Yes, I have a fever.
   b. Yes, I have constipation.
   c. Yes, I have a good appetite.

3. Do I have sinus trouble?

   a. No, you don't have frequent bowel movements.
   b. No, you don't have cramps.
   c. No, you have a cold.

4. Do you have itching?

   a. Yes, I'm dizzy.
   b. No, I don't have yellowish skin.
   c. Yes, I have hives.

5. Do you have hemorrhoids?

   a. No, I don't have pain in the waist.
   b. Yes, I have piles.
   c. Yes, I'm nauseated.

6. Do you have a headache?

   a. No, I don't have a headache.
   b. No, I don't have pain in my muscles.
   c. No, I don't have blood in my urine.

7. Are you weak?

   a. Yes, and I have itching.
   b. Yes, and I feel dizzy.
   c. Yes, and I feel burning when I urinate.

B. ¿Qué palabra no está relacionada con la palabra subrayada?

1. to urinate: burning, pain, irritation, cough

2. chest: lung, breast, finger, bust

3. stomach: intestine, diarrhea, leg, indigestion

4. foot: nail, hip, toe, heel

LECCIÓN 3

A. Choose the best answer or response to each question.

1. ¿Tiene usted tos?

   a. Sí, tengo catarro.
   b. Sí, tengo urticaria.
   c. Sí, tengo ardor al orinar.

2. ¿Tiene sudores?

   a. Sí, tengo fiebre.
   b. Sí, tengo constipación.
   c. Sí, tengo buen apetito.

3. ¿Tengo sinusitis?

   a. No, usted no tiene evacuaciones frecuentes.
   b. No, usted no tiene calambres.
   c. No, usted tiene un resfriado.

4. ¿Tiene picazón?

   a. Sí, tengo mareo.
   b. No, no tengo la piel amarilla.
   c. Sí, tengo urticaria.

5. ¿Tiene hemorroides?

   a. No, no tengo dolor en la cintura.
   b. Sí, tengo almorranas.
   c. Sí, tengo náuseas.

6. ¿Tiene dolor de cabeza?

   a. No, no tengo jaqueca.
   b. No, no tengo dolor en los músculos.
   c. No, no tengo sangre en la orina.

7. ¿Tiene usted debilidad?

   a. Sí, y tengo picazón.
   b. Sí, y siento mareo.
   c. Sí, y siento ardor al orinar.

B. What word is not related to the one underlined?

1. orinar: ardor, dolor, irritación, tos

2. pecho: pulmón, seno, dedo, busto

3. estómago: intestino, diarrea, pierna, indigestión

4. pie: uña, cadera, dedo, talón

C. Identifique la palabra o frase en la columna B que tiene significado semejante a una en la columna A.

	A			B
1.	How do you feel?	___	a.	It's delicious.
2.	How's everything?	___	b.	How's it going?
3.	See you later.	___	c.	Come in.
4.	Come in.	___	d.	I'm very sorry.
5.	My deepest sympathy.	___	e.	Don't mention it.
6.	You're welcome.	___	f.	How are you?
7.	It's very good.	___	g.	Good-bye.

LESSON 4

A. Escoja la hora correcta en la columna B para cada hora indicada en la columna A.

	A			B
1.	11:30	___	a.	It's eleven forty.
2.	5:15	___	b.	It's five fifteen.
3.	10:40	___	c.	It's one ten.
4.	1:20	___	d.	It's ten forty.
5.	6:45	___	e.	It's six forty.
			f.	It's one twenty.
			g.	It's eleven thirty.
			h.	It's twelve thirty.
			i.	It's quarter till seven.

B. Diga al paciente a qué hora debe tomar la medicina. Escoja la palabra o expresión que falta para completar la columna A de las que se dan en la columna B.

   At what time do I take the medicine?

	A		B
1.	At 2:00, at 4:00, at 6:00 -- or every ___ hours.	a.	after
		b.	noon
2.	___ meals.	c.	two
3.	Before bedtime, at ___ P.M.	d.	ten
4.	Every four hours -- at 10:00, at 2:00, at ___.	e.	twenty
		f.	five
		g.	now
		h.	six

C. Identify the word or expression in column B that has a similar meaning to each one in Column A.

    A   B

    1. ¿Cómo se siente?   ___   a. Está deliciosa.

    2. ¿Qué tal?   ___   b. ¿Cómo le va?

    3. Hasta la vista.   ___   c. Adelante.

    4. Pase.   ___   d. Lo siento mucho.

    5. Mi sentido pésame. ___   e. No hay de qué.

    6. De nada.   ___   f. ¿Cómo está usted?

    7. Está muy rica.   ___   g. Adiós.

LECCION 4

A. Choose the correct time in words from Column B for each hour in Column A.

    A   B

    1. 11:30   ___   a. Son las once y cuarto.

    2. 5:15   ___   b. Son las cinco y quince.

    3. 10:40   ___   c. Es la una y diez.

    4. 1:20   ___   d. Son las diez y cuarenta.

    5. 6:45   ___   e. Son las seis y cuarenta.

                                        f. Es la una y veinte.

                                        g. Son las once y media.

                                        h. Son las doce y treinta.

                                        i. Son las siete menos cuarto.

B. Tell the patient at what time he is to take medicine. choose the correct word or expression from Column B to complete each item in Column A.

    A   B

    ¿A qué hora tomo la medicina?

    1. A las dos, a las cuatro, a las seis --   a. después
        cada ___ horas.
                                                    b. mediodía
    2. ___ de las comidas.
                                                    c. dos
    3. Antes de acostarse, a las ___ de la noche.
                                                    d. diez
    4. Cada cuatro horas -- a las diez, a las dos,
        y a las ___.   e. veinte

                                                    f. cinco

                                                    g. ahora

                                                    h. seis

C. Encuentre en la columna B la palabra o frase de sentido opuesto a una en la
    columna A.

	A				B
1.	Hi!	___		a.	Stupendous!
2.	Good morning.	___		b.	Put this on.
3.	I feel better.	___		c.	Good night.
4.	I'm sorry.	___		d.	Stand up, please.
5.	Sit down, please.	___		e.	I feel worse.
6.	Take this off.	___		f.	See you later!

REVIEW OF LESSONS 1-5

Escoja la respuesta que mejor complete la oración.

1. The elbow and the wrist are joints of the ___.
    a. arm   b. leg   c. knee

2. The ankle and the knee are joints of the ___.
    a. leg   b. heel   c. hip

3. The nails and the ___ are similar parts of the hands and feet.
    a. arms   b. breasts   c. fingers and toes

4. The palm of the hand is similar to the ___ of the foot.
    a. sole   b. nose   c. back (of the trunk)

5. The liver and ___ are parts of the digestive system.
    a. the testicles   b. the stomach   c. the foot

6. ___ are organs of the reproductive system.
    a. The arms   b. The eyes   c. The genitals

7. ___ is not a reproductive organ.
    a. The womb   b. The penis   c. The bladder

8. You have diarrhea. Probably you have an infection in ___.
    a. the mouth   b. the intestines   c. the ear

9. You have an obstruction in the ___.
    a. cough   b. cranium   c. esophagus

10. You have hives. And you have ___.
    a. itching   b. good appetite   c. cramps

11. You have indigestion and ___.
    a. belching   b. phlegm   c. nervousness

12. ___ blood in your urine?
    a. Do you have   b. Do you feel   c. Fever

13. At what time do I take the medicine? Every ___ hours.
    a. 28   b. 3   c. 11:15

C. Find the word or expression in Column B that has an opposite meaning to the one given in Column A.

	A		B
1.	¡Hola! ___	a.	¡Estupendo!
2.	Buenos días. ___	b.	Póngase esto.
3.	Me siento mejor. ___	c.	Buenas noches.
4.	Lo siento. ___	d.	Levántese, por favor.
5.	Siéntese, por favor. ___	e.	Me siento peor.
6.	Quítese esto. ___	f.	¡Hasta luego!

REPASO DE LAS LECCIONES 1-5

Choose the answer that best completes each statement.

1. El codo y la muñeca son articulaciones del ___.

   a. brazo   b. pierna   c. rodilla

2. El tobillo y la rodilla son coyunturas de la ___.

   a. pierna   b. talón   c. cadera

3. Las uñas y los ___ son partes similares de las manos y los pies.

   a. brazos   b. pechos   c. dedos

4. La palma de la mano es similar a la ___ del pie.

   a. planta   b. nariz   c. espalda

5. El hígado y ___ son partes del aparato digestivo.

   a. los testículos   b. el estómago   c. el pie

6. ___ son órganos del aparato reproductivo.

   a. Los brazos   b. Los ojos   c. Los genitales

7. ___ no es un órgano reproductivo.

   a. La matriz   b. El pene   c. La vejiga

8. Tiene diarrea. Probablemente tiene infección en ___.

   a. la boca   b. los intestinos   c. el oído

9. **Tiene obstrucción en el ___.**

   a. tos   b. cráneo   c. esófago

10. Tiene urticaria. Y tiene ___.

    a. picazón   b. buen apetito   c. calambres

11. Tiene indigestión y ___.

    a. eructos   b. flema   c. nerviosidad

12. ¿___ sangre en la orina?

    a. Tiene   b. Siente   c. Fiebre

13. ¿A qué hora tomo la medicina? Cada ___ horas.

    a. veinteocho   b. tres   c. once y quince

14. What time is it? It's ___.

    a. 3   b. 25   c. before going to bed

15. It's 12:00. It's ___.

    a. noon   b. 35   c. 13

16. At what time do I take the medicine? ___.

    a. Each   b. Gladly   c. In the afternoon

17. 30 grams and 100 grams are ___ grams.

    a. 40   b. 130   c. 1300

18. Two portions of 100 calories have ___ calories.

    a. 150   b. 200   c. 1000

19. One liter is ___.

    a. 500 cc   b. 1000 cc   c. 1500 cc

20. One teaspoonful is ___.

    a. 1 yard   b. 1 gram   c. 1 dram

LESSON 6

A. Escoja la respuesta que mejor complete la oración.

1. The brother of your father is your ___.

    a. grandmother   b. uncle
    c. cousin   d. brother-in-law

2. The mother of your husband is your ___.

    a. grandmother   b. aunt
    c. mother-in-law   d. daughter-in-law

3. The father of your son is your ___.

    a. brother-in-law   b. husband
    c. cousin   d. relative

4. My granddaughter is the daughter of my ___.

    a. son   b. friend
    c. neighbor   d. cousin

5. The mother of my mother is my ___.

    a. daughter   b. grandmother
    c. daughter-in-law   d. sister-in-law

B. Dé la forma feminina de las siguientes palabras.

1. married   2. son-in-law

3. neighbor   4. father

5. relative   6. boy

14. ¿Qué hora es? Son ___.

    a. las tres   b. las veinticinco   c. antes de acostarse

15. Son las doce. Es ___.

    a. mediodía   b. treinta y cinco   c. trece

16. ¿A qué hora tomo la medicina? ___.

    a. Cada   b. Con mucho gusto   c. Por la tarde

17. Treinta gramos y cien gramos son ___ gramos.

    a. cuarenta   b. ciento treinta   c. mil trece

18. Dos porciones de cien calorías tienen ___ calorías.

    a. ciento cincuenta   b. doscientas   c. mil

19. Un litro es ___.

    a. quinientos cen-   b. mil centímetros   c. mil quinientos
       tímetros cúbicos   cúbicos   centímetros cúbicos

20. Una cucharadita es ___.

    a. una vara   b. un gramo   c. un dracma

LECCIÓN 6

A. Select the answer that best completes the sentence.

1. El hermano de su padre es su ___.

    a. abuelo   b. tío
    c. primo   d. cuñado

2. La madre de su esposo es su ___.

    a. abuela   b. tía
    c. suegra   d. nuera

3. El padre de su hijo es su ___.

    a. cuñado   b. esposo
    c. primo   d. pariente

4. Mi nieta es la hija de mi ___.

    a. hijo   b. amigo
    c. vecino   d. primo

5. La madre de mi madre es mi ___.

    a. hija   b. abuela
    c. nuera   d. cuñada

B. Give the feminine form of the following words.

1. casado   2. yerno

3. vecino   4. padre

5. pariente   6. niño

C. Escoja la palabra o frase que pueda ser sustituida por la palabra subrayada.

1. You want aspirin. You have a <u>headache</u>. ___

2. You have a pain in the <u>joint</u>. ___

3. Do you have a bad <u>taste</u> in your mouth? ___

4. Does your <u>breast</u> hurt? ___

5. I have blood when I have a bowel movement. Do I have <u>piles</u>? ___

a. joint

b. headache

c. hemorrhoids

d. taste

e. chest

LESSON 7

A. Escoja la mejor respuesta a cada pregunta.

1. What is your name?

   a. Juan.
   c. Call the doctor.
   b. I'm the patient.
   d. He's my husband.

2. Do you have a family?

   a. Yes, I have a pain here.
   c. I'm 25 years old.
   b. Yes, I have 3 children.
   d. I want to introduce you to
       my husband.

3. What work does your husband do?

   a. Housewife.
   c. Carpenter.
   b. He's on vacation.
   d. He's Protestant.

4. How is she related to you?

   a. He's not my neighbor.
   c. She's my sister.
   b. It's private.
   d. He's a student.

5. What religion are you?

   a. It's double.
   b. He's the patient.
   b. I'm Catholic.
   d. He doesn't have an insurance
       policy.

B. Dé la palabra interrogativa que complete cada pregunta.

1. _____ is the responsible   It's my husband, Fernando García.
   party?

2. _____ is the nurse's name?   Her name is María.

3. _____ does one pay?   In the office.

4. _____ does a private room $90.00.
   cost?

5. _____ is the matter with you?   I have a pain in my back.

6. _____ are you from?   I'm from Mexico.

7. _____ is the number of your   It's Main Street, Number 1513.
   house?

C. Choose the word or phrase that could be substituted for the one underlined.

1. Desea aspirina. Tiene <u>dolor de cabeza</u>. ___   a. articulación

2. Tiene dolor en la <u>coyuntura</u>.   ___   b. jaqueca

3. ¿Tiene mal <u>gusto</u> en la boca?   ___   c. hemorroides

4. ¿Le duele el <u>seno</u>?   ___   d. sabor

5. Tengo sangre al defecar. ¿Tengo   e. pecho
   <u>almorranas</u>?   ___

LECCION 7

A. Select the best answer to each question.

1. ¿Cómo se llama?

   a. Juan.   b. Soy el paciente.
   c. Llame al médico.   d. Es mi esposo.

2. ¿Tiene usted familia?

   a. Sí, tengo un dolor aquí.   b. Sí, tengo tres hijos.
   c. Tengo veinticinco años.   d. Quiero presentarle a mi
                                       esposo.

3. ¿Qué trabajo hace su esposo?

   a. Ama de casa.   b. Está de vacaciones.
   c. Carpintero.   d. Es protestante.

4. ¿Qué parentezco tiene con Ud.?

   a. No es mi vecino.   b. Es privado.
   c. Es mi hermana.   d. Es estudiante.

5. ¿Qué religión tiene?

   a. Es doble.   b. Soy católico.
   c. Es el paciente.   d. No tiene póliza de seguro.

B. Give the interrogative word that best completes each question.

1. ¿_____ es el responsable?   Es mi esposo, Fernando García.

2. ¿_____ se llama la enfermera?   Se llama María.

3. ¿_____ hay que pagar?   En la oficina.

4. ¿_____ cuesta un cuarto   Cuesta $90.00.
   privado?

5. ¿_____ le pasa?   Tengo dolor de espalda.

6. ¿De _____ es Ud.?   Soy de México.

7. ¿_____ es la dirección de   Es Calle Principal, número
   su casa?   quince trece.

C. Escoja la mejor respuesta a la pregunta. Escriba la letra al lado de la
   pregunta.

1. Do you have itching?   ___
2. Do you have pain in
   your chest?   ___
3. Do you have an infection?___
4. Do you want something?   ___
5. What's the matter?   ___

a. Yes, it's my heart.
b. Yes, food, please.
c. The equipment isn't working.
d. Yes, here on my skin.
e. Yes, in the kidneys.

LESSON 8

A. Escoja la mejor respuesta para cada pregunta.

1. How much must I pay now?

   a. It's a private hospital.
   c. In the office.
   b. The cashier.
   d. A minimum deposit.

2. How should I pay? Cash or ___?

   a. the rest
   c. dismissal
   b. on terms
   d. vacant

3. Can I have a private room?

   a. Yes, in order to leave.
   c. Yes, for hospitalization.
   b. No, there aren't any vacant.
   d. No, it's a clinic.

4. On ___ and Sundays the doctor doesn't have office hours.

   a. Tuesdays
   c. Wednesdays
   b. Saturdays
   d. Mondays

5. Today is Wednesday. Come back tomorrow. Come back ___.

   a. Tuesday
   c. Monday
   b. Thursday
   d. Friday

6. The day before Monday is ___.

   a. Tuesday
   c. Saturday
   b. Sunday
   d. Friday

7. The month after March is ___.

   a. February
   c. April
   b. May
   d. January

8. The month before May is ___.

   a. April
   c. March
   b. July
   d. June

C. Choose the best answer to each question. Write the letter beside the question.

1. ¿Tiene picazón? ___

2. ¿Tiene dolor en el pecho?___

3. ¿Tiene infección? ___

4. ¿Desea algo? ___

5. ¿Qué pasa? ___

a. Sí, es el corazón.

b. Sí, comida, por favor.

c. El aparato está malo.

d. Sí, aquí en la piel.

e. Sí, en los riñones.

LECCION 8

A. Choose the best answer to each question.

1. ¿Cuánto hay que pagar ahora?

   a. Es un hospital privado.
   c. En la oficina.
   b. A la cajera.
   d. Un depósito mínimo.

2. ¿Cómo tengo que pagar?   Al contado o ___?

   a. el resto
   c. de alta
   b. a plazos
   d. vacante

3. ¿Puedo tener un cuarto privado?

   a. Sí, para salir.
   c. Sí, de hospitalización.
   b. No, no hay vacante.
   d. No, es una clínica.

4. Los ___ y los domingos no hay consulta.

   a. martes
   c. miércoles
   b. sábados
   d. lunes

5. Hoy es miércoles. Vuelva mañana. Vuelva el ___.

   a. martes
   b. lunes
   b. jueves
   d. viernes

6. El día antes del lunes es el ___.

   a. martes
   c. sábado
   b. domingo
   d. viernes

7. El mes después de marzo es ___.

   a. febrero
   c. abril
   b. mayo
   d. enero

8. El mes antes de mayo es ___.

   a. abril
   c. marzo
   b. julio
   d. junio

B. Dé en español el número de días que tiene cada mes usando las expresiones siguientes.

	31 days		less than 30
1. August	_____	2. February	_____
3. October	_____	4. January	_____
5. June	_____	6. September	_____
7. April	_____	8. March	_____
9. November	_____	10. May	_____
11. December	_____	12. July	_____

(30 days)

C. Escoja la mejor respuesta para cada pregunta.

1. Do you have pain in your heel?

   a. No, on the sole of my foot.
   c. No, in the spleen.

   b. No, in the armpit.
   d. No, it's the neck.

2. When do I take the medicine?

   a. Before going to bed.
   c. Get up.

   b. Sit down.
   d. It's 4:00 p.m.

3. What time is it?

   a. It's 15 till 8:00.
   c. It weighs 20 grams.

   b. It has 100 calories.
   d. At midnight.

4. How do you say inglés?

   a. Please speak more slowly.
   c. You say English.

   b. Yes, a little.
   d. It means English.

5. Where is the bathroom?

   a. He's all right.
   c. It's the address of my house.

   b. It's here.
   d. It's delicious.

B. Give in Spanish the number of days that each month has, using the following expressions.

treinta y un días   treinta días   menos de treinta

1. agosto   _____   2. febrero   _____

3. octubre   _____   4. enero   _____

5. junio   _____   6. septiembre   _____

7. abril   _____   8. marzo   _____

9. noviembre   _____   10. mayo   _____

11. diciembre   _____   12. julio

C. Choose the best answer to each question.

1. ¿Tiene dolor en el talón?

   a. No, en la planta del pie.   b. No, en la axila.
   c. No, en el bazo.   d. No, es el cuello.

2. ¿Cuándo tomo la medicina?

   a. Antes de acostarse.   b. Siéntese.
   c. Levántese.   d. Son las cuatro de la tarde.

3. ¿Qué hora es?

   a. Son las ocho menos quince.   b. Tiene cien calorías.
   c. Pesa veinte gramos.   d. A medianoche.

4. ¿Cómo se dice inglés?

   a. Favor de hablar más despacio.   b. Sí, un poco.
   c. Se dice English.   d. Quiere decir English.

5. ¿Dónde está el baño?

   a. Está muy bien.   b. Está aquí.
   c. Es la dirección de mi casa.   d. Está muy rico.

LESSON 9

A. Escoja la respuesta que complete mejor la oración.

1. A man does not use ___.
   a. a vest
   c. men's shorts
   b. a bra
   d. a belt

2. If you're going to wear a suit, you might also wear ___.
   a. a tie
   c. pajamas
   b. a skirt
   d. a robe

3. If a woman is going to the hospital, she doesn't need to take ___.
   a. a nightgown
   c. robe
   b. slippers
   d. earrings

4. If you're going to the bathroom, you can put on your ___.
   a. bracelet
   c. checkbook
   b. slippers
   d. glasses

5. You have your money in ___.
   a. your billfold
   c. your wig
   b. your ring
   d. your watch

B. Encuentre una palabra en la columna B que se relacione de algún modo con una palabra en la columna A.

A		B
1. men's shorts	___	a. purse
2. coat	___	b. blouse
3. girdle	___	c. contact lenses
4. hose	___	d. bra
5. shirt	___	e. ring
6. jeweled ring	___	f. scarf
7. glasses	___	g. undershirt
8. handbag	___	h. shoes

C. Dé la hora indicada menos treinta minutos.

1. At 12:00.

2. At 11:30.

3. At 10:15.

4. At 8:20.

5. It's 5:35.

6. It's 1:05.

7. It's 18 till 4:00.

<u>LECCION 9</u>

A. Select the best answer to complete each sentence.

    1. Un hombre no usa ___.
        a. chaleco
        c. calzoncillos
        b. sostén
        d. cinturón

    2. Si va a ponerse el traje, puede ponerse también ___.
        a. la corbata
        c. las pijamas
        b. la falda
        d. la bata

    3. Si una señora va al hospital no necesita llevar ___.
        a. camisa de noche
        c. bata
        b. zapatillas
        d. aretes

    4. Si va al baño puede ponerse ___.
        a. la pulsera
        c. el libro de cheques
        b. las zapatillas
        d. los anteojos

    5. Ud. tiene el dinero en ___.
        a. la billetera
        c. la peluca
        b. el anillo
        d. el reloj

B. Find a word in column B that is related in some way with each word in Column A.

	A			B
1.	calzoncillos	___	a.	bolsa
2.	abrigo	___	b.	blusa
3.	faja	___	c.	lentes de contacto
4.	medias	___	d.	sostén
5.	camisa	___	e.	anillo
6.	sortija	___	f.	bufanda
7.	anteojos	___	g.	camiseta
8.	cartera	___	h.	zapatos

C. Give the time half an hour earlier than each one given.

    1. A las doce.

    2. A las once y media.

    3. A las diez y cuarto.

    4. A las ocho y veinte.

    5. Son las cinco y treinta y cinco.

    6. Es la una y cinco.

    7. Son las cuatro menos dieciocho.

REVIEW OF LESSONS 6-10

A. Escoja la respuesta que mejor complete cada pregunta u oración.

1. What work does your husband do? He's ___.

   a. the patient
   b. a businessman
   c. my husband

2. I want a ___ room.

   a. private
   b. every 2 hours
   c. on terms

3. Who is the patient? She's ___.

   a. the insurance policy
   b. the responsible party
   c. my husband's mother

4. Why have you come to the hospital? Because ___.

   a. I'm Protestant
   b. my husband isn't here
   c. I have pains in my abdomen

5. Please sign ___.

   a. the anesthesia
   b. the doctor
   c. the permit

6. Visiting hours are ___.

   a. from 2:00 to 4:00 P.M.
   b. from 2:00 to 4:00 A.M.
   c. from 11:00 to 12:00 P.M.

7. Is he your husband's brother? Yes, he's my ___.

   a. nephew
   b. brother-in-law
   c. cousin

B. Escriba la letra al lado de la categoría a que cada artículo pertenece.

1. slippers ___	a.	A woman uses
2. undershirt ___	b.	A man uses
3. girdle ___	c.	A man and a woman both use
4. watch ___		
5. toothpaste ___		
6. undershorts ___		
7. bra ___		
8. earrings ___		

REPASO DE LAS LECCIONES 6-10

A. Select the most suitable completion for the following statements or questions.

1. ¿Qué trabajo hace su esposo? Es ___.

   a. el paciente
   b. hombre de negocios
   c. mi esposo

2. Deseo un cuarto ___.

   a. privado
   b. cada dos horas
   c. a plazos

3. ¿Quién es la paciente? Es ___.

   a. la póliza de seguros
   b. el responsable
   c. la madre de mi esposo

4. ¿Por qué viene al hospital? Porque ___.

   a. soy protestante
   b. mi esposo no está aquí
   c. tengo dolores en el abdomen

5. Favor de firmar ___.

   a. la anestesia
   b. el médico
   c. el permiso

6. Las horas de visita son ___.

   a. de dos a cuatro de la tarde
   b. de dos a cuatro de la mañana
   c. de once a doce de la noche

7. ¿Es el hermano de su esposo? Sí, es mi ___.

   a. sobrino
   b. cuñado
   c. primo

B. Next to each article write the letter of the category to which the article belongs.

1. las zapatillas ___   a. La señora usa

2. la camiseta ___   b. El señor usa

3. la faja ___   c. El señor y la señora usan

4. el reloj ___

5. la pasta de dientes ___

6. los calzoncillos ___

7. el sostén ___

8. los aretes ___

C. ¿Qué palabra no pertenece a cada serie?

1. zip code, pain, address, street, apartment

2. family, doctor, nurse, teacher, therapist, housewife

3. emergency room, office, laboratory, room, telephone

4. married, single, widower, son, divorced

5. grandfather, brother, uncle, cousin, neighbor

LESSON 11

A. Escoja la mejor respuesta a la pregunta u oración.

1. Is it necessary to pay cash?

   a. If you feel well.
   b. If you have the permit.
   c. No, you can pay by the month.

2. May one see the patient?

   a. Yes, after 2:00.
   b. Yes, if you wear a vest.
   c. Yes, if you don't go to the bathroom.

3. When may one visit in the hospital?

   a. On the dresser.
   b. Gladly.
   c. In the afternoon.

4. You need to sleep.

   a. Well, I'm going to turn out the light.
   b. Well, I'm going to turn on the light.
   c. Well, I'm going to turn on the television.

5. Where shall I put the flowers?

   a. From 11:00 to 12:00.
   b. On the pillow.
   c. Outside.

6. When will the meal be served?

   a. Gladly.
   b. Lie down.
   c. Right away.

B. ¿Qué pregunta corresponde mejor a cada respuesta?

1. Then you have to pay cash.

   a. May I have visitors?
   b. What are the rules?
   c. And if I don't have insurance?

C. In each series, what does not belong?

   1. la zona postal, el dolor, la dirección, la calle, el apartamento

   2. familia, médico, enfermera, profesor, terapista, ama de casa

   3. la sala de emergencia, la oficina, el laboratorio, el cuarto, el teléfono

   4. casado, soltero, viudo, hijo, divorciado

   5. abuelo, hermano, tío, primo, vecino

LECCION 11

A. Select the best answer to each question or statement.

   1. ¿Es necesario pagar al contado?

      a. Si Ud. se siente bien.
      b. Si Ud. tiene el permiso.
      c. No, puede pagar por meses.

   2. ¿Se puede ver al paciente?

      a. Sí, después de las dos.
      b. Sí, si llevan el chaleco.
      c. Sí, si no van al baño.

   3. ¿Cuándo se puede visitar en el hospital?

      a. En el tocador.
      b. Con mucho gusto.
      c. Por la tarde.

   4. Ud. necesita dormir.

      a. Pues, voy a apagar la luz.
      b. Pues, voy a encender la luz.
      c. Pues, voy a poner el televisor.

   5. ¿Dónde pongo las flores?

      a. De once a doce.
      b. En la almohada.
      c. Afuera.

   6. ¿Cuándo se sirve la comida?

      a. Con mucho gusto.
      b. Acuéstese.
      c. En seguida.

B. Which question is most appropriate for each statement?

   1. Entonces tiene que pagar al contado.

      a. ¿Puedo tener visitas?
      b. ¿Cuáles son las reglas?
      c. ¿Y si no tengo seguro?

2. They're comfortable, with telephone and television.

    a. What information do you wish?
    b. How much does a private room cost?
    c. What are the rooms like?

3. I need to change the bed.

    a. What time is it?
    b. What do you need?
    c. When may I see the patient?

C. Escoja la mejor respuesta a la pregunta u oración.

1. I want to introduce you to Dr. Sánchez.

    a. You must go to the office.   b. Glad to know you.
    c. At 6:00.   d. Gladly.

2. At what time are they going to operate on me?

    a. At 8:00 A.M.   b. 1000 cc.
    c. 44 grams.   d. Every 3 hours.

3. Good morning. How do you feel?

    a. Better, thanks.   b. It's there.
    c. Nothing, thanks.   d. Sit down.

4. How many calories does a serving of cereal have?

    a. It has 13 calories.   b. It has 3000 calories.
    c. It has 130 calories.   d. It has millions of calories.

5. Do you have any brothers and sisters?

    a. Yes, I have 3 children.   b. Yes, I have one brother and one sister.

    c. Yes, they're my cousins.   d. Yes, they're my mother's brothers (and sisters).

6. Who is your sister-in-law?

    a. María is my brother's mother.   b. María is my brother's mother-in-la

    c. María is my brother's daughter.   d. María is my brother's wife.

LESSON 12

A. Escoja la respuesta que mejor complete cada oración.

1. Are you going to wear ___, sir?

    a. your skirt   b. your bra
    c. your girdle   d. your tie

2. Please make a ___.

    a. head   b. smear
    c. elbow   d. fist

2. Son amplios, con teléfono y televisor.

    a. ¿Qué información desea?
    b. ¿Cuánto cuesta un cuarto privado?
    c. ¿Cómo son los cuartos?

3. Necesito cambiar la cama.

    a. ¿Qué hora es?
    b. ¿Qué necesita usted?
    c. ¿Cuándo se puede ver al paciente?

C. Select the best answer or response to each question or statement.

1. Quiero presentarle al doctor Sánchez.

    a. Hay que ir a la oficina.   b. Mucho gusto.
    c. A las seis.   d. Con mucho gusto.

2. ¿A qué hora me van a operar?

    a. A las ocho de la mañana.   b. Mil centímetros cúbicos.
    c. Cuarenta y cuatro gramos.   d. Cada tres horas.

3. Buenos días. ¿Cómo se siente?

    a. Mejor, gracias.   b. Está allí.
    c. Nada, gracias.   d. Siéntese.

4. ¿Cuántas calorías tiene una porción de cereal?

    a. Tiene trece calorías.   b. Tiene tres mil calorías.
    c. Tiene ciento treinta calorías.   d. Tiene millones de calorías.

5. ¿Tiene Ud. hermanos?

    a. Sí, tengo tres hijos.   b. Sí, tengo un hermano y una hermana.
    c. Sí, son mis primos.   d. Sí, son los hermanos de mi madre.

6. ¿Quién es su cuñada?

    a. María es la madre de mi hermano.   b. María es la suegra de mi hermano.
    c. María es la hija de mi hermano.   d. María es la esposa de mi hermano.

LECCIÓN 12

A. Choose the best word to complete each sentence.

1. ¿Va Ud. a llevar ___, señor?

    a. la falda   b. el sostén
    c. la faja   d. la corbata

2. Favor de cerrer ___.

    a. la cabeza   b. el unto
    c. el codo   d. el puño

3. I'm going to measure ___.

    a. the albumin   b. the rabbit
    c. the count   d. the microscope

4. Please roll up ___.

    a. the bathroom   b. the sputum
    c. your sleeve   d. the urine

5. This examination is to find out if you're ___.

    a. in the bathroom   b. happy
    c. pregnant   d. pressure

B. Encuentre la palabra relacionada.

1. toilet   ___   a. anesthesia

2. gestation   ___   b. pregnant

3. relative   ___   c. on terms

4. heart   ___   d. cousin

5. laboratory   ___   e. circulation

6. operation   ___   f. bathroom

7. syringe   ___   g. analysis

8. to pay   ___   h. injection

C. Encuentre en la columna B la respuesta correcta a la pregunta en la columna A.

             A   B

1. What is your address?   a. I'm a businessman.

2. What is your telephone number?   b. 628-1113.

3. What is your insurance company?   c. 22 Main Street.

4. What is your religion?   d. My name is Juan Pérez.

5. What work do you do?   e. I'm Jewish.

6. What is your name?   f. I don't have a hospitalization
                                policy.

LESSON 13

A. Escoja la expresión que tenga significado semejante a las subrayadas.

1. My head aches.

    a. I have to take aspirin.
    b. I have a headache.
    c. Every 4 hours.

2. Do you have good elimination?

    a. Do you urinate normally?
    b. Do you drink enough water?
    c. Is your urine concentrated?

3. Voy a medir ___.

    a. la albúmina   b. el conejo
    c. el recuento   d. el microscopio

4. Favor de levantarse ___.

    a. el baño   b. el esputo
    c. la manga   d. la orina

5. Este examen es para saber si está ___.

    a. en el baño   b. contenta
    c. embarazada   d. presión

B. Match the related words.

1. el inodoro   ___   a. la anestesia

2. gestación   ___   b. embarazada

3. el pariente   ___   c. a plazos

4. el corazón   ___   d. el primo

5. el laboratorio   ___   e. la circulación

6. la operación   ___   f. el baño

7. la jeringuilla   ___   g. el análisis

8. pagar   ___   h. la inyección

C. Select the best answer in Column B to each question in Column A.

                A   B

1. ¿Cuál es la dirección de su casa?   a. Soy hombre de negocios.

2. ¿Cuál es el número de su telé-   b. Seis dos ocho, once trece.
    fono?

3. ¿Cuál es su compañía de segu-   c. Calle Principal veintidós.
    ros?

4. ¿Cuál es su religión?   d. Me llamo Juan Pérez.

5. ¿Cuál es su trabajo?   e. Soy judío.

6. ¿Cómo se llama Ud.?   f. No tengo póliza de hospitaliza-
                                    ción.

LECCION 13

A. Select the expression closest in meaning to the one underlined.

1. <u>Me duele la cabeza.</u>

    a. Tengo que tomar aspirina.
    b. Tengo jaqueca.
    c. Cada cuatro horas.

2. <u>¿Elimina Ud. bien?</u>

    a. ¿Orina Ud. normalmente?
    b. ¿Toma bastante agua?
    c. ¿Tiene Ud. la orina concentrada?

3. <u>I have difficulty with my vision</u>.

    a. I don't see dark spots.
    b. I see very well.
    c. I don't see very well.

4. <u>Do you rest well</u>?

    a. Do you sleep well?
    b. Do you feel well today?
    c. Does your back ache?

B. Complete con la mejor respuesta.

1. How long have you had yellowish skin? For ___.

    a. 3 weeks   b. heat   c. the bed

2. What other symptoms do you have? I have ___.

    a. 2 months   b. x-rays   c. little appetite

3. When can I go home?

    a. Yesterday.   b. Tuesday.   c. In 1965.

4. What analysis are they going to do?

    a. Irregular pulse. b. Stuffy nose.   c. Blood.

C. Escoja la frase que complete mejor la oración.

1. ___ the checkbook.

    a. Please put away b. I'm going to   c. Gladly
                               visit

2. I have a pain in my abdomen. I'm not going to wear ___.

    a. my bra   b. my glasses   c. my girdle

3. How cold! I'm going to wear ___.

    a. my shirt   b. my tie   c. my coat

LESSON 14

A. Escoja la palabra o frase semejante en significado a la que se subraya.

1. <u>I have tonsillitis</u>.

    a. arthritis
    b. paralysis
    c. inflammation of the tonsils.

2. <u>Do you rest well</u>?

    a. Do you sleep well?
    b. Do you feel good today?
    c. Does your waist hurt?

3. It's an analysis to see if you have <u>diabetes</u>.

    a. concentrated urine.
    b. cholesterol in the blood
    c. sugar in the blood

3. <u>Tengo trastornos en la vista.</u>

    a. No veo obscuro.
    b. Veo muy bien.
    c. No veo muy bien.

4. <u>¿Descansa Ud. bien?</u>

    a. ¿Duerme Ud. bien?
    b. ¿Se siente bien hoy?
    c. ¿Le duele la espalda?

B. Complete each statement with the best answer.

1. ¿Desde cuándo tiene Ud. la piel amarilla? Hace ___.

    a. tres semanas   b. calor   c. la cama

2. ¿Qué otros síntomas tiene? Tengo ___.

    a. dos meses   b. los rayos X   c. poco apetito

3. ¿Cuándo puedo ir a casa?

    a. Ayer.   b. El martes.   c. En mil novecientos sesenta y cinco.

4. ¿Qué análisis van a hacer?

    a. El pulso alterado.   b. La nariz tupida.   c. De sangre.

C. Choose the best completion for each statement.

1. ___ el libro de cheques.

    a. Favor de guardar   b. Voy a visitar   c. Con mucho gusto

2. Tengo dolor en el abdomen. No voy a ponerme ___.

    a. el sostén   b. los lentes   c. la faja

3. ¡Qué frío! Voy a ponerme ___.

    a. la camisa   b. la corbata   c. el abrigo

LECCION 14

A. Select the word or expression closest in meaning to the one underlined.

1. Tengo <u>amigdalitis</u>.

    a. artritis
    b. parálisis
    c. tonsilitis

2. <u>¿Descansa Ud. muy bien?</u>

    a. ¿Duerme Ud. bien?
    b. ¿Se siente bien hoy?
    c. ¿Le duele la cintura?

3. Es un análisis para ver si tiene <u>diabetes</u>.

    a. la orina concentrada
    b. colesterol en la sangre
    c. azúcar en la sangre

4. How long have you had <u>yellowish skin</u>?

    a. jaundice
    b. hives
    c. whooping cough

5. Do you <u>have</u> heart disease?

    a. have pain
    b. suffer from
    c. have swelling

6. <u>Have you had</u> pain in your legs?

    a. Have you slept
    b. Have you eliminated
    c. Have you felt

B. Encuentre la palabra relacionada y escriba la letra en el espacio en blanco.

1. weakness	___	a. skin
2. sore throat	___	b. malignant tumor
3. shortness of breath	___	c. blood
4. palpitations	___	d. heart
5. cancer	___	e. joints
6. rheumatism	___	f. difficulty breathing
7. acne	___	g. intestine
8. epilepsy	___	h. attacks
9. diverticulitis	___	i. tiredness
10. high blood pressure	___	j. tonsillitis.

C. Escoja la frase que mejor complete la oración.

1. I need water. I don't have a ___.	a. to put away
2. I'm nauseated. I need the ___.	b. to go to the bathroom
3. Where is the ___ and the toothpaste?	c. glass
4. Do you need ___ or do you need to use the bedpan?	d. to write
	e. brush
5. I need ___ my money before the operation.	f. basin for vomit
6. You need ___ your name and address.	

4. ¿Desde cuándo tiene <u>la piel amarilla</u>?

   a. ictericia
   b. urticaria
   c. tos ferina

5. ¿<u>Padece</u> del corazón?

   a. Tiene dolor
   b. Sufre
   c. Tiene hinchazón

6. ¿<u>Ha tenido</u> dolor en las piernas?

   a. Ha dormido
   b. Ha eliminado
   c. Ha sentido

B. Find the related word and write the letter in the blank.

   1. debilidad ___   a. la piel

   2. dolor de garganta ___   b. tumor maligno

   3. respiración corta ___   c. la sangre

   4. palpitaciones ___   d. el corazón

   5. cáncer ___   e. las articulaciones

   6. reumatismo ___   f. dificultad al respirar

   7. acné ___   g. el intestino

   8. epilepsia ___   h. ataques

   9. diverticulitis ___   i. cansancio

   10. alta presión ___   j. amigdalitis

C. Choose the best completion for each statement.

   1. Necesito agua. No tengo ___.   a. guardar

   2. Tengo náuseas. Necesito la ___.   b. ir al baño

   3. ¿Dónde está el ___ y la pasta de dientes?   c. vaso

   4. ¿Necesita Ud. ___ o necesita usar el bidet?   d. escribir

                                            e. cepillo

   5. Necesito ___ el dinero antes de la operación.   f. vasija para vómito

   6. Ud. necesita ___ su nombre y su dirección.

REVIEW OF LESSONS 11-15

A. Complete cada pregunta u oración con la mejor respuesta.

 1. How long have you had ___ when you cough?

    a. nervousness   b. expectora-   c. weakness   d. digestion
                         tion

 2. Please ___ on the table.

    a. pain   b. know   c. measure   d. get up

 3. For 3 days I've had ___ when I swallow.

    a. difficulty   b. air   c. colic   d. **tonsillitis.**

 4. Do you need a ___ for vomit?

    a. glass   b. machine   c. handbag   d. basin

 5. I've been ___ a lot, and I need to change my gown.

    a. sweating   b. instruments c. belching   d. colds

 6. What drink do you prefer? I prefer ___.

    a. ice   b. onion   c. lettuce   d. milk

 7. My brother likes hot ___.

    a. beer   b. chocolate   c. ice cream d. cream

 8. I love cottage ___.

    a. broth   b. bread   c. cheese   d. sugar

 9. My ___ ache.

    a. head   b. legs   c. foot   d. back

10. A drink that is a stimulant is ___.

    a. milk   b. coffee   c. water   d. juice

11. I like toast and ___.

    a. butter   b. oats   c. water   d. potatoes

12. Please pass the ___ cheese.

    a. sugar   b. sauce   c. cream   d. juice

13. For breakfast I'm going to have ___ juice.

    a. soda pop   b. beer   c. coffee   d. orange

14. I like cereal with ___.

    a. pepper   b. peanut   c. vinegar   d. honey
                         butter

15. My favorite fruits are strawberries and ___.

    a. garlic   b. sauces   c. mangos   d. ice

REPASO DE LAS LECCIONES 11-15

A. Complete each statement or question with the best answer.

1. ¿Desde cuándo tiene Ud. ___ al toser?

   a. nerviosidad   b. expectora-   c. debilidad   d. digestión
   ción

2. Favor de ___ a la mesa.

   a. dolor   b. saber   c. medir   d. subir

3. Hace tres días que tengo ___ al tragar.

   a. dificultad   b. aire   c. cólicos   d. tonsilitis

4. ¿Necesita Ud. ___ para vomitar?

   a. un vaso   b. una máquina   c. una bolsa   d. una vasija

5. Tengo muchos ___ y necesito cambiarme la bata.

   a. sudores   b. instrumen-   c. eructos   d. resfriados
   tos

6. ¿Qué bebida prefiere? Prefiero ___.

   a. hielo   b. cebolla   c. lechuga   d. leche

7. A mi hermano le gusta el ___ caliente.

   a. cerveza   b. chocolate   c. helado   d. crema

8. Me encanta el ___ requesón.

   a. caldo   b. pan   c. queso   d. azúcar

9. Me duelen ___.

   a. la cabeza   b. las piernas   c. el pie   d. la espalda

10. Una bebida estimulante es ___.

    a. la leche   b. el café   c. el agua   d. el jugo

11. Me gusta el pan tostado con ___.

    a. mantequilla   b. avena   c. agua   d. patatas

12. Favor de pasar el queso ___.

    a. azúcar   b. salsa   c. crema   d. jugo

13. De desayuno voy a tomar jugo de ___.

    a. soda   b. cerveza   c. café   d. naranja

14. Me gusta el cereal con ___.

    a. pimienta   b. crema de   c. vinagre   d. miel
    cacahuete

15. Mis frutas favoritas son las fresas y ___.

    a. el ajo   b. las salsas   c. los man-   d. el hielo
    gos

B. Escoja la expresión de significado semejante a la subrayada.

1. I have a headache.

   a. My waist aches.
   b. My head aches.
   c. I have an obstruction in the esophagus.

2. Do you have the written order?

   a. May I sign now?
   b. Are you right?
   c. Do you have the permit?

3. I'm not hemorrhaging now.

   a. I have enough blood.
   b. I have high blood pressure.
   c. I'm not bleeding now.

4. I have burning when I urinate.

   a. I urinate frequently.
   b. I have burning in the urethra.
   c. I have sugar in the urine.

5. The meal is served now.

   a. One may visit now.
   b. Supper is served late.
   c. Lunch is served right away.

LESSON 16

A. Complete cada oración con la mejor palabra o frase.

1. How do you want your steak? I want it ___.

a. raw	b. rare
c. frozen	d. soft-boiled

2. My son prefers fried ___.

a. salads	b. lettuce
c. strawberries	d. shrimp

3. I like ___ eggs.

a. scrambled	b. roasted
c. raw	d. peas

4. For supper they're serving ___.

a. pepper, garlic, and butter	b. peaches, raisins, and grapefruit
c. roast beef, **vege**tables, and fruit	d. onion, sauce, and dark bread

5. I want to make ___ peppers.

a. Brussels	b. hard
c. pork	d. stuffed

B. Choose the expression most similar in meaning to the one underlined.

1. Tengo jaqueca.

   a. Tengo dolor de cintura.
   b. Tengo dolor de cabeza.
   c. Tengo obstrucción en el esófago.

2. ¿Tiene Ud. la orden escrita?

   a. ¿Puedo firmar ahora?
   b. ¿Tiene Ud. razón?
   c. ¿Tiene Ud. el permiso?

3. Ya no tengo hemorragia.

   a. Tengo bastante sangre.
   b. Tengo la presión alta.
   c. Ya no tengo flujo de sangre.

4. Tengo ardor al orinar.

   a. Orino con frecuencia.
   b. Tengo ardor en la uretra.
   c. Tengo azúcar en la orina.

5. Se sirve la comida ahora.

   a. Se visita ahora.
   b. Se sirve la cena tarde.
   c. Se sirve el almuerzo en seguida.

LECCIÓN 16

A. Complete each statement with the best word or phrase.

1. ¿Cómo quiere el biftec? Lo quiero ___.

   a. crudo
   c. helado
   b. poco asado
   d. pasado por agua

2. Mi hijo prefiere los ___ fritos.

   a. ensaladas
   c. fresas
   b. lechuga
   d. camarones

3. Me gustan los huevos ___.

   a. revueltos
   c. crudos
   b. asados
   d. chícharos

4. Para la cena sirven ___.

   a. pimienta, ajo y mantequilla
   c. carne asada, verduras y frutas
   b. melocotones, pasas y toronjas
   d. cebolla, salsa y pan moreno

5. Quiero preparar chiles ___.

   a. de Bruselas
   c. de puerco
   b. duros
   d. rellenos

B. Escriba en la primera línea la clasificación a que pertenece cada grupo (fruits, fish, vegetables, drinks, meats, seasonings). En la última línea escriba otro ejemplo de alimentos en cada grupo.

1. _____, tuna, salmon, sardine, _____

2. _____, broccoli, endive, cauliflower, _____

3. _____, coffee, chocolate, tea, _____

4. _____, steak, ham, hamburger, _____

5. _____, melon, lemon, pear, _____

6. _____, salt, pepper, garlic, _____

C. Tache un síntoma que no pertenezca a cada serie.

1. For two days I've had nausea, dizziness, diarrhea, and constipation.

2. For several days I've had a cough, phlegm, cramps, and a sore throat.

D. Complete cada respuesta con una expresión de tiempo.

1. How long have you had insomnia? For _____.

2. How long have you been nervous? For _____.

3. How long have you had a poor appetite? For _____.

4. How long have you had sinus trouble? For _____.

5. How long have you had sweating? For _____.

LESSON 17

A. Escoja la respuesta que mejor complete la oración.

1. Please give me the glass of ___.

   a. water   b. biscuit   c. dessert   d. cake

2. When is breakfast served? It's served at ___.

   a. the saucer b. about 7:00   c. nothing   d. at night

3. Do you like ___ fruit?

   a. skimmed   b. carbonated   c. wheat   d. canned

4. I need to choose my ___.

   a. cooked   b. meal   c. favorite d. frozen

5. What should I do to lose ___?

   a. breakfast b. tray   c. sherbet d. weight

B. ¿Qué palabra no pertenece a cada serie?

1. breakfast, menu, snack, lunch

2. knife, spoon, fork, canned

3. ice cream, gelatin, soup, lemon pie

4. tray, napkin, table, supper

5. cakes, fresh, frozen, cooked

B. Write on the first line the classification to which each group belongs (frutas, pescados, vegetales, bebidas, carnes, condimentos). On the last line write one more example of the foods in each group.

1. _____, atún, salmón, sardina, _____

2. _____, bróculi, endibia, coliflor, _____

3. _____, café, chocolate, té, _____

4. _____, biftec, jamón, hamburguesa, _____

5. _____, melón, limón, pera, _____

6. _____, sal, pimienta, ajo, _____

C. Cross out one symptom that does not belong in each series.

1. Hace dos días que tengo náuseas, mareo, diarrea y constipación.

2. Hace unos días que tengo tos, flema, calambres y dolor de garganta.

D. Complete each answer with any appropriate time expression.

1. ¿Desde cuándo tiene Ud. insomnio? Hace _____.

2. ¿Desde cuándo tiene nerviosidad? Hace _____.

3. ¿Desde cuándo tiene mal apetito? Hace _____.

4. ¿Desde cuándo tiene sinusitis? Hace _____.

5. ¿Desde cuándo tiene sudores? Hace _____.

LECCION 17

A. Complete each statement with the best choice.

1. Me permite el vaso de ___.

    a. agua   b. bizcocho   c. postre   d. torta

2. ¿Cuándo se sirve el desayuno? Se sirve ___.

    a. el plati-   b. a eso de las   c. nada   d. por la noche
       llo   siete

3. ¿Le gustan las frutas ___?

    a. descrema-   b. gaseosas   c. de trigo   d. en lata
       das

4. Necesito seleccionar mi ___.

    a. cocida   b. comida   c. preferida   d. congelada

5. ¿Qué debo hacer para perder ___?

    a. desayuno   b. la bandeja   c. nieve   d. peso

B. Which word does not belong in each series?

1. desayuno, menú, merienda, almuerzo

2. cuchillo, cucharilla, tenedor, enlatada

3. helado, gelatina, sopa, pastel de limón

4. la bandeja, la servilleta, la mesa, la cena

5. queques, frescos, congelados, cocidos

C. Conteste cada pregunta en la forma negativa.

Ejemplo: <u>Have you had</u> tonsillitis? <u>No</u>, Doctor, <u>I haven't had</u> tonsillitis.
Sir
Ma'am
Miss

1. Have you had scarlet fever?

2. Have you had diphtheria?

3. Have you had measles?

4. Have you had whooping cough?

5. Have you had rheumatic fever?

6. Have you had heart disease?

7. Have you had epilepsy?

8. Have you had diabetes?

9. Have you had cancer?

LESSON 18

A. Complete cada oración con la mejor respuesta.

1. If you are having kidney trouble, you shouldn't have much ___.

   a. salt   b. sugar
   c. milk   d. water

2. A good diet should be rich in ___.

   a. balanced   b. proteins
   c. fats   d. spices

3. Besides minerals, a good diet should have ___.

   a. vitamins   b. ulcers
   c. aluminum   d. diabetes

4. To gain weight, you should eat ___.

   a. less   b. more
   c. water   d. coffee

5. You shouldn't lose much weight ___.

   a. before going to bed   b. every morning
   c. before sleeping   d. rapidly

B. Tache la palabra o frase que <u>no pueda</u> completar la oración.

1. A person who has heart trouble can have ___.

   a. fruit juice   b. alcoholic beverages
   c. coffee   d. skim milk

2. Eggs do not contain ___.

   a. milk   b. fat
   c. minerals   d. protein

C. Answer each question in the negative.

Example: ¿Ha tenido Ud. amigdalitis?   No, doctor, no he tenido amigdalitis.
                                        señor
                                        señora
                                        señorita

1. ¿Ha tenido Ud. escarlatina?

2. ¿Ha tenido Ud. difteria?

3. ¿Ha tenido Ud. sarampión?

4. ¿Ha tenido Ud. tos ferina?

5. ¿Ha tenido Ud. fiebre reumática?

6. ¿Ha tenido Ud. enfermedades del corazón?

7. ¿Ha tenido Ud. epilepsia?

8. ¿Ha tenido Ud. diabetes?

9. ¿Ha tenido Ud. cáncer?

LECCIÓN 18

A. Complete each statement with the best choice.

1. Si los riñones funcionan mal, no debe tomar mucha ___.

   a. sal   b. azúcar
   c. leche   d. agua

2. Una buena dieta debe ser rica en ___.

   a. balanceada   b. proteínas
   c. grasa   d. especias

3. Además de minerales, una buena dieta debe tener ___.

   a. vitaminas   b. úlceras
   c. aluminio   d. diabetes

4. Para aumentar de peso debe comer ___.

   a. menos   b. más
   c. agua   d. café

5. No debe perder mucho peso ___.

   a. antes de acostarse   b. todas las mañanas
   c. antes de dormir   d. rápidamente

B. Cross out the word or phrase that cannot fill each blank.

1. Una persona que padece del corazón puede tomar ___.

   a. jugo de frutas   b. bebidas alcohólicas
   c. café   d. leche descremada

2. El huevo no contiene ___.

   a. leche   b. grasa
   c. minerales   d. proteína

3. If a patient has a stomach ulcer, he shouldn't have ___.

    a. milk   b. greasy foods
    c. drinks that are stimulants   d. many spices

4. In order to lose weight it is necessary to exercise and ___.

    a. drink a lot of water   b. follow a low-carbohydrate diet

    c. eat a lot of vegetables   d. eat fried foods

5. For dessert you may have ___.

    a. meringue cookies   b. fresh fruit
    c. pudding   d. frozen fish

6. Of course you can eat ___.

    a. the napkin   b. lemon pie
    c. rice pudding   d. custard

7. What childhood illnesses have you had? Have you had ___?

    a. headache   b. measles
    c. whooping cough   d. scarlet fever

C. Conteste la pregunta en el afirmativo o el negativo.

    Ejemplo: Do you want soup?   Yes, Sir, I want soup.
                                 Miss
                                 Ma'am
                 No,   , I don't want soup.

    1. Do you want cheese?

    2. Do you want bread?

    3. Do you want fruit?

    4. Do you want water?

    5. Do you want coffee?

    6. Do you want hot tea?

    7. Do you want iced tea?

    8. Do you want a banana?

    9. Do you want strawberries?

    10. Do you want strawberry ice cream?

    11. Do you want chocolate ice cream?

LESSON 19

A. Escoja la respuesta que mejor complete cada oración.

    1. You should eat when you're _____.

    2. You should drink when you're _____.

    3. You should sleep when you're _____.

    4. Please turn on the air conditioning. I'm _____.

3. Si un paciente tiene una úlcera en el estómago, no debe tomar ___.

a. leche
b. alimentos grasosos
c. bebidas estimulantes
d. muchas especias

4. Para perder peso es necesario hacer ejercicios y ___.

a. tomar mucha agua
b. seguir una dieta baja en carbo-hidratos
c. comer muchos vegetales
d. comer alimentos fritos

5. De postre puede tomar ___.

a. merengues
b. frutas frescas
c. pudín
d. pescado congelado

6. Claro que puede comer ___.

a. la servilleta
b. pastel de limón
c. arroz con leche
d. flan

7. ¿Qué enfermedades de la infancia ha tenido Ud.? ¿Ha tenido ___?

a. dolor de cabeza
b. sarampión
c. tos ferina
d. escarlatina

C. Answer each question in the affirmative or negative.

Example: ¿Quiere Ud. sopa? Sí, señor, quiero sopa.
señorita
señora
No,   , no quiero sopa.

1. ¿Quiere Ud. queso?

2. ¿Quiere Ud. pan?

3. ¿Quiere Ud. frutas?

4. ¿Quiere Ud. agua?

5. ¿Quiere Ud. café?

6. ¿Quiere Ud. té caliente?

7. ¿Quiere Ud. té helado?

8. ¿Quiere Ud. un plátano?

9. ¿Quiere Ud. fresas?

10. ¿Quiere Ud. helado de fresas?

11. ¿Quiere Ud. helado de chocolate?

LECCION 19

A. Write the word that best completes each sentence.

1. Ud. debe comer cuando tiene _____.

2. Ud. debe beber cuando tiene _____.

3. Ud.· debe dormir cuando tiene _____.

4. Favor de poner el aire acondicionado, tengo _____.

B. Complete cada pregunta según el ejemplo.

Ejemplo: You have to go to bed. <u>Do I</u> have to go to bed?

1. You have to sit down. _____ have to sit down?

2. You have to shave. _____ have to shave?

3. You have to weigh yourself. _____ have to weigh _____?

4. You have to take care of yourself. _____ have to take care of _____?

C. Complete la oración con uno de los cuatro verbos siguientes.

<u>wash</u>   <u>bend</u>   <u>change</u>   <u>turn over</u>

1. You have to _____ in bed, to the left.

2. You have to _____ your knee.

3. You have to _____ your position.

4. You have to _____ your hands.

5. You have to _____ your elbow.

6. You have to _____ to the right.

7. You have to _____ clothes.

8. You have to _____ your leg.

9. You have to _____ your teeth.

10. You have to _____ your feet.

D. Conteste con la forma correcta del adjetivo según los ejemplos. (Recuerde que en inglés los adjetivos no tienen concordancia.)

Ejemplos: <u>Do you like</u> chicken (sing.)?   Yes, it's delicious (m.).
                       soup?   it's delicious (f.).
          <u>Do you like</u> peas (pl.)?   they're delicious (m., pl.).
                       fruit?   they're delicious (f., pl.).

1. <u>Do you like</u> rice?

2.   vegetables?

3.   salad?

4.   potatoes?

5.   milk?

6.   beverages?

B. Complete each question according to the example.

    Example: Ud. tiene que <u>acostarse</u>. ¿Tengo que <u>acostarme</u>?

    1. Ud. tiene que <u>sentarse</u>. ¿Tengo que _____?

    2. Ud. tiene que <u>afeitarse</u>. ¿Tengo que _____?

    3. Ud. tiene que <u>pesarse</u>. ¿Tengo que _____?

    4. Ud. tiene que <u>cuidarse</u>. ¿Tengo que _____?

C. Choose one of the four verbs that follow to complete each sentence.

    <u>lavarse</u>   <u>doblar</u>   <u>cambiarse</u>   <u>voltearse</u>

    1. Ud. tiene que _____ en la cama a la izquierda.

    2. Ud. tiene que _____ la rodilla.

    3. Ud. tiene que _____ de posición.

    4. Ud. tiene que _____ las manos.

    5. Ud. tiene que _____ el codo.

    6. Ud. tiene que _____ sobre el lado derecho.

    7. Ud. tiene que _____ de ropa.

    8. Ud. tiene que _____ la pierna.

    9. Ud. tiene que _____ los dientes.

    10. Ud. tiene que _____ los pies.

D. Answer each question with the correct form of the adjective, according to the examples.

    Examples: <u>Le gusta</u> el pollo?   Sí, es delicioso.
                        la sopa?   es deliciosa.
                <u>Le gustan</u> los guisantes?   son deliciosos.
                        las frutas?   son deliciosas.

    1. ¿Le gusta el arroz?

    2. ¿Le gustan los vegetales?

    3. ¿Le gusta la ensalada?

    4. ¿Le gustan las papas?

    5. ¿Le gusta la leche?

    6. ¿Le gusta la bebida?

GENERAL REVIEW OF LESSONS 1-20

A. Escoja la respuesta que mejor complete cada oración.

1. Miss, please open ___.

   a. the head
   c. the elbow
   b. the pillow
   d. the window

2. The patient is not going to wear ___.

   a. her skirt
   c. her girdle
   b. her bra
   d. her tie

3. I have to measure ___.

   a. the medicine
   c. the count
   b. the rabbit
   d. the thermometer

4. Please go to the ___ now.

   a. bathroom
   c. sleeve
   b. sputum
   d. door

5. In the laboratory they're going to ___ a sample of your blood.

   a. prick
   c. put away
   b. take
   d. call

6. The doctor wants to find out if you're ___.

   a. in the bathroom
   c. pregnant
   b. angry
   d. tired

7. You shouldn't worry. These are ___ examinations.

   a. routine
   c. bothersome
   b. complicated
   d. a lot of work

8. How do you feel today? I'm ___.

   a. worse
   c. come in
   b. you're welcome
   d. come in

9. May one have visitors? Yes, ___.

   a. never
   c. 2 times a day
   b. before breakfast
   d. at midnight

10. ___ circulates through the arteries and veins.

    a. Blood
    c. Coagulation
    b. Urine
    d. Air

11. The ___ is an endocrine gland.

    a. thyroid
    c. bladder
    b. lungs
    d. heart

12. The patient is sad because they're going to ___ him.

    a. observe
    c. consult
    b. eliminate
    d. operate on

13. You may have visitors, but you shouldn't ___ a lot.

    a. digest
    c. suffer
    b. talk
    d. weaken

REPASO GENERAL DE LAS LECCIONES 1-20

A. Complete each sentence with the best choice.

1. Señorita, favor de abrir ___.

    a. la cabeza   b. la almohada
    c. el codo   d. la ventana

2. La paciente no va a llevar ___.

    a. la falda   b. el sostén
    c. la faja   d. la corbata

3. Tengo que medir ___.

    a. la medicina   b. el conejo
    c. el recuento   d. el termómetro

4. Favor de ir al ___ ahora.

    a. baño   b. esputo
    c. manga   d. puerta

5. En el laboratorio le van a ___ una muestra de sangre.

    a. pinchar   b. sacar
    c. guardar   d. llamar

6. El médico quiere saber si usted está ___.

    a. en el baño   b. enojada
    c. embarazada   d. cansada

7. Ud. no debe estar preocupada. Estos son exámenes ___.

    a. de rutina   b. complicados
    c. molestos   d. de mucho trabajo

8. ¿Cómo se siente Ud. hoy? Me siento ___.

    a. peor   b. de nada
    c. adelante   d. pase

9. ¿Se puede tener visitas? Sí, ___.

    a. nunca   b. antes de desayuno
    c. dos veces al día   d. a medianoche

10. ___ circula por las arterias y las venas.

    a. La sangre   b. La orina
    c. La coagulación   d. El aire

11. La ___ es una glándula endocrina.

    a. tiroides   b. pulmones
    c. vejiga   d. corazón

12. El paciente está triste porque lo van a ___.

    a. observar   b. eliminar
    c. consultar   d. operar

13. Ud. puede tener visitas pero no debe ___ mucho.

    a. digerir   b. conversar
    c. sufrir   d. debilitar

14. I don't know if the doctor is going to use general ___.

    a. euthanasia   b. toxemia
    c. anesthesia   d. power

15. In order to lose weight you should follow instructions and weigh yourself ___.

    a. once a year   b. once a month
    c. once a day   d. every hour

16. You should follow a diet rich in ___.

    a. balanced   b. low roughage
    c. without fat   d. proteins

17. Egg yolk contains ___.

    a. egg white   b. cream
    c. cholesterol   d. whey

18. Are you going to leave? Here is your ___.

    a. soap   b. toothpaste
    c. coat   d. blanket

19. How long have you had ___ when you cough?

    a. obstruction   b. nervousness
    c. constipation   d. expectoration

20. I've had ___ when I swallow for several days now.

    a. air   b. colic
    c. tonsillitis   d. difficulty

21. Do you need ___ for vomiting?

    a. a glass   b. a sheet
    c. a bag   d. a pan

22. I need a better diet because I have to take a lot of ___.

    a. colds   b. syrups
    c. laxatives   d. Monday

23. Do you want to ___ your teeth before breakfast?

    a. comb   b. wash
    c. get up   d. bend

24. I'm going to put the ___ in the bathroom.

    a. swallow   b. razor
    c. keep   d. sleep

25. For how long have you had fever? ___ 2 days.

    a. For   b. I have
    c. When   d. Why

26. Would you close the drapes, please? I'm ___.

    a. sleepy   b. hungry
    c. hot   d. afraid

27. If you don't feel comfortable, you can ___.

    a. get weighed   b. shave
    c. put on makeup   d. turn over

14. No sé si el médico va a usar ___ general.

    a. eutanasia   b. toxemia
    c. anestesia   d. potencia

15. Para perder peso debe seguir las instrucciones y pesarse ___.

    a. una vez al año   b. una vez al mes
    c. una vez al día   d. cada hora

16. Debe seguir una dieta rica en ___.

    a. balanceada   b. residuo bajo
    c. sin grasa   d. proteínas

17. La yema del huevo contiene ___.

    a. clara   b. crema
    c. colesterol   d. suero

18. ¿Va a salir? Aquí tiene Ud. ___.

    a. el jabón   b. la pasta de dientes
    c. el abrigo   d. la frazada

19. ¿Desde cuándo tiene Ud. ___ al toser?

    a. obstrucción   b. nerviosidad
    c. estreñimiento   d. expectoración

20. Hace varios días que tengo ___ al tragar.

    a. aire   b. cólicos
    c. tonsilitis   d. dificultad

21. ¿Necesita Ud. ___ para vomitar?

    a. un vaso   b. una sábana
    c. una bolsa   d. una vasija

22. Necesito una dieta mejor porque tengo que tomar muchos ___.

    a. resfriados   b. jarabes
    c. laxantes   d. lunes

23. ¿Quiere Ud. ___ los dientes antes de desayuno?

    a. peinarse   b. lavarse
    c. levantarse   d. doblarse

24. Voy a poner la máquina de ___ en el baño.

    a. tragar   b. afeitar
    c. guardar   d. dormir

25. ¿Desde cuándo tiene Ud. fiebre? ___ dos días.

    a. Hace   b. Tengo
    c. Cuando   d. ¿Por qué?

26. ¿Quiere usted cerrar la cortina, por favor? Tengo ___.

    a. sueño   b. hambre
    c. calor   d. miedo

27. Si no se siente cómodo puede ___.

    a. pesarse   b. afeitarse
    c. maquillarse   d. voltearse

28. After a bath I feel ___ .

    a. more comfortable   b. sadder
    c. larger   d. fatter

29. Of course you can eat ___ .

    a. the cup   b. the napkin
    c. apple pie   d. the knife.

B. Escoja la mejor respuesta para cada pregunta.

1. Who's going to operate on me?

   a. The anesthesia.   b. The doctor.
   c. The patient.   d. The permit.

2. What is your religion?

   a. I'm a Protestant.   b. I'm the patient.
   c. I'm not Catholic.   d. I'm a housewife.

3. What's that?

   a. It's the insurance policy.   b. She's the mother of the patient.
   c. He's the responsible party. d. She's the nurse.

4. How are you going to pay?

   a. It's a private hospital.   b. On terms.
   c. I don't have insurance.   d. With a deposit.

5. Who is the patient?

   a. He's not from the United States. b. It's my grandfather.
   c. He's a student.   d. He's Jewish.

6. Is it necessary to walk in the hallways?

   a. If you feel well enough.   b. If you like your room.
   c. If you don't have the permit. d. If you can eliminate.

7. What are you going to do with the syringe?

   a. I'm going to take away the   b. I'm going to give you an
      bedpan.   injection.
   c. Tubes and microscopes.   d. I'm going to close the door.

C. Escoja la expresión de significado semejante a la expresión numerada.

1. I have a headache.

   a. I take aspirin.   b. It doesn't hurt.
   c. Every 4 hours.   d. My head hurts.

2. Can you write your name here?

   a. Can you sign this?   b. Do you have the permit?
   c. Do I need the permit?   d. Can you keep the authorization?

3. Are you drinking sufficient liquids?

   a. Do you urinate frequently?   b. Do you drink enough water?
   c. Is your urine concentrated? d. Do you feel burning when you
                                      urinate?

28. Después del baño me siento más ___.

   a. cómoda   b. triste
   c. grande   d. obesa

29. Claro que puede comer ___.

   a. la taza   b. la servilleta
   c. pastel de manzana   d. el cuchillo

B. Select the best answer to each question.

1. ¿Quién me va a operar?

   a. La anestesia.   b. El médico.
   c. El paciente.   d. El permiso.

2. ¿Cuál es su religión?

   a. Soy protestante.   b. Soy el enfermo.
   c. No soy católico.   d. Soy ama de casa.

3. ¿Qué es eso?

   a. Es la póliza de seguros.   b. Es la madre del paciente.
   c. Es el responsable.   d. Es la enfermera.

4. ¿Cómo va a pagar Ud.?

   a. Es un hospital privado.   b. A plazos.
   c. No tengo seguro.   d. Con un depósito.

5. ¿Quién es el paciente?

   a. No es de los Estados Unidos.   b. Es mi abuelo.
   c. Es estudiante.   d. Es judío.

6. ¿Es necesario caminar en los pasillos?

   a. Si Ud. se siente bien.   b. Si le gusta su cuarto.
   c. Si no tiene el permiso.   d. Si puede eliminar.

7. ¿Qué va a hacer con la jeringuilla?

   a. Voy a quitarle la chata.   b. Voy a ponerle una inyección.

   c. Tubos y microscopios.   d. Voy a cerrar la puerta.

C. Select the expression closest in meaning to the one numbered.

1. Tengo jaqueca.

   a. Tomo aspirina.   b. No me duele.
   c. Cada cuatro horas.   d. Me duele la cabeza.

2. ¿Puede escribir su nombre aquí?

   a. ¿Puede firmar esto?   b. ¿Tiene el permiso?
   c. ¿Necesito el permiso?   d. ¿Puede guardar la autorización?

3. ¿Toma Ud. sufiente líquido?

   a. ¿Orina usted con frecuencia?   b. ¿Toma bastante agua?
   c. ¿Tiene la orina concentrada?   d. ¿Siente ardor al orinar?

4. I have vision difficulties.

    a. I don't see dark spots.   b. I don't see well.
    c. I see very well.   d. I don't see anything.

5. Are you better now?

    a. Are you sleeping well?   b. Are you resting well?
    c. Do you feel well today?   d. Are you walking well?

6. I'm not hemorrhaging now.

    a. I have enough blood.   b. I don't have any blood flow now.
    c. I have high blood pressure. d. I don't have blood in my urine
                                   now.

7. You shouldn't drink alcoholic beverages or coffee.

    a. You shouldn't have milk or   b. You shouldn't drink anything
       stimulants.   with meals.
    c. You shouldn't drink much.   d. You shouldn't have stimulants
                                   or depressants.

D. Escriba una pregunta apropiada para cada respuesta.

1. P.
   R. I feel fine now, thanks.

2. P.
   R. No, you don't have very much fever.

3. P.
   R. That man is my patient.

4. P.
   R. Yes, I like eggs, but I don't want any now.

5. P.
   R. Of course! You can choose your menu for lunch.

6. P.
   R. I have cramps and poor circulation in my legs.

7. P.
   R. You can go home Sunday.

LESSON 21

A. Escoja en la columna B la mejor respuesta para cada expresión en la columna A.

A		B
1. My head aches.	___	a. You must use disinfectant powder.
2. I have a sore throat.	___	b. You have to take a laxative.
3. My back hurts.	___	c. You should use liniment.
4. My skin itches.	___	d. For a headache, you should take aspirin.
5. My eyes hurt.	___	e. You must gargle.
6. My incision hurts.	___	f. Do you need glasses?
7. I'm constipated.	___	g. If you have a lot of pain, you should take this pill.

4. Tengo trastornos en la vista.

    a. No veo obscuro.   b. No veo bien.
    c. Veo muy bien.   d. No veo nada.

5. ¿Está mejor ahora?

    a. ¿Duerme Ud. bien?   b. ¿Descansa Ud. bien?
    c. ¿Se siente Ud. bien hoy?   d. ¿Camina Ud. bien?

6. Ya no tengo hemorragia.

    a. Tengo bastante sangre.   b. Ya no tengo flujo de sangre.
    c. Tengo la presión alta.   d. Ya no tengo sangre en la orina.

7. No debe tomar bebidas alcohólicas ni café.

    a. No debe tomar leche ni   b. No debe beber nada con las
        estimulantes.   comidas.
    c. No debe beber mucho.   d. No debe tomar estimulantes ni
                                     depresantes.

D. Write a suitable question for each answer given.

1. Q.
    A. Me siento bien ahora, gracias.

2. Q.
    A. No, no tiene la fiebre muy alta.

3. Q.
    A. Ese señor es mi paciente.

4. Q.
    A. Sí, me gustan los huevos, pero no quiero ahora.

5. Q.
    A. ¡Cómo no! Puede seleccionar su menú para el almuerzo.

6. Q.
    A. Tengo calambres y mala circulación en las piernas.

7. Q.
    A. Puede volver a su casa el domingo.

LECCION 21

A. Select from Column B the best response to each statement in Column A.

A		B
1. Me duele la cabeza. ____		a. Hay que usar polvo desinfectante.
2. Me duele la garganta. ____		b. Tiene que tomar un purgante.
3. Me duele la espalda. ____		c. Debe usar linimento.
4. Me pica la piel. ____		d. Para jaqueca, tiene que tomar aspirina.
5. Me duelen los ojos. ____		e. Hay que hacer gárgaras.
6. Me duele la herida. ____		f. ¿Necesita anteojos?
7. Estoy constipado. ____		g. Si tiene mucho dolor, debe tomar esta pastilla.

B. Conteste cada pregunta con cualquier color apropiado según el ejemplo.

Ejemplo: What skirt are you going to wear? My red skirt.

1. What dress are you going to wear?

2. What robe are you going to wear?

3. What shoes are you going to wear?

4. What suit are you going to wear?

5. What uniform are you going to wear?

6. What shirt are you going to wear?

7. What tie are you going to wear?

8. What blouse are you going to wear?

9. What socks are you going to wear?

C. Conteste cada pregunta según los ejemplos.

Ejemplos: Do you like dessert?   Yes, I like dessert.
          Do you like cookies?   Yes, I like cookies.

1. Do you like gelatin?

2. Do you like cherries?

3. Do you like cherry pie?

4. Do you like apples?

5. Do you like apple pie?

6. Do you like ice cream?

7. Do you like desserts?

8. Do you like cake?

LESSON 22

A. Conteste cada pregunta con una expresión de significado opuesto a la que se subraya.

1. Do I need to raise my leg?

   No, you need to _____ your leg.

2. Do I need to move my leg to the right?

   No, you need to move your leg _____.

3. Is it necessary to give me an ice pack?

   No, it's necessary to give you _____.

4. Is it necessary to give me a hot bath?

   No, it's necessary to give you _____.

5. Is it necessary to give me a stimulant?

   No, it's necessary to give you _____.

B. Answer each question with any appropriate color, according to the example. Remember that the color will have an ending that corresponds to that of the article of clothing.

Example: ¿Qué falda va a ponerse?   La falda roja.

1. ¿Qué vestido va a ponerse?

2. ¿Qué bata va a ponerse?

3. ¿Qué zapatos va a ponerse?

4. ¿Qué traje va a ponerse?

5. ¿Qué uniforme va a ponerse?

6. ¿Qué camisa va a ponerse?

7. ¿Qué corbata va a ponerse?

8. ¿Qué blusa va a ponerse?

9. ¿Qué calcetines va a ponerse?

C. Answer each question according to the examples.

Examples: ¿Le gusta el postre?   Sí, me gusta el postre.
¿Le gustan las galletas?   Sí, me gustan las galletas.

1. ¿Le gusta la gelatina?

2. ¿Le gustan las cerezas?

3. ¿Le gusta el pastel de cereza?

4. ¿Le gustan las manzanas?

5. ¿Le gusta el pastel de manzana?

6. ¿Le gusta el helado?

7. ¿Le gustan los postres?

8. ¿Le gusta la torta?

LECCION 22

A. Answer each question by giving an expression opposite in meaning to the one underlined.

1. ¿Necesito <u>levantar</u> la pierna?

No, necesita _____ la pierna.

2. ¿Necesito mover la pierna <u>a la derecha</u>?

No, necesita mover la pierna _____ .

3. ¿Es necesario ponerme <u>una bolsa de hielo</u>?

No, es necesario ponerle _____ .

4. ¿Es necesario darme <u>un baño caliente</u>?

No, es necesario darle _____ .

5. ¿Es necesario darme <u>un estimulante</u>?

No, es necesario darle _____ .

B. Escoja la expresión de la columna A que se pueda usar correctamente con cada expresión de la columna B.

A		B
1 liter of glucose.	___	a. You have to
a bath.	___	b. We must give you (externally)
your leg.	___	c. You need to move
an ice pack.	___	d. We must give you (internally; place over or under)
your right arm.	___	
an injection.	___	
gargle.	___	
your fingers.	___	
exercise.	___	
your joints.	___	

C. Conteste cada pregunta usando <u>am</u>, <u>feel like</u>, <u>have</u>, según la pregunta.

Ejemplo: <u>Are you cold</u>? <u>Yes, I'm cold</u>.

1. Are you hot?

2. Are you thirsty?

3. Are you hungry?

4. Do you feel like sleeping?

5. Do you feel like eating?

6. Do you have to exercise?

7. Do you have to keep the money?

8. Do you have to rest now?

9. Do you have to wait now?

10. Do you have to leave now?

LESSON 23

A. Complete cada oración con el órgano o aparato afectado por cada enfermedad.

1. Hepatitis is a disease of the _____.

2. Impetigo is a disease of the _____.

3. Tuberculosis is a disease of the _____.

4. Dysentery is a disease of the _____.

5. Meningitis is a disease of the _____.

6. Glaucoma is a disease of the _____.

B. Choose the expression in Column A with which each item in Column B can be correctly used.

A		B
un litro de glucosa.	___	a. Tiene que hacer
un baño.	___	b. Hay que darle
la pierna.	___	c. Necesita mover
una bolsa de hielo.	___	d. Hay que ponerle
el brazo derecho.	___	
una inyección.	___	
gárgaras.	___	
los dedos.	___	
ejercicio.	___	
las articulaciones.	___	

C. Answer each question with <u>tener</u> according to the example.

Example: <u>Tiene Ud. frío? Sí, tengo frío.</u>

1. ¿Tiene Ud. calor?

2. ¿Tiene Ud. sed?

3. ¿Tiene Ud. hambre?

4. ¿Tiene Ud. ganas de dormir?

5. ¿Tiene Ud. ganas de comer?

6. ¿Tiene que hacer ejercicio?

7. ¿Tiene que guardar el dinero?

8. ¿Tiene que descansar ahora?

9. ¿Tiene que esperar ahora?

10. ¿Tiene que salir ahora?

LECCION 23

A. Complete each sentence by giving the organ or system affected by each disease.

1. La hepatitis es una enfermedad del _____.

2. El impétigo es una enfermedad de la _____.

3. La tuberculosis es una enfermedad de los _____.

4. La disentería es una enfermedad del _____.

5. La meningitis es una enfermedad del _____.

6. El glaucoma es una enfermedad de los _____.

B. Complete cada oración con la mejor respuesta.

1. A childhood disease is ___.

    a. anthrax   b. pneumonia
    c. rabies   d. whooping cough

2. This is <u>not</u> a disease of the respiratory system: ___.

    a. flu   b. influenza
    c. German measles   d. cold

3. One must ___ the patient if he has a contagious disease.

    a. isolate   b. have visitors
    c. see   d. operate

4. A synonym for mumps is ___.

    a. parotitis   b. encephalitis
    c. malaria   d. influenza

5. Shots against ___ are usually given in the stomach.

    a. smallpox   b. tetanus
    c. measles   d. rabies

C. Conteste cada pregunta según el ejemplo.

Ejemplo: <u>Should I get up</u>? <u>Yes, you should get up</u>.

1. Should I wash?

2. Should I bathe?

3. Should I shave?

4. Should I comb my hair?

5. Should I change my gown?

6. Should I sit down?

7. Should I take care of myself?

8. Should I brush my teeth?

9. Should I turn over?

10. Should I get weighed?

LESSON 24

A. Escoja una palabra entre las siguientes que pueda reemplazar la palabra
    subrayada en cada oración.

    equipment   clean   salve
    you need   dressing   an antiseptic
                                                solution

1. <u>It's necessary</u> to change the bandage.

2. I have to <u>wash</u> the wound with soap and water.

3. Should I put <u>ointment</u> on the wound?

4. I need to sterilize the <u>instrument</u> with alcohol.

B. Complete each sentence with the best choice.

1. Una enfermedad infantil es ___.

    a. el ántrax   b. la pulmonía
    c. la rabia   d. la tos ferina

2. Esta enfermedad no es del aparato respiratorio: ___.

    a. la gripe   b. la influenza
    c. la rubéola   d. el catarro

3. Hay que ___ al paciente si tiene una enfermedad contagiosa.

    a. aislar   b. tener visitas
    c. ver   d. operar

4. Un sinónimo de paperas es ___.

    a. parotiditis   b. encefalitis
    c. paludismo   d. gripe

5. Las inyecciones contra ___ generalmente se ponen en el estómago.

    a. la viruela   b. el tétano
    c. el sarampión   d. la rabia

C. Answer each question according to the example.

Example: ¿Debo levantarme? Sí, usted debe levantarse.

1. ¿Debo lavarme?

2. ¿Debo bañarme?

3. ¿Debo afeitarme?

4. ¿Debo peinarme?

5. ¿Debo cambiarme la bata?

6. ¿Debo sentarme?

7. ¿Debo cuidarme?

8. ¿Debo lavarme los dientes?

9. ¿Debo voltearme?

10. ¿Debo pesarme?

LECCION 24

A. Choose a word from those listed that can replace the one underlined in each sentence.

    aparato   limpiar   pomada
    necesita   el vendaje   una solución
                                                 antiséptica

1. Es necesario cambiar la venda.

2. Tengo que lavar la herida con agua y jabón.

3. ¿Debo ponerle ungüento en la herida?

4. Necesito esterilizar el instrumento con alcohol.

5. One must change the bandage.

6. You need to use a disinfectant.

B. Conteste cada pregunta según el ejemplo. Use it o them para reemplazar la palabra subrayada.

Ejemplo: Do you have to use bleach? Yes, I have to use it.

1. Do you have to use iodine?

2. Do you have to use medicine?

3. Do you have to use medicines?

4. Do you have to use bandages?

5. Do you have to use soap?

6. Do you have to use soap and water?

7. Do you have to use antiseptic solutions?

C. Seleccione en la columna B tantas respuestas como sea posible para cada pregunta en la columna A.

A	B
1. Why are you upset? _____	a. Because my family is here.
2. Why are you happy? _____	b. Because I'm afraid.
3. Why are you sad? _____	c. Because I don't like the food.
4. Why are you angry? _____	d. Because I don't have any money.
5. Why are you worried? _____	e. Because I don't have work.
	f. Because I feel like leaving.
	g. Because I feel like crying.
	h. Because I feel better.

REVIEW OF LESSONS 21-25

A. Escoja la mejor respuesta para cada oración o pregunta.

1. You shouldn't get up, but I'm going to give you a bath.

    a. A tub bath?   b. A sponge bath?
    c. A shower?   d. A steam bath?

2. I have a sore throat.

    a. You should use ointment.   b. Do your eyes hurt?
    c. You should gargle.   d. You have to take a laxative.

3. It itches.

    a. Yes, it's whooping cough.   b. Yes, it's pneumonia.
    c. Yes, it's measles.   d. Yes, it's cholera.

4. I'm constipated.

    a. You need milk of magnesia.   b. You have to use ointment.
    c. It's the yellow tablet.   d. I'm going to give you a bath.

5. Hay que cambiar la venda.

6. Necesita usar un desinfectante.

B. Answer each question according to the example. In your answer use lo, la, los, or las to replace the underlined words.

Example: ¿Tiene que usar cloro? Sí, tengo que usarlo.

1. ¿Tiene que usar yodo?

2. ¿Tiene que usar medicina?

3. ¿Tiene que usar medicinas?

4. ¿Tiene que usar vendajes?

5. ¿Tiene que usar jabón?

6. ¿Tiene que usar agua y jabón?

7. ¿Tiene que usar soluciones antisépticas?

C. Select from Column B all the answers that might be given for each question in Column A.

	A		B
1.	¿Por qué está usted mortificado?	_____	a. Porque mi familia está aquí.
2.	¿Por qué está usted contento?	_____	b. Porque tengo miedo.
3.	¿Por qué está usted triste?	_____	c. Porque no me gusta la comida.
4.	¿Por qué está usted enojado?	_____	d. Porque no tengo dinero.
5.	¿Por qué está usted preocupado?	_____	e. Porque no tengo trabajo.
			f. Porque tengo ganas de salir.
			g. Porque tengo ganas de llorar.
			h. Porque me siento mejor.

REPASO DE LAS LECCIONES 21-25

A. Choose the best response to each statement or question.

1. Ud. no debe levantarse, pero voy a darle un baño.

    a. ¿Un baño de tina?   b. ¿Un baño de esponja?
    c. ¿Un baño de ducha?   d. ¿Un baño de vapor?

2. Me duele la garganta.

    a. Debe usar ungüento.   b. ¿Le duelen los ojos?
    b. Debe hacer gárgaras.   d. Tiene que tomar un purgante.

3. Me pica.

    a. Sí, es la tos ferina.   b. Sí, es la pulmonía.
    c. Sí, es el sarampión.   d. Sí, es el cólera.

4. Estoy constipado.

    a. Necesita leche de magnesia.   b. Tiene que usar el ungüento.
    c. Es la tableta amarilla.   d. Le voy a dar un baño.

5. What pill should I take?

    a. The red liquid.   b. Disinfectant powder.
    c. Cough syrup.   d. The red tablet.

6. I'm hot and feverish.

    a. Do you want a bottle?   b. You need a hot water bottle.

    c. Do you want an alcohol bath?   d. You need to exercise.

7. I have a headache.

    a. She has to take your blood   b. You need to gargle.
       pressure.
    c. Yes, it itches.   d. You have to take aspirin.

8. When do I take the medicine?

    a. According to the label.   b. One tablespoonful.
    c. In a bottle.   d. Two pills.

9. It's meningitis.

    a. Yes, it's very serious.   b. I love it.
    c. Yes, it's nothing.   d. It itches.

10. Who's going to give me the physical therapy treatment?

    a. The surgeon.   b. The therapist.
    c. The doctor.   d. The bed.

11. Have you had childhood illnesses?

    a. Yes, cough and headache.   b. Yes, anthrax and typhoid.
    c. Yes, chicken pox and German   d. Yes, malaria and yellow fever.
       measles.

12. You shouldn't move your leg.

    a. Are you going to put it in   b. Should I walk?
       traction?
    c. Should I exercise more?   d. Do I need intravenous feeding?

B. Complete la oración con la mejor respuesta.

1. To avoid germs, you need to use ___.

    a. an instrument   b. a disinfectant
    c. a wound   d. the air

2. You have to use gauze and ___.

    a. adhesive tape   b. ammonia
    c. bed   d. bleach

3. You should wash the instrument and afterward ___.

    a. dry it   b. expose it
    c. change it   d. cure it

4. I haven't had my period and I think I'm ___.

    a. moderate   b. question
    c. weight   d. pregnant

5. ¿Qué pastilla debo tomar?

    a. El líquido rojo.   b. Polvo desinfectante.
    c. Jarabe para la tos.   d. La tableta roja.

6. Tengo calor y fiebre.

    a. ¿Quiere un frasco?   b. Necesita una bolsa de agua caliente.
    c. ¿Quiere un baño de alcohol?   d. Es necesario hacer ejercicios.

7. Me duele la cabeza.

    a. Tiene que tomarle la presión.   b. Necesita hacer gárgaras.

    c. Sí, tengo picazón.   d. Tiene que tomar aspirina.

8. ¿Cuándo tomo la medicina?

    a. Según la etiqueta.   b. Una cucharada.
    c. En una botella.   d. Dos pastillas.

9. Es la meningitis.

    a. Sí, es muy grave.   b. Me encanta.
    c. Sí, no es nada.   d. Me pica.

10. ¿Quién va a darme el tratamiento de fisioterapia?

    a. El cirujano.   b. El terapista.
    c. El médico.   d. La cama.

11. ¿Ha tenido enfermedades de la infancia?

    a. Sí, tos y dolor de cabeza.   b. Sí, antrax y tifoidea.
    c. Sí, viruelas locas y   d. Sí, paludismo y fiebre amarilla.
        rubéola.

12. No debe mover la pierna.

    a. ¿Va a ponerla en tracción?   b. ¿Debo caminar?

    c. ¿Debo hacer más ejercicios? d. ¿Necesito suero intravenoso?

B. Choose the best completion for each statement.

1. Para evitar microbios, usted necesita usar ___.

    a. un aparato   b. un desinfectante
    c. una herida   d. el aire

2. Hay que usar gasa y ___.

    a. tela adhesiva   b. amoníaco
    c. cama   d. cloro

3. Debe lavar el aparato y después ___.

    a. secarlo   b. exponerlo
    c. cambiarlo   d. curarlo

4. No tengo mi regla y creo que estoy ___.

    a. moderada   b. pregunta
    c. peso   d. embarazada

5. My legs are swollen, and I have ___ in my legs, too.

   a. heartburn
   c. nausea

   b. flow
   d. cramps

6. You should go to the hospital because you're having frequent ___.

   a. contractions
   c. headache

   b. acidity
   d. suitcases

7. If your bag of waters ___, you should go to the hospital.

   a. breaks
   c. sees

   b. danger
   d. brush

8. You can use water and ___.

   a. bandage
   c. ointment

   b. iodine
   d. soap

LESSON 26

A. Tache la palabra o expresión que <u>no pueda</u> completar la oración.

1. Take off ___, please.

   a. your blouse
   c. your coat

   b. the bed
   d. all your clothes

2. I want a ___ room.

   a. private
   c. floor

   b. double
   d. several person

3. Let's go to the ___ room.

   a. urinate
   c. labor

   b. maternity
   d. delivery

4. We must call the doctor. You have ___.

   a. **the bottle**
   c. **constant contractions**

   b. strong pains
   d. frequent contractions

5. She doesn't want the doctor to use ___ for the delivery.

   a. forceps
   c. spinal anesthetic

   b. general anesthetic
   d. thermometer

B. Escoja la palabra correcta para completar cada oración.

1. If the baby is not a boy, it's a ___.

2. If you have fever, you have high ___.

3. If you're asleep, you can ___.

4. If you can't have a normal delivery, you need ___.

5. If you lose water, you have to stay in ___.

6. If you don't want natural childbirth, you must have ___.

a. dyspepsia

b. anesthesia

c. temperature

d. cesarean section

e. girl

f. blood pressure

g. wake up

h. bed

i. aspirin

5. Tengo las piernas hinchadas y ___ en las piernas también.

   a. hervor   b. flujo
   c. náuseas   d. calambres

6. Debe ir al hospital porque tiene ___ frecuentes.

   a. contracciones   b. acidez
   c. dolor de cabeza   d. maletas

7. Si se le ___ la fuente debe ir al hospital.

   a. rompe   b. peligro
   c. ve   d. cepillo

8. Puede lavarse con agua y ___.

   a. vendaje   b. yodo
   c. ungüento   d. jabón

LECCIÓN 26

A. Cross out the word or expression that <u>cannot</u> complete the sentence.

1. Quítese ___, por favor.

   a. la blusa   b. la cama
   c. el abrigo   d. toda la ropa

2. Quiero un cuarto ___.

   a. privado   b. doble
   c. piso   d. múltiple

3. Vamos a la sala de ___.

   a. orinar   b. maternidad
   c. labor   d. partos

4. Hay que llamar al médico. Tiene ___.

   a. la botella   b. dolores fuertes
   c. pujos seguidos   d. contracciones frecuentes

5. No quiere que el médico use ___ en el parto.

   a. forceps   b. anestesia general
   c. raquidia   d. termómetro   .

B. Choose the correct word to complete each sentence.

1. Si el bebé no es un niño, es una ___.   a. dispepsia

2. Si tiene fiebre, Ud. tiene la ___ alta.   b. anestesia

3. Si Ud. está dormida, puede ___.   c. temperatura

4. Si no puede tener un parto normal, hay   d. cesárea
   que hacerle una ___.
                                                  e. niña
5. Si pierde agua, tiene que quedarse en la ___.
                                                  f. presión
6. Si no quiere un parto natural, hay que
   darle ___.   g. despertarse

                                                  h. cama

                                                  i. aspirina

C. Conteste las preguntas según los ejemplos.

Ejemplos: Does your waist hurt? Yes, my waist hurts.
Do your legs hurt? Yes, my legs hurt.

1. Does your chest hurt?

2. Does your wrist hurt?

3. Do your shoulders hurt?

4. Do your fingers hurt?

5. Does your finger hurt?

6. Does your back hurt?

7. Does your thigh hurt?

8. Do your thighs hurt?

9. Do your muscles hurt?

10. Does your stomach hurt?

11. Does your foot hurt?

LESSON 27

A. Escoja la mejor respuesta para completar la oración.

1. It's necessary to change the baby's ___.

   a. diaper   b. bottle
   c. clean   d. shower

2. It's necessary to give the baby ___.

   a. a room   b. water
   c. pills   d. a lamp

3. It's necessary to rinse ___.

   a. the milk   b. the formula
   c. the laxative   d. the bottles

4. A sedative is necessary ___.

   a. when you walk   b. at bedtime
   c. when you put on cream   d. on the perineum

5. It's necessary to put ___ on the incision.

   a. a laxative   b. the lamp
   c. cream   d. the stitches

C. Answer each question according to the examples.

Examples: ¿Le duele la cintura? Sí, me duele la cintura.
                    ¿Le duelen las piernas? Sí, me duelen las piernas.

1. ¿Le duele el pecho?

2. ¿Le duele la muñeca?

3. ¿Le duelen los hombros?

4. ¿Le duelen los dedos?

5. ¿Le duele el dedo?

6. ¿Le duele la espalda?

7. ¿Le duele el muslo?

8. ¿Le duelen los muslos?

9. ¿Le duelen los músculos?

10. ¿Le duele el estómago?

11. ¿Le duele el pie?

LECCION 27

A. Choose the best completion for each sentence.

1. Es necesario cambiar ___ a la niña.

   a. el pañal
   c. limpio

   b. la botella
   d. ducha

2. Es necesario dar ___ al bebé.

   a. cuarto
   c. píldoras

   b. agua
   d. lámpara

3. Es necesario enjuagar ___.

   a. la leche
   c. el laxante

   b. la fórmula
   d. las botellas

4. Es necesario un calmante ___.

   a. al andar
   c. al ponerse crema

   b. al acostarse
   d. en el perineo

5. Es necesario ponerle ___ en la herida.

   a. un laxante
   c. crema

   b. la lámpara
   d. las puntadas

B. ¿Qué verbos pueden completar solo la oración 1? ¿Cuáles pueden completar solo la oración 2? ¿Qué verbos pueden completar ambas 1 y 2?

1. It's necessary to ___ the bottles.

2. It's necessary to ___ the baby.

a. take care of

b. rinse

c. change

d. wash

e. sterilize

f. bathe

g. dry

h. put to bed

i. give water to

j. boil

C. ¿Qué color concuerda con cada artículo de vestir?

1. the robe (f.)   ___

2. the dress (m.)   ___

3. the slippers (f.)   ___

4. the shoes (m.)   ___

a. white (f., pl.)

b. red (f., sing.)

c. black (m., pl.)

d. purple (m., sing.)

e. yellow (f., pl.)

f. yellow (f., sing.)

g. white (m., sing.)

h. black (f., sing.)

LESSON 28

A. Complete cada oración con la mejor respuesta.

1. You must bathe the baby in ___ water.

a. warm   b. hot
c. icy   d. dirty

2. You can put the baby into the water after ___.

a. drying him well   b. wetting him well
c. preparing the formula   d. the umbilical cord falls off

3. You must sterilize ___.

a. the measuring cup   b. the sterilizer
c. the nipples   d. the child

4. Every three or four hours you can ___ the baby.

a. measure   b. feed
c. bathe   d. sleep

5. After having milk, the baby has to ___.

a. eliminate   b. burp
c. wash   d. change

B. Which verbs can complete only sentence 1? Which can complete only sentence 2?
    Which can complete both 1 and 2?

    1. Es necesario ___ las botellas.   a. cuidar

    2. Es necesario ___ al bebé.   b. enjuagar

                                                         c. cambiar

                                                         d. lavar

                                                         e. esterilizar

                                                         f. bañar

                                                         g. secar

                                                         h. acostar

                                                         i. dar agua

                                                         j. hervir

C. Which colors agree with each article of clothing?

    1. la bata   ___   a. blancas

    2. el vestido   ___   b. roja

    3. las zapatillas   ___   c. negros

    4. los zapatos   ___   d. morado

                                                         e. amarillas

                                                         f. amarilla

                                                         g. blanco

                                                         h. negra

LECCION 28

A. Complete each statement with the best choice.

    1. Hay que bañar al bebé en agua ___.

        a. tibia   b. caliente
        c. helada   d. sucia

    2. Puede sumergir al niño en agua después de ___.

        a. secarlo bien   b. mojarlo bien
        c. preparar la fórmula   d. caérsele el ombligo

    3. Hay que esterilizar ___.

        a. la taza de medir   b. el esterilizador
        c. las teteras   d. el niño

    4. Cada tres o cuatro horas puede ___ al niño.

        a. medir   b. alimentar
        c. bañar   d. dormir

    5. Después de tomar la leche el niño tiene que ___.

        a. eliminar   b. eructar
        c. lavarse   d. cambiar

B. Encuentre la palabra o expresión relacionada.

1.	eliminate	___	a. sterilizer
2.	breast	___	b. formula
3.	bath	___	c. measure
4.	milk	___	d. soap
5.	utensil	___	e. have a bowel movement
6.	cup	___	f. nipple
7.	bottle	___	g. baby bottle

C. Conteste la pregunta según el ejemplo.

Ejemplo: Is it necessary to call the doctor?
          Yes, ma'am, you need to call the doctor.

1. Is it necessary to call the nurse?

2. Is it necessary to call my husband?

3. Is it necessary to take down the information?

4. Is it necessary to change the baby?

5. Is it necessary to feed the baby?

6. Is it necessary to go to the laboratory?

7. Is it necessary to go to the bathroom?

8. Is it necessary to go to the delivery room?

LESSON 29

A. ¿Qué palabra no pertenece a esta serie?

1. diaphragm, cervical cap, shield, abortion

2. rhythm, jelly, coitus interruptus, withdrawal

3. vaginal douche, suppository, pill, spiral, loop

4. condom, rubber, prophylactic, IUD

B. Tache la palabra o frase que no se pueda poner en el blanco.

1. The pill can produce ___ .

   a. discharge of blood   b. loss of hair
   c. pain in the breasts   d. rings

2. Contraceptives try to prevent the joining of ___ and ovum.

   a. semen   b. condom
   c. sperm   d. sperm

3. I think that I'm pregnant because I haven't had ___ .

   a. my period   b. menstruation
   c. my monthly period   d. ova

4. Contraceptives that men can use are ___ .

   a. jellies   b. condoms
   c. prophylactics   d. coitus interruptus

B. Find the related word or expression.

1. eliminar   ___   a. el esterilizador
2. el pecho   ___   b. la fórmula
3. el baño   ___   c. medir
4. la leche   ___   d. el jabón
5. el utensilio   ___   e. defecar
6. la taza   ___   f. el pezón
7. la botella   ___   g. el biberón

C. Answer each question according to the example.

Example: ¿Es necesario llamar al médico?
         Sí, señora, usted necesita llamar al médico.

1. ¿Es necesario llamar a la enfermera?
2. ¿Es necesario llamar a mi esposo?
3. ¿Es necesario tomar la información?
4. ¿Es necesario cambiar al bebé?
5. ¿Es necesario dar de comer al niño?
6. ¿Es necesario ir al laboratorio?
7. ¿Es necesario ir al baño?
8. ¿Es necesario ir a la sala de partos?

LECCION 29

A. Which word does not belong in each series?

1. diafragma, gorro cervical, escudo, aborto
2. ritmo, jalea, interrupción del coito, la retirada
3. lavado vaginal, supositorio, la píldora, el espiral, el lazo
4. condón, una goma, un profiláctico, un dispositivo intrauterino

B. Cross out the word or phrase which <u>cannot</u> be used in each sentence.

1. La píldora puede producir ___.

   a. flujo de sangre   b. pérdida de pelo
   c. dolor en los senos   d. anillos

2. Los contraceptivos tratan de evitar el encuentro de ___ y el óvulo.

   a. el semen   b. el condón
   c. la semilla   d. el esperma

3. Creo que estoy embarazada porque no tengo ___.

   a. período   b. menstruación
   c. regla   d. óvulos

4. Anticonceptivos que pueden usar los hombres son ___.

   a. jaleas   b. condones
   c. profilácticos   d. interrupción de coito

5. ___ is not a very effective method of birth control.

   a. Withdrawal   b. Vaginal douche
   c. Sterilization   d. Vaginal spermicides

C. Conteste cada grupo de preguntas según los ejemplos.

    Ejemplo: <u>What does the doctor say</u>? Should I rest?
              <u>He says that you should rest</u>.

1.   Can I rest?

2.   Must I rest?

3.   Is it necessary to rest?

4.   Do I need to rest?

5.   Am I going to rest?

6.   Do I have to rest?

    Ejemplo: <u>He says that</u> when you rest, <u>you'll get well</u>.
              <u>When I rest</u>?

7.   when you walk

8.   when you sleep

9.   when you eat well

10.   when you have medicine

11.   when you exercise

REVIEW OF LESSONS 26-30

A. Escoja la pregunta para la respuesta dada.

1. In order to contract the uterus.

   a. What should I do?
   b. May I sit down?
   c. Why is it necessary?
   d. Where?

2. A spinal.

   a. What happened?
   b. What anesthesia are they going to give you?
   c. What did he suffer?
   d. Do you have the authorization?

3. No, I don't need to urinate.

   a. Do you want to go to the bathroom?
   b. Who is your doctor?
   c. Here? Thanks.
   d. Have you lost water?

4. The baby has to burp.

   a. And before delivery?
   b. And before nursing him?
   c. And after giving him milk?
   d. And after the umbilical cord falls off?

5. ___ es un método anticonceptivo no muy eficaz.

    a. La retirada   b. La ducha vaginal
    c. Esterilización   d. Espermicidas vaginales

C. Answer each group of sentences according to the examples.

    Example: ¿Qué dice el médico? ¿Debo descansar?
              Dice que debe descansar.

    1.   ¿Puedo descansar?

    2.   ¿Hay que descansar?

    3.   ¿Es necesario descansar?

    4.   ¿Necesito descansar?

    5.   ¿Voy a descansar?

    6.   ¿Tengo que descansar?

    Example: Dice que al descansar, se cura.
              ¿Al descansar?

    7.   al caminar

    8.   al dormir

    9.   al comer bien

   10.   al tomar medicinas

   11.   al hacer ejercicio

REPASO DE LAS LECCIONES 26-30

A. Choose the question for the answer given.

    1. Para contraer el útero.

        a. ¿Qué debo hacer?
        b. ¿Puedo sentarme?
        c. ¿Para qué es necesario?
        d. ¿Dónde?

    2. Raquídea.

        a. ¿Qué pasó?
        b. ¿Qué anestesia le van a dar?
        c. ¿Qué sufrió?
        d. ¿Tiene la autorización?

    3. No, no necesito orinar.

        a. ¿Quiere ir al baño?
        b. ¿Quién es su médico?
        c. ¿Aquí? Gracias.
        d. ¿Ha perdido agua?

    4. El niño tiene que eructar.

        a. ¿Y antes del parto?
        b. ¿Y antes de darle el pecho?
        c. ¿Y después de darle leche?
        d. ¿Y después de caérsele el ombligo?

5. With your elbow.

   a. Dry him well?
   b. Bathe him?
   c. How do I test the water?
   d. When can I put him into water?

6. Every fifteen minutes.

   a. How often?
   b. What kind of anesthesia do you want?
   c. Am I going to have a difficult delivery?
   d. Very strong?

7. You should decide it with your husband.

   a. What do contraceptives do?
   b. What effect can it have on the woman?
   c. Are they effective?
   d. What method is best for me?

8. We're going to put in a catheter.

   a. And if I can't eat?
   b. And if I am nauseated?
   c. And if my bag of waters breaks?
   d. And if I can't urinate?

9. 8 pounds and 3 ounces.

   a. When is he coming?
   b. Why are you worried?
   c. How much does he weigh?
   d. Are you hungry?

10. The permit is on the table.

   a. Where is the authorization?
   b. How many children do you have?
   c. Who is your husband?
   d. When are you going to sign the permit?

B. Tache la palabra que no se pueda usar para completar la oración.

1. We're going to do ___.

   a. a rectal exam
   b. a physical exam
   c. a blood count
   d. the blood pressure

2. It's necessary to ___ to the baby.

   a. give water
   b. breastfeed
   c. nurse
   d. give a shower

3. Take off ___, please.

   a. your scar
   b. your wig
   c. your rings
   d. (out) your dentures

5. Con el codo.

   a. ¿Secarlo bien?
   b. ¿Bañarlo?
   c. ¿Cómo hay que probar el agua?
   d. ¿Cuándo puede sumergirlo en agua?

6. Cada quince minutos.

   a. ¿Con qué frecuencia?
   b. ¿Qué clase de anestesia quiere?
   c. ¿Voy a tener un parto difícil?
   d. ¿Muy fuertes?

7. Debe decidirlo con su esposo.

   a. ¿Qué hacen los anticonceptivos?
   b. ¿Qué efecto puede tener en la mujer?
   c. ¿Son eficaces?
   d. ¿Qué método es mejor para mí?

8. Vamos a ponerle una sonda.

   a. ¿Y si no puedo comer?
   b. ¿Y si tengo náuseas?
   c. ¿Y si se me rompe la fuente?
   d. ¿Y si no puedo orinar?

9. Ocho libras y tres onzas.

   a. ¿Cuándo viene?
   b. ¿Por qué se preocupa?
   c. ¿Cuánto pesa?
   d. ¿Tiene hambre?

10. El permiso está en la mesa.

    a. ¿Dónde está la autorización?
    b. ¿Cuántos hijos tiene?
    c. ¿Quién es su esposo?
    d. ¿Cuándo va a firmar el permiso?

B. Cross out the word that does not fit in the blank in each statement.

   1. Vamos a hacerle ___.

      a. un tacto rectal
      b. un reconocimiento
      c. un recuento
      d. la presión

   2. Es necesario dar ___ al bebé.

      a. agua
      b. el pecho
      c. de mamar
      d. un baño de regadera

   3. Quítese ___, por favor.

      a. la cicatriz
      b. la peluca
      c. los anillos
      d. los dientes postizos

4. We're going to give you ___.

   a. an analgesic
   b. general anesthesia
   c. gas
   d. high blood pressure

5. We must put a lamp ___.

   a. on the stitches
   b. on the incision
   c. on the stitches
   d. on the bottle

6. You should sterilize ___ in hot water.

   a. nipples (baby bottle)
   b. nipples (baby bottle)
   c. nipples (mother)
   d. baby bottles

7. A contraceptive that a man can use is ___.

   a. the diaphragm
   b. the condom
   c. the rubber
   d. the prophylactic

8. The baby's going to be born soon. We're going to take you ___.

   a. to the pre-delivery room
   b. to the labor room
   c. to dismiss you
   d. to the delivery room

9. It's necessary to ___ the baby bottles.

   a. rinse
   b. sterilize
   c. hang
   d. wash

10. You have to use ___ for the formula.

   a. bottles
   b. a measuring cup
   c. a diaper
   d. baby bottles

4. Vamos a darle ___.

   a. un analgésico
   b. anestesia general
   c. gas
   d. alta presión

5. Hay que ponerle una lámpara ___.

   a. en los puntos
   b. en la herida
   c. en las puntadas
   d. en la botella

6. Debe esterilizar ___ en agua caliente.

   a. las teteras
   b. los tetos
   c. los pezones
   d. los biberones

7. Un anticonceptivo que puede usar el hombre es ___.

   a. el diafragma
   b. el condón
   c. la goma
   d. el profiláctico

8. Ya el niño va a nacer. Vamos a llevarla ___.

   a. a la sala prenatal
   b. a la sala de labor
   c. a darle de alta
   d. a la sala de partos

9. Es necesario ___ los biberones.

   a. enjuagar
   b. esterilizar
   c. colgar
   d. lavar

10. Usted tiene que usar ___ para la fórmula.

    a. botellas
    b. una taza de medir
    c. un pañal
    d. biberones

LESSON 31

A. Escriba la letra del grupo a que pertenece cada palabra.

1. tracheotomy	____	a. a kind of operation
2. operation	____	b. a procedure
3. ovary	____	c. a gland
4. prostate	____	d. an organ
5. analysis	____	
6. appendectomy	____	
7. mastectomy	____	
8. kidney	____	
9. uterus	____	
10. cauterization	____	
11. pancreas	____	

B. Complete cada oración con la palabra apropiada.

1. An operation on the uterus is called _____.

2. The gallbladder is part of the _____.

3. We're going to take out your appendix if you have _____.

4. To close the incision it is necessary to take 12 _____.

5. When a surgeon operates for cataracts, it is an operation on the

_____.

C. Conteste cada pregunta según el ejemplo. Emplee _it_ y _them_ en sus respuestas.
Ejemplo: Have you taken the medicine? Yes, I've taken _it_ (f.).

1. Have you taken the pill?

2. Have you taken the liquid?

3. Have you taken the tablets?

4. Have you taken the pills?

5. Have you taken the laxative?

6. Have you taken the lozenge?

7. Have you taken the liquids?

8. Have you taken the medicines?

LESSON 32

A. Si la oración es verdad escriba _true_, si no, escriba _false_.

1. If your temperature is 98.6, you have normal temperature.

2. A sty is a foreign body in the ear.

3. Worms are internal parasites.

4. Merthiolate is used for coughing.

LECCION 31

A. Write the letter of the group to which each word belongs.

1. traqueotomía _____   a. una clase de operación
2. operación _____   b. un procedimiento
3. ovario _____   c. una glándula
4. próstata _____   d. un órgano
5. análisis
6. apendectomía _____
7. mastectomía
8. riñón _____
9. útero _____
10. cauterización _____
11. páncreas _____

B. Complete each statement with the correct word.

1. La operación del útero se llama _____.
2. La vesícula es una parte del _____.
3. Le vamos a sacar el apéndice si usted tiene _____.
4. Para cerrar la incisión es necesario darle doce _____.
5. Cuando el cirujano opera las cataratas, es una operación en los
   _____.

C. Answer each question according to the example. Use lo, la, los, las as needed.
   Example: ¿Ha tomado la medicina? Sí, la he tomado.

1. ¿Ha tomado la píldora?
2. ¿Ha tomado el líquido?
3. ¿Ha tomado las tabletas?
4. ¿Ha tomado las píldoras?
5. ¿Ha tomado el laxante?
6. ¿Ha tomado la pastilla?
7. ¿Ha tomado los líquidos?
8. ¿Ha tomado las medicinas?

LECCION 32

A. Mark each statement sí or no.

1. Si su temperatura es noventa y ocho seis, Ud. tiene temperatura normal.
2. Un orzuelo es un cuerpo extraño en el oído.
3. Las lombrices son parásitos intestinales.
4. El mertiolato se usa para la tos.

5. If you have heatstroke, you are sunburned.

6. Crab lice are parasites in the pubic hair.

7. If a person has lice, he should take bicarbonate.

8. You can buy a flea at the drugstore.

9. You don't need a prescription to buy bandages and iodine.

10. In the supermarket, there are Band-aids, aspirin, and ticks.

B. Relacione las palabras que representen ideas opuestas.

1. heatstroke	___	a.	microbe
2. diarrhea	___	b.	cotton
3. astringent	___	c.	antidote
4. poison	___	d.	constipation
5. antibody	___	e.	laxative
		f.	frostbite

C. Conteste las preguntas según el ejemplo. Emplee _it_ y _them_ en sus respuestas.
Ejemplo: Can I eat bread? No, you can't eat _it_ (m.).

1. Can I eat fried chicken?

2. Can I eat butter?

3. Can I eat beans?

4. Can I eat potatoes?

5. Can I eat carrots?

6. Can I eat ice cream?

7. Can I eat shrimp?

8. Can I eat tomatoes?

9. Can I eat corn?

10. Can I eat lettuce?

LESSON 33

A. Escoja una palabra de significado semejante a la palabra subrayada.

1. The girl has <u>convulsions</u>.	a.	light
2. You need rest; you're <u>fatigued</u>.	b.	grave
3. We've got to ask for <u>help</u>.	c.	fits
4. He has a <u>serious</u> illness.	d.	tired
5. The injury is <u>minor</u>.	e.	assistance
6. The baby has a <u>rash</u> on his back.	f.	eruption
7. He has a <u>cut</u> on his arm.	g.	broken
8. He's <u>fractured</u> a bone.	h.	injury

5. Si Ud. tiene insolación, está quemado del sol.

6. Las ladillas son parásitos en el pelo de la región púbica.

7. Si una persona tiene piojos, debe tomar bicarbonato.

8. Ud. puede comprar una pulga en la farmacia.

9. Ud. no necesita receta para comprar vendas y yodo.

10. En el supermercado hay curitas, aspirinas y garrapatas.

B. Choose the opposite of each word.

1. insolación	___	a. microbio
2. diarrea	___	b. algodón
3. astringente	___	c. antídoto
4. veneno	___	d. constipación
5. anticuerpo	___	e. laxante
		f. congelado

C. Answer each question according to the example. Use <u>lo</u>, <u>la</u>, <u>los</u>, <u>las</u> as needed.

Example: ¿Puedo comer pan? No, Ud. no puede comer<u>lo</u>.

1. ¿Puedo comer pollo frito?

2. ¿Puedo comer mantequilla?

3. ¿Puedo comer frijoles?

4. ¿Puedo comer papas?

5. ¿Puedo comer zanahorias?

6. ¿Puedo comer helado?

7. ¿Puedo comer camarones?

8. ¿Puedo comer tomates?

9. ¿Puedo comer maíz tierno?

10. ¿Puedo comer lechuga?

LECCION 33

A. Choose the word most similar in meaning to the one underlined.

1. La muchacha tiene <u>convulsiones</u>.	a. leve
2. **Necesita descanso; tiene <u>fatiga</u>.**	b. grave
3. Hay que pedir <u>ayuda</u>.	c. ataques
4. Tiene una enfermedad <u>seria</u>.	d. cansancio
5. La lesión es <u>menor</u>.	e. socorro
6. El bebé tiene <u>salpullido</u> en la espalda.	f. erupción
7. Tiene una <u>cortada</u> en el brazo.	g. quebrado
8. Se ha <u>fracturado</u> un hueso.	h. herida

B. Llene el espacio en blanco con la palabra correspondiente, según el ejemplo.

Ejemplo: I'm going to give you the tourniquet. I'm going to give it to you.

1. I'm going to give you the label.   I'm going to give _____ to you.

2. I'm going to give you the treatments. I'm going to give _____ to you.

3. I'm going to give you the medicine.   I'm going to give _____ to you.

4. I'm going to give you the antidote.   I'm going to give _____ to you.

5. You're going to give me the pills.   You're going to give _____ to me.

6. You're going to give me the
    bandage.   You're going to give _____ to me.

7. You're going to give me the
    small bottles.   You're going to give _____ to me.

8. You're going to give me the bottle.   You're going to give _____ to me.

9. You're going to give me the alcohol. You're going to give _____ to me.

C. Conteste las preguntas según el ejemplo. Emplee it y them en su respuesta.

Ejemplo: Have you taken the medicine? No, I haven't taken it.

1. Have you taken the pill?

2. Have you taken the aspirins?

3. Have you taken the laxative?

4. Have you taken the liquids?

5. Have you taken the liquid?

6. Have you taken the tablets?

LESSON 34

A. Tache la palabra que no se pueda usar en cada oración.

1. He has a ___ fracture.

    a. multiple   b. hot
    c. complete   d. compound

2. We must take him to the ___ room.

    a. emergency   b. emergency
    c. intensive care   d. ambulance

3. He has a bean in ___.

    a. his nose   b. his throat
    c. his face   d. his ear

4. We must give him the antidote because he took ___.

    a. a reaction   b. lye
    c. poison   d. carbon tetrachloride

5. The child swallowed ___.

    a. a pin   b. an accident
    c. a coin   d. a marble

B. Fill the blank with the correct word, according to the example.

Example: Le voy a dar el torniquete. Se lo voy a dar.

1. Le voy a dar la etiqueta.   Se _____ voy a dar.

2. Le voy a dar los tratamientos.   Se _____ voy a dar.

3. Le voy a dar la medicina.   Se _____ voy a dar.

4. Le voy a dar el antídoto.   Se _____ voy a dar.

5. Me va a dar las píldoras.   Me _____ va a dar.

6. Me va a dar la venda.   Me _____ va a dar.

7. Me va a dar los frascos.   Me _____ va a dar.

8. Me va a dar la botella.   Me _____ va a dar.

9. Me va a dar el alcohol.   Me _____ va a dar.

C. Answer the questions according to the example. Use lo, la, los, las as needed.

Example: ¿Ha tomado la medicina? No, no la he tomado.

1. ¿Ha tomado la píldora?

2. ¿Ha tomado las aspirinas?

3. ¿Ha tomado el laxante?

4. ¿Ha tomado los líquidos?

5. ¿Ha tomado el líquido?

6. ¿Ha tomado las tabletas?

LECCION 34

A. Cross out the word that cannot be used to complete each sentence.

1. Tiene una fractura ___.

   a. múltiple   b. caliente
   c. completa   d. compuesta

2. Hay que llevarlo a la sala de ___.

   a. urgencia   b. emergencia
   c. cuidado intenso   d. ambulancia

3. Tiene un frijol en ___.

   a. la nariz   b. la garganta
   c. la cara   d. el oído

4. Hay que darle el antídoto porque tomó ___.

   a. una reacción   b. lejía
   c. veneno   d. tetracloruro de carbón

5. El niño tragó ___.

   a. un alfiler   b. un accidente
   c. una moneda   d. un mármol

B. Si la información es verdad, escriba <u>true</u>. Escriba <u>false</u> si no es verdad.

1. A person who is unconscious has lost his senses.

2. Turpentine is a cough medicine.

3. Lye, bleach, and ice cream are poisonous.

4. Reaction against a substance can be fatal.

5. If you are in an accident, you are dehydrated.

C. Conteste la pregunta según el ejemplo. Emplee <u>it</u> y <u>them</u> en su respuesta.

Ejemplo: How long has he had worms? <u>He's had</u> them <u>for</u> two weeks.

1. How long has he had a tick?

2. How long has he had lice?

3. How long has he had fleas?

4. How long has he had an eruption?

5. How long has he had pain?

6. How long has he had a headache?

7. How long has he had nausea?

8. How long has he had that scar?

REVIEW OF LESSONS 31-35

A. Escoja la expresión de significado semejante a la que se subraya.

1. <u>He's pale.</u>

    a. He has bad color.   b. He has a rapid pulse.
    c. We must take his blood   d. He has a graft on the aorta.
       pressure.

2. He has <u>high blood pressure</u>.

    a. varicose veins   b. rhythmic pulse
    c. hypotension   d. hypertension

3. He has <u>rapid heartbeat</u>.

    a. arteriosclerosis   b. an embolus
    c. tachycardia   d. an infarct

4. She has <u>varicose veins</u>.

    a. coronary   b. varices
    c. hypotension   d. various

5. The girl has <u>sunstroke</u>.

    a. indisposition   b. scab
    c. heatstroke   d. nosebleed

6. He has to take medicine for <u>worms</u>.

    a. parasites   b. salve
    c. bites   d. blisters

B. If the information is true, write <u>sí</u>; write <u>no</u> if it is false.

1. Una persona que está inconsciente ha perdido el sentido.

2. La trementina es una medicina para la tos.

3. La lejía, el cloro y el helado son venenosos.

4. La reacción contra una substancia puede ser fatal.

5. **Si Ud. está en un accidente está deshidratado.**

C. Answer each question according to the example. Use <u>lo</u>, <u>la</u>, <u>los</u>, <u>las</u> in your answer.

Example: ¿Desde cuándo tiene lombrices? <u>Hace</u> dos semanas <u>que</u> las <u>tiene</u>.

1. ¿Desde cuándo tiene una garrapata?

2. ¿Desde cuándo tiene piojos?

3. **¿Desde cuándo tiene pulgas?**

4. ¿Desde cuándo tiene erupción?

5. ¿Desde cuándo tiene dolor?

6. **¿Desde cuándo tiene jaqueca?**

7. ¿Desde cuándo tiene náuseas?

8. ¿Desde cuándo tiene esa cicatriz?

REPASO DE LAS LECCIONES 31-35

A. Choose the expression that has a similar meaning to the one underlined in each statement.

1. <u>Está pálido.</u>

    a. Tiene mal color.   b. Tiene el pulso rápido.
    c. Hay que tomarle la presión.   d. Tiene un injerto en la aorta.

2. Tiene <u>la presión alta.</u>

    a. várices   b. el pulso rítmico
    c. hipotensión   d. hipertensión

3. Tiene <u>palpitación rápida.</u>

    a. arterioesclerosis   b. embolia
    c. taquicardia   d. infarto

4. Tiene <u>venas varicosas.</u>

    a. coronaria   b. várices
    c. hipotensión   d. varias

5. La muchacha tiene una <u>insolación.</u>

    a. destemplanza   b. postilla
    c. postración del calor   d. hemorragia nasal

6. Tiene que **tomar** la medicina para <u>las lombrices.</u>

    a. los parásitos   b. la pomada
    c. las picaduras   d. las ampollas

7. You must avoid excessive <u>tiredness</u>.

    a. attacks   b. acidosis
    c. tourniquet   d. fatigue

8. He has to <u>blow</u> his nose.

    a. blow   b. take
    c. sit down   d. bend

B. Complete cada oración con la mejor respuesta.

1. You have to sign the permit ___.

    a. to disinfect me   b. to shave me
    c. nothing   d. to operate

2. We're going to give you ___.

    a. an injection   b. a poison
    c. allergy   d. high blood pressure

3. You need to fasten your ___ with adhesive tape.

    a. teeth   b. rings
    c. wig   d. oxygen

4. They're going to do a trepanation ___.

    a. of the ovaries   b. of the appendix
    c. of the skull   d. of the uterus

5. They're going to take out ___.

    a. my brain   b. a fibroma
    c. a foot   d. my throat

6. You should read ___.

    a. the scab   b. the pharmacy
    c. the label   d. the drops

7. Poor thing! He can't walk. He has ___ nail.

    a. an infected   b. a straw
    c. on his toe   d. a sty

C. Conteste la pregunta según el ejemplo.

Ejemplo: Do you <u>work</u> much? No, doctor, I don't <u>work</u> a lot.

1. Do you walk much?

2. Do you drink much coffee?

3. Do you smoke much?

4. Do you drive much?

5. Do you need much rest?

7. Hay que evitar el exceso de <u>cansancio</u>.

    a. ataques   b. acidosis
    c. torniquete   d. fatiga

8. Tiene que <u>soplarse</u> la nariz.

    a. sonarse   b. tomarse
    c. sentarse   d. doblarse

B. Complete each statement with the best choice.

1. Tiene que firmar el permiso para ___.

    a. desinfectarme   b. afeitarme
    c. nada   d. operar

2. Vamos a ponerle ___.

    a. una inyección   b. un veneno
    c. alergia   d. alta presión

3. Hay que asegurar ___ con tela adhesiva.

    a. los dientes   b. los anillos
    c. la peluca   d. el oxígeno

4. Le van a hacer una trepanación ___.

    a. de los ovarios   b. del apéndice
    c. del cráneo   d. del útero

5. Me van a sacar ___.

    a. el cerebro   b. un fibroma
    c. un pie   d. la garganta

6. Ud. debe leer ___.

    a. la postilla   b. la farmacia
    c. la etiqueta   d. las gotas

7. ¡Pobrecito! No puede andar. Tiene una uña ___.

    a. infectada   b. paja
    c. en el dedo   d. orzuelo

C. Answer each question according to the example.

Example: ¿<u>Trabaja</u> Ud. mucho? No, doctor, no <u>trabajo</u> mucho.

1. ¿Camina Ud. mucho?

2. ¿Toma Ud. mucho café?

3. ¿Fuma Ud. mucho?

4. ¿Maneja Ud. mucho?

5. ¿Necesita Ud. mucho descanso?

LESSON 36

A. Si la información es verdad, escriba _true_. Escriba _false_ si no es verdad.

1. Cancer is a catastrophic disease.

2. Gangrene is very contagious.

3. Leukemia is a disease of the digestive system.

4. Hemophilia is a hereditary disease.

5. Poor nutrition can cause anemia.

6. Diabetes is an endocrine disease.

7. Congenital means hereditary.

8. A person who is blind doesn't hear well.

B. Complete la oración con la clasificación que mejor corresponda a cada enfermedad.

1. Mongolism is ___.   a. a contagious disease

2. Epilepsy is ___.   b. a degenerative disease

3. Arthritis is ___.   c. a hereditary defect

4. Arteriosclerosis is ___.   d. an endocrine disease

5. Diabetes is ___.   e. a nervous illness

6. Tuberculosis is ___.

7. Hemophilia is ___.

C. Conteste cada pregunta según los ejemplos. Emplee _it_ y _them_ en su respuesta.

Ejemplos: Do you want potatoes? Yes, I want them (f.).
          Do you want to eat potatoes? Yes, I want to eat them (f.).

1. Do you want beans?

2. Do you want to eat beans?

3. Do you want ham?

4. Do you want to eat ice cream?

5. Do you want to eat bread?

6. Do you want fruit?

7. Do you want dessert?

8. Do you want to eat peas?

9. Do you want to eat fruit?

LECCION 36

A. If the information is true, write sí; write no if it is false.

1. El cáncer es una enfermedad catastrófica.

2. La gangrena es muy contagiosa.

3. La leucemia es una enfermedad del aparato digestivo.

4. La hemofilia es una enfermedad hereditaria.

5. La mala nutrición puede causar anemia.

6. La diabetes es una enfermedad endocrina.

7. Congénita quiere decir hereditaria.

8. El que está ciego no oye bien.

B. Complete each sentence with the classification that best corresponds to each illness.

1. El mongolismo es ___.   a. una enfermedad contagiosa

2. La epilepsia es ___.   b. una enfermedad degenerativa

3. La artritis es ___.   c. un defecto hereditario

4. La arterioesclerosis es ___.   d. una enfermedad endocrina

5. La diabetes es ___.   e. una enfermedad nerviosa

6. La tuberculosis es ___.

7. La hemofilia es ___.

C. Answer each question according to the examples. Use lo, la, los, las in your answer.

Examples: ¿Quiere papas? Sí, las quiero.
           ¿Quiere comer papas? Sí, las quiero comer.

1. ¿Quiere frijoles?

2. ¿Quiere comer frijoles?

3. ¿Quiere jamón?

4. ¿Quiere comer helado?

5. ¿Quiere comer pan?

6. ¿Quiere fruta?

7. ¿Quiere postre?

8. ¿Quiere comer chícharos?

9. ¿Quiere comer frutas?

LESSON 37

A. Dé la categoría a que pertenece cada palabra o expresión.

1. Aureomycin   ___   a. symptom of a venereal disease
2. discharge of pus   ___   b. antibiotic
3. gonorrhea   ___   c. venereal disease
4. sulfa   ___
5. chancre on the genitals   ___
6. streptomycin   ___
7. syphilis   ___
8. mental deterioration   ___
9. a sore that does not heal   ___
10. penicillin   ___

B. Si la información es verdad, escriba _true_. Escriba _false_ si no es verdad.

1. Inflammation of the glands of the groin can be a symptom of venereal disease.
2. One should avoid sexual relations in order not to have venereal disease.
3. If syphilis is not treated, it can produce insanity.
4. Gonorrhea is more obvious in women than in men.
5. After a while, symptoms of syphilis disappear without the patient's having treatment.
6. Venereal diseases are usually acquired by direct contact with a person who has the disease.
7. If you have gonorrhea, you don't need to go to the doctor.

C. Conteste cada pregunta según el ejemplo. Emplee _it_ y _them_ en la respuesta.

Ejemplo: Are they going to take out _my appendix_? Yes, they're going to take _it_ out.

1. Are they going to operate on _a finger_?
2. Are they going to operate on _two cysts_?
3. Are they going to take out _a fibroma_?
4. Are they going to operate on _my leg_?
5. Are they going to operate on _my tonsils_?
6. Are they going to operate on _a foot_?
7. Are they going to operate on _my throat_?

LECCION 37

A. Give the category to which each word or expression belongs.

    1. aureomicina   ___   a. síntoma de una enfermedad venérea
    2. flujo purulento   ___   b. antibiótico
    3. gonorrea   ___   c. enfermedad venérea
    4. sulfa   ___
    5. chancro en los genitales ___
    6. estreptomicina   ___
    7. sífilis   ___
    8. deterioración mental   ___
    9. un grano que no se cura ___
    10. penicilina   ___

B. If the information is true, write <u>sí</u>; write <u>no</u> if it is false.

    1. La inflamación de las glándulas de la ingle puede ser un síntoma de una enfermedad venérea.
    2. Hay que evitar las relaciones sexuales para no tener enfermedades venéreas.
    3. La sífilis que no se trata puede producir locura.
    4. La gonorrea es más evidente en la mujer que en el hombre.
    5. Después de cierto tiempo, los síntomas de la sífilis desaparecen sin que el paciente tome tratamiento.
    6. Las enfermedades venéreas se adquieren generalmente por contagio directo con una persona enferma.
    7. Si Ud. tiene gonorrea no necesita ir al médico.

C. Answer each question according to the example. Use <u>lo</u>, <u>la</u>, <u>los</u>, <u>las</u> in your answer.

    Example: ¿Me van a sacar <u>el apéndice</u>? Sí, se <u>lo</u> van a sacar.

    1. ¿Me van a operar <u>un dedo</u>?
    2. ¿Me van a operar <u>dos quistes</u>?
    3. ¿Me van a sacar <u>un fibroma</u>?
    4. ¿Me van a operar <u>la pierna</u>?
    5. ¿Me van a operar <u>las amígdalas</u>?
    6. ¿Me van a operar <u>un pie</u>?
    7. ¿Me van a operar <u>la garganta</u>?

LESSON 38

A. Tache la palabra que no complete cada frase.

1. He took an overdose of ___.

   a. barbiturates   b. cocaine
   c. morphine   d. alienation

2. What symptoms does he have? ___.

   a. Hallucinations   b. Heroin
   c. Dryness in the mouth   d. Vomiting

3. What does he use? ___.

   a. Needle marks   b. He inhales glue
   c. He smokes marijuana   d. Cocaine

4. ___ is a hallucinatory drug.

   a. LSD   b. Mescaline
   c. Penicillin   d. Marijuana

5. What happened to the young man? ___.

   a. He's very happy   b. He speaks incoherently
   c. He's lethargic   d. He has suicidal tendencies

6. What do I have to do? ___.

   a. You have to watch him   b. You have to stop using drugs
   c. You have to go shopping   d. You have to take methadone

B. Conteste la pregunta según el ejemplo.

Ejemplo: What do you take? I don't take anything.

1. What do you use?

2. What do you buy?

3. What do you eat?

4. What do you have?

5. What do you want?

6. What do you need?

C. Conteste la pregunta según el ejemplo.

Ejemplo: Does the patient want to rest? No, the patient doesn't want to rest.

1. Can the lady rest?

2. Can the patient walk?

3. Does your friend have children?

4. Does the nurse have a family?

5. Can the young lady speak Spanish?

LECCION 38

A. Cross out the word that does <u>not</u> complete each sentence.

1. Tomó una dosis excesiva de ___.

   a. barbiturato
   c. morfina

   b. cocaína
   d. alienación

2. ¿Qué síntomas tiene? ___.

   a. Alucinaciones
   c. Sequedad en la boca

   b. Heroína
   d. Vómitos

3. ¿Qué usa? ___.

   a. Marcas de aguja
   c. Fuma marihuana

   b. Inhala goma
   d. Cocaína

4. La ___ es una droga alucinatoria.

   a. LSD
   c. penicilina

   b. mescalina
   d. marihuana

5. ¿Qué le pasó al joven? ___.

   a. Está muy contento
   c. Está aletargado

   b. Habla incoherentemente
   d. Tiene tendencias suicidas

6. ¿Qué tengo que hacer? ___.

   a. Tiene que vigilarlo
   c. Tiene que ir de compras

   b. Tiene que dejar de usar drogas
   d. Tiene que tomar metadona

B. Answer each question according to the example.

Example: ¿Qué <u>toma</u> Ud.? No <u>tomo</u> nada.

1. ¿Qué usa Ud.?

2. ¿Qué compra Ud.?

3. ¿Qué come Ud.?

4. ¿Qué tiene Ud.?

5. ¿Qué quiere Ud.?

6. ¿Qué necesita Ud.?

C. Answer each question according to the example.

Example: ¿Quiere descansar el paciente? No, el paciente no quiere descansar.

1. ¿Puede descansar la señora?

2. ¿Puede andar el paciente?

3. ¿Tiene hijos su amigo?

4. ¿Tiene familia la enfermera?

5. ¿Puede hablar español la señorita?

LESSON 39

A. Escoja la palabra de sentido opuesto a la subrayada.

1. Please <u>raise</u> your head.   a. close
2. Please <u>open</u> your mouth.   b. inflamed
3. Please brush your teeth <u>before</u> eating.   c. lower
4. You have <u>good</u> teeth.   d. cold
5. John has <u>healthy</u> gums.   e. left
6. I don't have pain on the <u>right</u> side.   f. bad
7. Do <u>hot</u> things on your teeth bother you?   g. after

B. Complete cada oración con la palabra que respresenta la especialidad, la profesión o el lugar de empleo. (Vea las listas en las páginas 529 y 531.)

1. The pharmacist works in the _____.
2. The surgeon practices _____.
3. A radiologist is an expert in _____.
4. The specialty of the cardiologist is _____.
5. A psychologist is an expert in _____.
6. The specialty of the gynecologist is _____.
7. The anesthesiologist is the doctor who gives _____ to the patient.

C. Escoja la mejor respuesta a la pregunta.

1. What was it?   a. It was my brother-in-law.
2. What did your father take?   b. He had measles.
3. What did the boy swallow?   c. She tried to commit suicide.
4. Who was it?   d. He swallowed a pin.
5. What happened to you?   e. He took medicine.
6. What was the matter with your son?   f. It was a disaster.
7. What did she try to do?   g. Me? An accident?

LESSON 40

A. Escoja la mejor respuesta para completar la pregunta u oración.

1. Listen, darling, give me a ___.

   a. pretty   b. hug
   c. eye   d. quietly

2. Come here, honey, be ___ and open your mouth.

   a. that   b. "ah"
   c. cute   d. good

LECCIÓN 39

A. Choose the word opposite in meaning from the one underlined in each sentence.

1. Favor de <u>levantar</u> la cabeza.   a. cerrar

2. Favor de <u>abrir</u> la boca.   b. inflamadas

3. Favor de cepillarse los dientes <u>antes</u> de comer. c. bajar

4. Ud. tiene una dentadura <u>buena</u>.   d. frío

5. Juan tiene las encías <u>sanas</u>.   e. izquierdo

6. No tengo dolor en el lado <u>derecho</u>.   f. mala

7. ¿Le molesta lo <u>caliente</u> en la boca?   g. después

B. Complete each statement with the word that gives the appropriate specialty, profession, or place of work. (See the cognate lists on pp. 529 and 531.)

1. El farmacéutico trabaja en la _____.

2. El cirujano practica la _____.

3. Un radiólogo es un experto en _____.

4. La especialidad del cardiólogo es la _____.

5. Un psicólogo es un experto en _____.

6. La especialidad del ginecólogo es _____.

7. El anestesiólogo es el médico que da la _____ al paciente.

C. Choose the best answer for each question.

1. ¿Qué fue?   a. Fue mi cuñado.

2. ¿Qué tomó su padre?   b. Tuvo sarampión.

3. ¿Qué tragó el niño?   c. Trató de suicidarse.

4. ¿Quién fue?   d. Tragó un alfiler.

5. ¿Qué tuvo Ud.?   e. Tomó medicina.

6. ¿Qué tuvo su hijo?   f. Fue un desastre.

7. ¿Qué trató de hacer?   g. ¿Yo? Un accidente.

LECCIÓN 40

A. Choose the best answer to complete each statement or question.

1. Oye, precioso, hazme un ___.

    a. bonito   b. cariñito
    c. ojito   d. tranquilito

2. Ven, nené, sé ___ y abre la boquita.

    a. que   b. "ah"
    c. mono   d. bueno

3. Do you want your ___ now?

    a. while   b. play
    c. toys   d. will

4. Did you take your medicine? No, I ___.

    a. forgot   b. of course
    c. urinated   d. something

5. Do you want to rest a ___?

    a. with me   b. little while
    c. fear   d. now

6. Let me fasten your ___.

    a. bed   b. nurse
    c. book   d. shirt

B. Escoja la expresión de significado semejante a la que se subraya.

1. Come, dear one, close your eyes.   a. get up
2. Son, stand up, please.   b. little while
3. I don't feel like it, mommy.   c. brave
4. Wait just a minute.   d. be quiet
5. Where do you have pain?   e. go to sleep
6. Don't cry; you should be strong.   f. want to
7. Be nice and don't talk, darling.   g. does it hurt

C. Conteste cada pregunta en el tiempo usado en la pregunta.

1. Do you have sinusitis? No, I don't _____.
2. Have you had sinusitis? No, I _____.
3. Did your father have an accident? No, my father _____.
4. Was Mary a nurse here? Yes, she _____.
5. Have you had seizures? No, I _____.
6. Did the boy take drugs? No, he _____.
7. Do you have heart trouble? Yes, I _____.

FINAL EVALUATION OF LESSONS 1-41

A. Useful phrases, oral part. Escoja la mejor respuesta a la pregunta o expresión.

1. Good morning.

    a. Good morning.   b. And you?
    c. See you later.   d. Good afternoon.

2. How do you feel today?

    a. Hi!   b. So-so.
    c. It's nothing.   d. How's it going?

3. ¿Quieres tus ___ ahora?

   a. raticos   b. jugar
   c. juguetes   d. ganas

4. ¿Tomaste la medicina? No, se me ___.

   a. olvidó   b. cómo no
   c. orinó   d. algo

5. ¿Quieres descansar un ___?

   a. conmigo   b. ratico
   c. miedo   d. ahora

6. Déjame abrocharte la ___.

   a. cama   b. enfermera
   c. librito   d. camisa

B. Choose the expression most similar in meaning to the one underlined.

1. Vamos, chiquitín, <u>cierra los ojitos</u>.   a. párate

2. Mi hijito, <u>levántate</u>, por favor.   b. ratito

3. No <u>tengo ganas</u>, mamá.   c. valiente

4. Espérate un <u>momentico</u>.   d. cállate

5. ¿Dónde <u>tienes el dolor</u>?   e. duérmete

6. No llores, debes ser <u>fuerte</u>.   f. quiero

7. Sé bueno y <u>no hables</u>, nené.   g. te duele

C. Answer each question in the tense used in the question.

1. ¿Tiene sinusitis? No, yo no _____.

2. ¿Ha tenido sinusitis? Sí, yo _____.

3. ¿Tuvo un accidente su padre? No, mi padre no _____.

4. ¿Fue María enfermera aquí? Sí, ella _____.

5. ¿Ha sufrido ataques? No, yo no _____.

6. ¿Tomó drogas el muchacho? No, él no _____.

7. ¿Sufre Ud. del corazón? Sí, yo _____.

EVALUACION FINAL DE LAS LECCIONES 1-41

A. <u>Frases útiles, parte oral</u>. Choose the best answer or response to the question or statement.

1. Buenos días.

   a. Buenos días.   b. ¿Y Ud.?
   c. Hasta luego.   d. Buenas tardes.

2. ¿Cómo se siente hoy?

   a. ¡Hola!   b. Así así.
   c. No es nada.   d. ¿Cómo le va?

3. How goes it?

    a. What's the matter with you?   b. Come in.
    c. Please   d. Fine, thanks.

4. I'm sorry.

    a. It's nothing.   b. Come in.
    c. You're welcome.   d. Excuse me.

5. Thanks.

    a. Please.   b. My deepest sympathy.
    c. It's nothing.   d. Don't mention it.

6. Do you understand Spanish?

    a. Good luck.   b. Delicious.
    c. Yes, a little.   d. Gladly.

7. How do you say "enfermera"?

    a. It means nurse.   b. She's the nurse.
    c. You say nurse.   d. She's studying nursing.

8. The food is just great.

    a. Yes, it's delicious.   b. What a shame!
    c. Poor thing.   d. No, I don't have money.

9. Good luck.

    a. Do you understand Spanish?   b. Thanks, same to you.
    c. Gladly.   d. Yes, a little.

10. Where's the bathroom?

    a. He's not well.   b. What's the matter?
    c. It's here.   d. It's okay.

11. Do you need something?

    a. How goes it?   b. It's nothing.
    c. Nothing, thanks.   d. I don't know.

12. Take this off.

    a. The robe?   b. The bed?
    c. Slower.   d. The table?

13. Go to bed, please.

    a. Don't mention it.   b. The head.
    c. It doesn't cost anything.   d. Now, so early?

14. This thing isn't working.

    a. You're right, it isn't.   b. I don't know.
    c. It's here.   d. Do you want something?

15. I feel worse.

    a. I'm sorry.   b. Fantastic.
    c. Yes, she's the nurse.   d. It's not all right.

16. Put on your sweater.

    a. Yes, I'm afraid.   b. Yes, I'm hot.
    c. Yes, I'm cold.   d. Yes, I'm right.

3. ¿Qué tal?

    a. ¿Qué le pasa?   b. Pase.
    c. Por favor.   d. Bien, gracias.

4. Lo siento.

    a. No es nada.   b. Pase.
    c. De nada.   d. Con permiso.

5. Gracias.

    a. Por favor.   b. Mi sentido pésame.
    c. No es nada.   d. No hay de qué.

6. ¿Comprende Ud. español?

    a. Buena suerte.   b. Deliciosa.
    c. Sí, un poco.   d. Con mucho gusto.

7. ¿Cómo se dice "nurse"?

    a. Quiere decir enfermera.   b. Es la enfermera.
    c. Se dice enfermera.   d. Estudia enfermería.

8. La comida está muy rica.

    a. Sí, está deliciosa.   b. ¡Qué lástima!
    c. Pobrecito.   d. No, no tengo dinero.

9. Buena suerte.

    a. ¿Comprende español?   b. Gracias, igualmente.
    c. Con mucho gusto.   d. Sí, un poco.

10. ¿Dónde está el baño?

    a. No está bien.   b. ¿Qué pasa?
    c. Está aquí.   d. Está bien.

11. ¿Necesita algo?

    a. ¿Qué tal?   b. No es nada.
    c. Nada, gracias.   d. No sé.

12. Quítese esto.

    a. ¿La bata?   b. ¿La cama?
    c. Más despacio.   d. ¿La mesa?

13. Acuéstese, por favor.

    a. No hay de qué.   b. La cabeza.
    c. No cuesta nada.   d. ¿Ahora, tan temprano?

14. El aparato está malo.

    a. Sí, no está bien.   b. No sé.
    c. Está aquí.   d. ¿Desea algo?

15. Me siento peor.

    a. Lo siento.   b. Fantástico.
    c. Sí, es la enfermera.   d. No está bien.

16. Póngase el suéter.

    a. Sí, tengo miedo.   b. Sí, tengo calor.
    c. Sí, tengo frío.   d. Sí, tengo razón.

17. Please speak more slowly.

    a. Yes, gladly.   b. It's just delicious.
    c. I feel bad.   d. It means doctor.

18. Get up, please.

    a. Yes, I want to go to bed.   b. Sit down.
    c. Yes, I'm in traction.   d. Thanks. I want to walk.

19. Repeat, please.

    a. Don't you understand?   b. Poor thing.
    c. Stupendous.   d. Thanks a million.

20. Excuse me.

    a. Same to you.   b. So-so.
    c. Certainly.   d. My deepest sympathy.

B.   Completar. Escoja la respuesta que mejor complete cada pregunta u oración.

1. Do you have an infection in your ___?

    a. ear   b. pan
    c. bedpan   d. hair

2. I have my razor, but I don't have ___.

    a. scissors   b. the pitcher
    c. blades   d. brushes

3. The mother of your husband is your ___.

    a. sister-in-law   b. cousin
    c. niece   d. mother-in-law

4. How long have you had a cough? ___ some days.

    a. When   b. For
    c. How much   d. There are

5. There are ___ in a yard.

    a. 3 pounds   b. 36 inches
    c. 1/2 pound   d. 100 cc

6. I'm worried because ___.

    a. I don't have work   b. they're going to dismiss me
    c. it's okay   d. I don't have pain

7. Here's the pitcher and ice, but there isn't any ___.

    a. vase   b. pan
    c. glass   d. gauze

8. 200 and 300 are ___.

    a. 15   b. 500
    c. hot   d. who

9. Miss, please ___ the air conditioning. I'm cold.

    a. turn on   b. turn off
    c. close   d. open

17. Favor de hablar más despacio.

    a. Sí, con mucho gusto.   b. Está muy rica.
    c. Me siento mal.   d. Quiere decir médico.

18. Levántese, por favor.

    a. Sí, quiero acostarme.   b. Siéntese.
    c. Sí, estoy en tracción.   d. Gracias. Quiero caminar.

19. Repita, por favor.

    a. ¿No comprende?   b. Pobrecito.
    c. Estupendo.   d. Un millón de gracias.

20. Con permiso.

    a. Igualmente.   b. Así, así.
    c. Ud. lo tiene.   d. Mi sentido pésame.

B. Completion. Select the answer which best completes each statement or question.

1. ¿Tiene infección en el ___?

    a. oído   b. tazón
    c. bacín   d. pelo

2. Tengo la máquina de afeitar pero no tengo ___.

    a. tijeras   b. la jarra
    c. cuchillos   d. cepillos

3. La madre de su esposo es su ___.

    a. cuñada   b. prima
    c. sobrina   d. suegra

4. ¿Desde cuándo tiene Ud. tos? ___ unos días.

    a. Cuándo   b. Hace
    c. Cuánto   d. Hay

5. Hay ___ en una vara.

    a. tres libras   b. treinta y seis pulgadas
    c. medio libro   d. cien centímetros

6. Estoy preocupado porque ___.

    a. no tengo trabajo   b. me van a dar de alta
    c. está bien   d. no tengo dolor

7. Aquí está la jarra de agua con hielo pero no hay ___.

    a. florero   b. tazón
    c. vaso   d. gasa

8. Doscientos y trescientos son ___.

    a. quince   b. quinientos
    c. calientes   d. quienes

9. Señorita, favor de ___ el aireacondicionado. Tengo frío.

    a. poner   b. apagar
    c. cerrar   d. abrir

10. You have hospitalization ___.

    a. room   b. certain
    c. insurance   d. police

11. I have to change ___.

    a. the pound   b. the sheets
    c. the comb   d. the tonsils

12. I feel like laughing. I'm ___.

    a. sad   b. upset
    c. happy   d. tired

13. I'm nauseated. I need ___.

    a. the spitting pan   b. the bedpan
    c. the thermometer   d. the head

14. The son of your son is your ___.

    a. little son   b. son-in-law
    c. uncle   d. grandson

15. My ___ hurt.

    a. gargle   b. eyes
    c. hours   d. spoonfuls

16. When do I have to take ___?

    a. the ointment   b. the cough
    c. the liniment   d. the laxative

17. ___ treatments are necessary.

    a. Cobalt   b. Sponge
    c. Blood   d. Duty

18. I have itching on my skin. I have ___.

    a. yellow fever   b. flu
    c. poliomyelitis   d. hives

19. For going to the hospital you should take ___.

    a. the fountain   b. the contractions
    c. the navel   d. personal articles

20. You have pain and frequent ___.

    a. breasts   b. contractions
    c. strong   d. deep

21. You must put the bottles in a ___.

    a. sterilizer   b. baby bottle
    c. nipple   d. navel

22. Do you have ___ trouble?

    a. dentures   b. kidneys
    c. spinal anesthesia   d. scars

23. We're going to do an ___ operation.

    a. pharmacy   b. measles
    c. German measles   d. exploratory

10. Ud. tiene el ___ de hospitalización.

    a. cuarto   b. cierto
    c. seguro   d. policía

11. Tengo que cambiar ___.

    a. la libra   b. las sábanas
    c. el peine   d. las amígdalas

12. Tengo ganas de reír. Estoy ___.

    a. triste   b. mortificada
    c. contenta   d. cansada

13. Tengo naúseas. Necesito ___.

    a. la vasija   b. el bidet
    c. el termómetro   d. la cabecera

14. El hijo de su hijo es su ___.

    a. hijito   b. yerno
    c. tío   d. nieto

15. Me duelen ___.

    a. las gárgaras   b. los ojos
    c. las horas   d. las cucharadas

16. ¿Cuándo tengo que tomar ___?

    a. el ungüento   b. la tos
    c. el linimento   d. el purgante

17. Los tratamientos de ___ son necesarios.

    a. cobalto   b. esponja
    c. sangre   d. turno

18. Tengo picazón en la piel. Tengo ___.

    a. fiebre amarilla   b. gripe
    c. poliomielitis   d. urticaria

19. Para ir al hospital debe llevar ___.

    a. la fuente   b. las contracciones
    c. el ombligo   d. artículos personales

20. Tiene dolores y ___ frecuentes.

    a. pechos   b. pujos
    c. fuertes   d. profundos

21. Hay que poner las botellas en ___.

    a. el esterilizador   b. el biberón
    c. la tetera   d. el ombligo

22. ¿Padece Ud. de ___?

    a. dientes postizos   b. los riñones
    c. raquídea   d. cicatrices

23. Le vamos a hacer una operación ___.

    a. farmacia   b. sarampión
    c. rubéola   d. exploratoria

24. If you need cotton, you can ___ in the pharmacy.

   a. sell them   b. buy them
   c. buy it   d. buy him

25. We must ask for ___, because it's very serious.

   a. patient   b. help
   c. fatigue   d. fracture

26. Do you have ___ insufficiency?

   a. varicose   b. embolism
   c. arterial   d. aortic

27. ___ is a hereditary disease.

   a. Gangrene   b. Hemophilia
   c. The common cold   d. Tonsilitis

28. His ___ are bleeding.

   a. bridge   b. gums
   c. front   d. fillings

29. Please take off your ___.

   a. head   b. cup
   c. cavity   d. wig

30. You must burp the baby ___ giving him milk.

   a. before   b. quickly
   c. after   d. also

C. Respuestas. Escoja la mejor respuesta a cada pregunta o expresión.

   1. Do you feel burning when you urinate?

      a. Yes, I have a kidney infection.
      b. Yes, I have a cough.
      c. Yes, I have a tonsil infection.
      d. Yes, I have chills.

   2. Can I have a private room?

      a. No, there aren't any wards.
      b. No, there aren't any doubles.
      c. No, there aren't any vacant.
      d. No, they don't have a bath.

   3. Do you like fruit?

      a. Yes, especially bread and cheese.
      b. Yes, especially strawberries and raspberries.
      c. Yes, I like garlic and onion.
      d. Yes, I need a fork and a spoon.

   4. What would you like for dessert?

      a. Sausage.
      b. Cottage cheese.
      c. Ice cream.
      d. Pickles.

24. Si necesita algodón puede ___ en la farmacia.

    a. venderlos   b. comprarlos
    c. comprarlo   d. comprarle

25. Hay que pedir ___ porque está muy grave.

    a. paciente   b. socorro
    c. fatiga   d. fractura

26. ¿Tiene Ud. insuficiencia ___?

    a. varicosa   b. embolia
    c. arteria   d. aórtica

27. ___ es una enfermedad hereditaria.

    a. La gangrena   b. La hemofilia
    c. El catarro   d. La amigdalitis

28. Le sangran ___.

    a. el puente   b. las encías
    c. el frente   d. los empastes

29. Favor de quitarse ___.

    a. la cabeza   b. la taza
    c. la carie   d. la peluca

30. Hay que hacer eructar al niño ___ de darle la leche.

    a. antes   b. pronto
    c. después   d. también

C. _Responses_. Choose the best answer or response to each question or statement.

  1. ¿Siente ardor al orinar?

    a. Sí, tengo infección en los riñones
    b. Sí, tengo tos.
    c. Sí, tengo infección en las amígdalas.
    d. Sí, tengo escalofríos.

  2. ¿Puedo tener un cuarto privado?

    a. No, no hay múltiple.
    b. No, no hay doble.
    c. No, no hay vacante.
    d. No, no tienen baño.

  3. ¿Le gustan las frutas?

    a. Sí, especialmente pan y queso.
    b. Sí, especialmente fresas y frambuesas.
    c. Sí, me gustan el ajo y la cebolla.
    d. Sí, necesito tenedor y cuchara.

  4. ¿Qué quiere de postre?

    a. Salchica.
    b. Requesón.
    c. Helado.
    d. Pepinillo.

5. Are you single?

    a. My husband isn't here.
    b. Yes, I don't have a husband.
    c. Yes, I'm married.
    d. Yes, I have a family.

6. How would you like your eggs?

    a. Shrimp, please.
    b. Salad, thanks.
    c. Scrambled, please.
    d. Jam and butter.

7. Do you have a headache?

    a. No, I don't have a cough.
    b. No, I don't have pain when I urinate.
    c. No, I don't have tingling.
    d. No, I don't have a headache.

8. What is your religion?

    a. I'm a housewife.
    b. I'm from Mexico.
    c. I'm Jewish.
    d. I'm a nurse.

9. Have you had colitis?

    a. Yes, I've had intestinal inflammation.
    b. Yes, I've had whooping cough.
    c. Yes, I've had pain in the area of my heart.
    d. No, I haven't had measles.

10. You have an infection in the respiratory system.

    a. Is it my womb?
    b. Is it in my bronchial tubes?
    c. Is it in the joint?
    d. Is it my fingers?

11. I'm very hungry.

    a. Yes, very hot.
    b. You may visit now.
    c. They'll serve the meal soon.
    d. The food is very bad.

12. I think I'm pregnant.

    a. We'll give you a rabbit test.
    b. Do you have the written order?
    c. It hurts a lot.
    d. We'll do a Pap smear.

13. What time is it?

    a. It's 2:30.
    b. It's time.
    c. There are 4 weeks in a month.
    d. He weighs 8 pounds.

5. ¿Es Ud. soltera?

    a. Mi esposo no está aquí.
    b. Sí, no tengo esposo.
    c. Sí, soy casada.
    d. Sí, tengo familia.

6. ¿Cómo quiere los huevos?

    a. Camarones, por favor.
    b. Ensalada, gracias.
    c. Revueltos, por favor.
    d. Mermelada y mantequilla.

7. ¿Tiene jaqueca?

    a. No, no tengo tos.
    b. No, no tengo dolor al orinar.
    c. No, no tengo hormigueo.
    d. No, no tengo dolor de cabeza.

8. ¿Qué religión tiene?

    a. Soy ama de casa.
    b. Soy de México.
    c. Soy judío.
    d. Soy enfermera.

9. ¿Ha tenido Ud. colitis?

    a. Sí, he tenido inflamación intestinal.
    b. Sí, he tenido tos ferina.
    c. Sí, he tenido dolor en la región del corazón.
    d. No, no he tenido sarampión.

10. Tiene infección en el aparato respiratorio.

    a. ¿Es la matriz?
    b. ¿Es en los bronquios?
    c. ¿Es en la coyuntura?
    d. ¿Son los dedos?

11. Tengo mucha hambre.

    a. Sí, mucho calor.
    b. Se visita ahora.
    c. Se sirve la comida pronto.
    d. La comida está muy mala.

12. Creo que estoy embarazada.

    a. Le vamos a hacer el examen del conejo.
    b. ¿Tiene usted la orden escrita?
    c. Le duele mucho.
    d. Le vamos a hacer el examen de los untos de Papanicolaou.

13. ¿Qué hora es?

    a. Son las dos y media.
    b. Es la hora.
    c. Hay cuatro semanas en un mes.
    d. Pesa ocho libras.

14. Is it necessary to do exercises?

   a. Yes, I need a liter of glucose.
   b. Yes, you need to bend your leg.
   c. No, an ice pack.
   d. You need an alcohol bath.

15. Should I let air get to the incision?

   a. Yes, to dry it.
   b. Yes, you need to clean the instrument.
   c. Yes, you can avoid germs.
   d. Yes, I have to use bleach.

16. Why do you think you're pregnant?

   a. Because I have piles.
   b. Because I'm in a bad mood.
   c. Because I'm not having a discharge of blood.
   d. Because my breasts are normal.

17. Are you going to do a cesarean section?

   a. If you have a normal delivery.
   b. If you have a difficult delivery.
   c. If your bag of waters breaks.
   d. If you lose water.

18. Why do I need to take pills?

   a. Every 6 hours.
   b. To take many liquids.
   c. You can dangle your legs.
   d. To sleep well.

19. Can I nurse the baby?

   a. Yes, I'm going to bring the baby.
   b. It's necessary to give you an enema.
   c. You should dry the bottles.
   d. You should prepare the formula.

20. When can I put the baby in water?

   a. You must bathe him in warm water.
   b. You must avoid drafts.
   c. After drying him well.
   d. After his umbilical cord falls off.

21. What effects can the pill have?

   a. Some women are efficient.
   b. You should decide it with your husband.
   c. Some methods are efficient.
   d. Some women lose hair.

22. What anesthesia are they going to give me?

   a. We're going to give you an enema.
   b. We're going to prepare you.
   c. We're going to give you sodium pentothal.
   d. We're going to take you to the operating room.

14. ¿Es necesario hacer ejercicios?

    a. Sí, necesito un litro de glucosa.
    b. Sí, necesita doblar la pierna.
    c. No, una bolsa de hielo.
    d. Hay que darle un baño de alcohol.

15. ¿Hay que exponer la herida al aire?

    a. Sí, para secarla.
    b. Sí, necesita limpiar el aparato.
    c. Sí, puede evitar microbios.
    d. Sí, tengo que usar cloro.

16. ¿Por qué cree que está embarazada?

    a. Porque tengo almorranas.
    b. Porque tengo mal humor.
    c. Porque no tengo flujo de sangre.
    d. Porque tengo los senos normales.

17. ¿Van a hacerme una operación cesárea?

    a. Si tiene un parto normal.
    b. Si tiene un parto difícil.
    c. Si se le rompe la fuente.
    d. Si pierde agua.

18. ¿Para qué necesito tomar píldoras?

    a. Cada seis horas.
    b. Para tomar muchos líquidos.
    c. Puede colgar las piernas.
    d. Para dormir bien.

19. ¿Puedo darle el pecho al niño?

    a. Sí, voy a traer al bebé.
    b. Es necesario ponerle una enema.
    c. Debe enjuagar las botellas.
    d. Debe preparar la fórmula.

20. ¿Cuándo puedo sumergir al niño en agua?

    a. Hay que bañarlo en agua tibia.
    b. Hay que evitar la corriente de aire.
    c. Después de secarlo bien.
    d. Después de caérsele el ombligo.

21. ¿Qué efectos puede tener la píldora?

    a. Algunas mujeres son eficaces.
    b. Debe decidirlo con su esposo.
    c. Algunos métodos son eficaces.
    d. Algunas mujeres pierden pelo.

22. ¿Qué anestesia me van a dar?

    a. Le vamos a poner un lavado.
    b. Vamos a prepararlo.
    c. Le vamos a dar pentotal de sodio.
    d. Vamos a llevarlo a la sala de operaciones.

23. Where can I get a Band-Aid?

    a. On the label.
    b. In the medicine cabinet.
    c. In the prescription.
    d. On the bandage.

24. He must have mouth-to-mouth resuscitation.

    a. Yes, he almost drowned.
    b. Yes, he almost had an accident.
    c. Yes, he almost had an attack.
    d. Yes, he almost had a tourniquet.

25. We've got to call an ambulance.

    a. No, it's the emergency room.
    b. Yes, he's bleeding badly.
    c. Yes, he has a coin.
    d. No, it's not a very serious injury.

26. How long have you felt bad?

    a. For 100 years.
    b. For several days.
    c. I don't have symptoms.
    d. No, never.

27. What symptoms does he have?

    a. He has a good appetite.
    b. He has 5 fingers.
    c. He has suicidal tendencies.
    d. He has a lot of money.

28. Did you take your medicine?

    a. Yes, tomorrow.
    b. No, I forgot.
    c. Yes, he's very nice.
    d. You slept well.

D. Tache la palabra que no se pueda usar para completar la frase.

1. We're going to shave ___.

    a. your hair   b. your body hair
    c. your beard   d. your ankle

2. We're going to do an analysis of your ___.

    a. blood   b. sleeve
    c. sputum   d. urine

3. Do you have a swelling in the area of your ___?

    a. legs   b. eyes
    c. kidneys   d. hands

4. You can pay ___.

    a. with permission   b. on terms
    c. cash   d. in December

23. ¿Dónde puedo obtener una curita?

    a. En la etiqueta.
    b. En el botiquín.
    c. En la receta.
    d. En la venda.

24. Hay que darle respiración boca a boca.

    a. Sí, por poco se ahoga.
    b. Sí, por poco tiene un accidente.
    c. Sí, por poco tiene ataque.
    d. Sí, por poco tiene un torniquete.

25. Hay que llamar la ambulancia.

    a. No, es la sala de urgencia.
    b. Sí, está sangrando mucho.
    c. Sí, tiene una moneda.
    d. No, es una herida muy grave.

26. ¿Desde cuándo se siente mal?

    a. Hace cien años.
    b. Hace unos días.
    c. No tengo síntomas.
    d. No, nunca.

27. ¿Qué síntomas tiene?

    a. Tiene buen apetito.
    b. Tiene cinco dedos.
    c. Tiene tendencias suicidas.
    d. Tiene mucho dinero.

28. ¿Tomaste la medicina?

    a. Sí, mañana.
    b. No, se me olvidó.
    c. Sí, es muy simpático.
    d. Dormiste bien.

D. Cross out the word that __cannot__ be used to complete the sentence.

1. Vamos a rasurarle ___ .

    a. el pelo   b. el vello
    c. la barba   d. el tobillo

2. Le vamos a hacer un análisis de ___ .

    a. sangre   b. manga
    c. esputo   d. orina

3. ¿Tiene Ud. hinchazón en ___?

    a. las piernas   b. los ojos
    c. los riñones   d. las manos

4. Ud. puede pagar ___ .

    a. con permiso   b. a plazos
    c. al contado   d. en diciembre

5. You should follow a diet for ___.

    a. gaining weight   b. losing weight
    c. washing your back   d. lowering the cholesterol level

6. Ma'am, please take off your ___.

    a. undershorts   b. panties
    c. stockings   d. bra

7. I'm Jewish, and I don't want to eat ___.

    a. ham   b. veal
    c. pork   d. bacon

8. You have an infection around the ___ of your foot.

    a. toe   b. toenail
    c. sole   d. palm

9. I don't want ___ with my meal.

    a. wine   b. coffee
    c. oven   d. milk

10. I think I have sinus trouble, because I have ___.

    a. headache   b. hives
    c. mucus   d. a stopped up nose

11. In the hospital you need ___.

    a. a robe   b. a nightgown or nightshirt
    c. a coat   d. slippers

12. When do I take the medicine?

    a. Every 2 hours   b. According to the label.
    c. Before you go to bed.   d. Don't mention it.

13. He must have immunization against ___.

    a. dysentery   b. tuberculosis
    c. whooping cough   d. smallpox

14. ___ is (are) a very contagious disease.

    a. Impetigo   b. German measles
    c. Tetanus   d. Mumps

15. I have to use ___.

    a. soap   b. injuries
    c. adhesive tape   d. boiled water

16. You can ___ from the first day.

    a. get up   b. bathe
    c. especially   d. sit down

17. If you want to urinate, we're going to give you ___.

    a. the bedpan   b. the bedpan
    c. the bedpan   d. the flow

5. Debe seguir una dieta para ___.

    a. aumentar de peso   b. bajar de peso
    c. lavarse la espalda   d. bajar el nivel del colesterol

6. Señora, favor de quitarse ___.

    a. los calzoncillos   b. las pantaletas
    c. las medias   d. el sostén

7. Soy judío, y no quiero comer ___.

    a. jamón   b. ternera
    c. puerco   d. tocino

8. Tiene infección en ___ del pie.

    a. el dedo   b. la uña del dedo
    c. la planta   d. la palma

9. No quiero tomar ___ con la comida.

    a. vino   b. café
    c. horno   d. leche

10. Creo que tengo sinusitis, porque tengo ___.

    a. dolor de cabeza   b. urticaria
    c. mucosidad   d. la nariz tapada

11. En el hospital, Ud. necesita ___.

    a. bata   b. camisa de noche
    c. abrigo   d. zapatillas

12. ¿Cuándo tomo la medicina?

    a. Cada dos horas.   b. Según la etiqueta.
    c. Antes de acostarse.   d. No hay de qué.

13. Hay que inmunizarlo contra la ___.

    a. disentería   b. tuberculosis
    c. tos ferina   d. viruela

14. ___ es una enfermedad muy contagiosa.

    a. El impétigo   b. La rubéola
    c. El tétano   d. La parotiditis

15. Tengo que usar ___.

    a. jabón   b. las heridas
    c. tela adhesiva   d. agua hervida

16. Ud. puede ___ desde el primer día.

    a. levantarse   b. bañarse
    c. especialmente   d. sentarse

17. Si quiere orinar vamos a ponerle ___.

    a. la chata   b. el bacín
    c. la cuña   d. el flujo

18. Some women use ___.

    a. the condom   b. the cervical cap
    c. the diaphragm   d. jellies

19. They're going to operate on my ___.

    a. jaw   b. eyelash
    c. nose   d. throat

20. What happened to him? He got ___.

    a. burned   b. a broken foot
    c. frostbitten   d. careful

21. What's the matter? He has a ___ fracture.

    a. better   b. serious
    c. minor   d. compound

22. Let me fasten your ___.

    a. hair   b. shirt
    c. shoes   d. pants

18. Algunas mujeres usan ___.

    a. el condón
    c. el diafragma
    b. el gorro cervical
    d. jaleas

19. Me van a operar de la ___.

    a. mandíbula
    c. nariz
    b. pestaña
    d. garganta

20. ¿Qué le pasó? Se ha ___.

    a. quemado
    c. congelado
    b. fracturado un pie
    d. cuidado

21. ¿Qué tiene? Tiene una fractura ___.

    a. mejor
    c. menor
    b. mayor
    d. compuesta

22. Déjame abrocharte ___.

    a. el pelo
    c. los zapatos
    b. la camisa
    d. el pantalón

Vocabularies

The vocabularies include words from the New Material in the lessons supplemented by other useful words and verb forms. Words from the pronunciation section and the identification exercises in the lessons are not necessarily included since these may not be frequently used words. Listed separately immediately preceding the vocabularies are tables of numbers and time units, and this section begins with lists of cognate words with the following terminations:

English	Spanish
(cognate infinitives)	-ar, -er, -ir
-ion	-ión
-ance, -ence, -ia, -y	-ancia, -encia, -ia
-y	-ía*
-in, -ine	-ina, -ino
-ic, -ical	-ico
-ry	-rio
-ism	-ismo
-ous	-oso
-ant, -ent	-ante, -ente
-ent	-ento
-ble	-ble
-ty	-dad
-sis, -lis	-sis, -lis
-itis	-itis

Cognates that are not included in these lists but are of particular medical importance or that are pronounced very differently are listed in the vocabularies, however.

Nouns that are not obviously masculine (-o) or feminine (-a) are marked in the vocabularies (m.) or (f.). In the English-Spanish Vocabulary, if nouns and verbs have the same form in English, the Spanish noun is given first, followed by the infinitive (which ends in -ar, -er, or -ir). In the Spanish-English Vocabulary, the first and third person singular forms of frequently used irregular verbs are given, either under the infinitive or, if the spelling is very different from the infinitive, as a separate entry.

---

*Cognates ending in -ia and -ía are separated because of the pronunciation problems they pose for English-speaking students.

Cognate Words

to absorb	to contract	to facilitate	to precipitate
to accept	to control	to form	to preoccupy
to acquire	to converse	to fracture	to prepare
to affirm	to convert	to function	to prevent
to adjust	to cost	to imagine	to proceed
to alienate	to cure	to include	to progress
to alter	to debilitate	to indicate	to prohibit
to amputate	to decide	to infect	to prolong
to analyze	to declare	to inform	to pronounce
to annul	to depend	to inhibit	to propagate
to appreciate	to describe	to immunize	to propose
to arrest	to discover	to inoculate	to protect
to articulate	to disinfect	to inspect	to protest
to authorize	to destroy	to interest	to provoke
to balance	to determine	to interpret	to project
to calm	to diagnose	to investigate	to purify
to cause	to digest	to maintain	to recommend
to circulate	to dilate	to masticate	to recognize
to coagulate	to discuss	to masturbate	to recuperate
to compensate	to diminish	to note	to reduce
to communicate	to dissolve	to observe	to refer
to concede	to distinguish	to obstruct	to relate
to concentrate	to distribute	to occur	to remedy
to conclude	to divide	to offend	to renovate
to conserve	to eliminate	to omit	to repair
to consider	to sterilize	to operate	to repeat
to consist	to evacuate	to urinate	to represent
to constipate	to evaluate	to penetrate	to resent
to consult	to examine	to perceive	to resolve
to contaminate	to exist	to permit	to respect
to contain	to explore	to practice	to respire

Palabras cognadas

INFINITIVOS

absorber	contraer	facilitar	precipitar
aceptar	controlar	formar	preocupar
adquirir	conversar	fracturar	preparar
afirmar	convertir	funcionar	prevenir
ajustar	costar	imaginar	proceder
alienar	curar	incluir	progresar
alterar	debilitar	indicar	prohibir
amputar	decidir	infectar	prolongar
analizar	declarar	informar	pronunciar
anular	depender	inhibir	propagar
apreciar	describir	inmunizar	proponer
arrestar	descubrir	inocular	proteger
articular	desinfectar	inspeccionar	protestar
autorizar	destruir	interesar	provocar
balancear	determinar	interpretar	proyectar
calmar	diagnosticar	investigar	purificar
causar	digerir	mantener	recomendar
circular	dilatar	masticar	reconocer
coagular	discutir	masturbar	recuperar
compensar	disminuir	notar	reducir
comunicar	disolver	observar	referir
conceder	distinguir	obstruir	relatar
concentrar	distribuir	ocurrir	remediar
concluir	dividir	ofender	renovar
conservar	eliminar	omitir	reparar
considerar	esterilizar	operar	repetir
consistir	evacuar	orinar	representar
constipar	evaluar	penetrar	resentir
consultar	examinar	percibir	resolver
contaminar	existir	permitir	respetar
contener	explorar	practicar	respirar

to restore	to revise	to suspend	to ventilate
to resuscitate	to select	to transmit	to visit
to result	to separate	to ulcerate	to vomit
to resume	to suffer	to use	to vote
to retire	to suppurate	to utilize	

ENDINGS: -ion

action	construction	evacuation	indisposition
administration	contamination	evaluation	infection
admission	contraction	evasion	inflammation
alienation	contraception	evolution	information
alimentation	conversation	expectation	infraction
alteration	convulsion	expectoration	inhalation
hallucination	deception	explication	immersion
amplification	decision	exploration	immunization
application	declaration	explosion	inoculation
articulation	defecation	extraction	inspection
association	depression	ejaculation	installation
attention	description	fecundation	institution
authorization	desertion	fibrillation	instruction
calcification	malnutrition	flexion	interaction
cauterization	deterioration	formation	interpretation
certification	determination	friction	interruption
cession	digestion	function	intoxication
circulation	direction	gestation	investigation
coagulation	discretion	hospitalization	injection
commission	discussion	hypertension	irritation
comparison	distribution	hyperventilation	lesion
complication	division	hypotension	limitation
compression	duration	hypoventilation	lotion
communication	education	identification	locomotion
concentration	elevation	illusion	mastication
condition	elimination	incision	masturbation
conservation	emotion	incubation	menstruation
consideration	eruption	indecision	moderation
constipation	station	indication	mortification
constitution	sterilization	indigestion	nutrition

restaurar	revisar	suspender	ventilar
resucitar	seleccionar	transmitir	visitar
resultar	separar	ulcerar	vomitar
resumir	sufrir	usar	votar
retirar	supurar	utilizar	

TERMINACIONES: -ión

acción	construcción	evacuación	indisposición
administración	contaminación	evaluación	infección
admisión	contracción	evasión	inflamación
alienación	contracepción	evolución	información
alimentación	conversación	expectación	infracción
alteración	convulsión	expectoración	inhalación
alucinación	decepción	explicación	inmersión
amplificación	decisión	exploración	inmunización
aplicación	declaración	explosión	inoculación
articulación	defecación	extracción	inspección
asociación	depresión	eyaculación	instalación
atención	descripción	fecundación	institución
autorización	deserción	fibrilación	instrucción
calcificación	desnutrición	flexión	interacción
cauterización	deterioración	formación	interpretación
certificación	determinación	fricción	interrupción
cesión	digestión	función	intoxicación
circulación	dirección	gestación	investigación
coagulación	discreción	hospitalización	inyección
comisión	discusión	hipertensión	irritación
comparación	distribución	hiperventilación	lesión
complicación	división	hipotensión	limitación
compresión	duración	hipoventilación	loción
comunicación	educación	identificación	locomoción
concentración	elevación	ilusión	masticación
condición	eliminación	incisión	masturbación
conservación	emoción	incubación	menstruación
consideración	erupción	indecisión	moderación
constipación	estación	indicación	mortificación
constitución	esterilización	indigestión	nutrición

observation	promotion	religion	signification
obsession	propensity	repetition	situation
obstruction	protection	reputation	solution
occupation	provision	resolution	suggestion
omission	projection	respiration	suppuration
operation	pulsation	restriction	tension
palpitation	ration	resuscitation	temptation
perception	radiation	retention	traction
portion	reaction	revision	transformation
position	recreation	revolution	transfusion
prostration	recuperation	salivation	transmission
preoccupation	reduction	satisfaction	trepanation
preparation	reflection	section	ulceration
presentation	refraction	secretion	union
prevention	region	selection	variation
privation	rehabilitation	separation	ventilation
profession	relation	session	vision
prohibition			

ENDINGS: -ance, -ence, -ia, -y

abstinence	clemency	elegance	flatulence
acromegaly	competency	embolism	phobia
adolescence	conscience	emergency	frequency
allergy	constancy	eminence	hemophilia
ambulance	convalescence	epilepsy	hemorrhage
analgesia	decency	essence	hernia
anemia	deficiency	spice	hydrophobia
anesthesia	dementia	euphoria	hydrotherapy
anorexia	diathermy	eugenics	hysteria
anuria	diphtheria	euthanasia	idiosyncrasy
arrogance	discrepancy	evidence	ignorance
assistance	dyspepsia	excellence	importance
asthenia	distance	existence	incontinence
atrophy	dystrophy	experience	independence
autopsy	eclampsia	family	indigence
biopsy	efficiency	pharmacy	indulgence

observación	promoción	religión	significación
obsesión	propensión	repetición	situación
obstrucción	protección	reputación	solución
ocupación	provisión	resolución	sugestión
omisión	proyección	respiración	supuración
operación	pulsación	restricción	tensión
palpitación	ración	resucitación	tentación
percepción	radiación	retención	tracción
porción	reacción	revisión	transformación
posición	recreación	revolución	transfusión
postración	recuperación	salivación	transmisión
preocupación	reducción	satisfacción	trepanación
preparación	reflexión	sección	ulceración
presentación	refracción	secreción	unión
prevención	región	selección	variación
privación	rehabilitación	separación	ventilación
profesión	relación	sesión	visión
prohibición			

TERMINACIONES: -ancia, -encia, -ia

abstinencia	clemencia	elegancia	flatulencia
acromegalia	competencia	embolia	fobia
adolescencia	conciencia	emergencia	frecuencia
alergia	constancia	eminencia	hemofilia
ambulancia	convalescencia	epilepsia	hemorragia
analgesia	decencia	esencia	hernia
anemia	deficiencia	especia	hidrofobia
anestesia	demencia	euforia	hidroterapia
anorexia	diatermia	eugenesia	histeria
anuria	difteria	eutanasia	idiosincracia
arrogancia	discrepancia	evidencia	ignorancia
asistencia	dispepsia	excelencia	importancia
astenia	distancia	existencia	incontinencia
atrofia	distrofia	experiencia	independencia
autopsia	eclampsia	familia	indigencia
biopsia	eficiencia	farmacia	indulgencia

infancy	negligence	prominence	therapy
imminence	neuralgia	rabies	tolerance
instance	neurasthenia	reference	toxemia
insufficiency	orthopedics	residence	transcendence
interference	patience	resistance	transparency
laparoscopy	permanence	resonance	uremia
leukemia	polycythemia	septicemia	urgency
malaria	potency	sufficiency	vehemence
memory	presence	tendency	violence
menopause			

ENDINGS: -y

anatomy	empathy	laparotomy	pleurisy
anesthesiology	endocrinology	lobectomy	police
anomaly	infirmary	mastectomy	proctology
bacteriology	epidemiology	microbiology	psychology
biology	episiotomy	myopia	psychiatry
bronchopneumonia	pharmacology	neonatology	pneumonia
calorie	physiology	neurology	radiography
cardiology	gastroenterology	odontology	radiology
surgery	geography	ophthalmology	roentgenology
citizenry	geriatrics	optometry	sympathy
colectomy	gynecology	orthodontics	sociology
company	hematology	osteopathy	technology
accounting	hypochondria	otorhinolaryngology	tracheotomy
courtesy	hysterectomy	parasitology	urology
dermatology	engineering	pathology	vasectomy
dysentery	immunology	pediatrics	zoology
ecology			

ENDINGS: -in, -ine

Achromycin	cholesterol	scarlet fever	gelatin
adrenaline	curtain	streptomycin	glycerin
amphetamine	discipline	strychnine	insulin
angina	Dramamine	extrauterine	intestine
aspirin	ephedrine	gamma globulin	intrauterine
calamine	endocrine	gasoline	margarine

infancia	negligencia	prominencia	terapia
inminencia	neuralgia	rabia	tolerancia
instancia	neurastenia	referencia	toxemia
insuficiencia	ortopedia	residencia	transcendencia
interferencia	paciencia	resistencia	transparencia
laparoscopia	permanencia	resonancia	uremia
leucemia	policitemia	septicemia	urgencia
malaria	potencia	suficiencia	vehemencia
memoria	presencia	tendencia	violencia
menopausia			

TERMINACIONES: -ía

anatomía	empatía	laparotomía	pleuresía
anestesiología	endocrinología	lobectomía	policía
anomalía	enfermería	mastectomía	proctología
bacteriología	epidemiología	microbiología	psicología
biología	episiotomía	miopía	psiquiatría
bronconeumonía	farmacología	neonatología	pulmonía
caloría	fisiología	neurología	radiografía
cardiología	gastroenterología	odontología	radiología
cirugía	geografía	oftalmología	roentgenología
ciudadanía	geriatría	optometría	simpatía
colectomía	ginecología	ortodontología	sociología
compañía	hematología	osteopatía	tecnología
contaduría	hipocondría	otorrinolaringología	traqueotomía
cortesía	histerectomía	parasitología	urología
dermatología	ingeniería	patología	vasectomía
disentería	inmunología	pediatría	zoología
ecología			

TERMINACIONES: -ina, -ino

acromicina	colesterina	escarlatina	gelatina
adrenalina	cortina	estreptomicina	glicerina
anfetamina	disciplina	estricnina	insulina
angina	dramamina	extrauterino	intestino
aspirina	efedrina	gamaglobulina	intrauterino
calamina	endocrina	gasolina	margarina

medicine
melamine
mescaline
mine
office

urine
penicillin
protein
quinine
resin

routine
saccharin
sardine
tetramycin

toxin
vagina
Vaseline
vitamin

ENDINGS: -ic, -ical

alcoholic
anaphylactic
analgesic
analytic
antibiotic
antispasmodic
antiseptic
antitetanic
aortic
barbaric

bubonic
characteristic
Catholic
clinic
cosmetic
cubic
diabetic
ectopic
emetic

spasmodic
physical
genetic
mechanical
narcotic
orthopedic
paralytic
plastic
prophylactic

pubic
public
rheumatic
rhythmic
technical
therapeutic
tetanic
tubal
uric

ENDINGS: -ry

adversary
agrarian
ambulatory
anniversary
circulatory
commentary
compensatory
consulting
  (office)
contrary
criterion

dictionary
dormitory
exploratory
functionary
funerary
gregarious
hereditary
laboratory
lavatory
mystery

necessary
ordinary
ovary
preparatory
primary
regulatory
revolutionary
rudimentary
sanatorium

sanitary
secretary
solitary
suppository
territory
transitory
various
veterinary
vibratory

ENDINGS: -ism

activism
albinism
alcoholism
altruism
anachronism
aneurysm

anglicism
asceticism
astigmatism
baptism
botulism
conventionalism

cretinism
dramatization
egotism
embolism
strabismus
fatalism

favoritism
feudalism
humanism
humorousness
illusionism
intellectualism

medicina	orina	rutina	toxina
melamina	penicilina	sacarina	vagina
mescalina	proteína	sardina	vaselina
mina	quinina	tetramicina	vitamina
oficina	resina		

TERMINACIONES: -ico

alcohólico	bubónico	espasmódico	púbico
anafiláctico	característico	físico	público
analgésico	católico	genético	reumático
analítico	clínico	mecánico	rítmico
antibiótico	cosmético	narcótico	técnico
antiespasmódico	cúbico	ortopédico	terapeútico
antiséptico	diabético	paralítico	tetánico
antitetánico	ectópico	plástico	tubárico
aórtico	emético	profiláctico	úrico
barbárico			

TERMINACIONES: -rio

adversario	diccionario	necesario	sanitario
agrario	dormitorio	ordinario	secretario
ambulatorio	exploratorio	ovario	solitario
aniversario	funcionario	preparatorio	supositorio
circulatorio	funerario	primario	territorio
comentario	gregario	regulatorio	transitorio
compensatorio	hereditario	revolucionario	vario
consultorio	laboratorio	rudimentario	veterinario
	lavatorio	sanatorio	vibratorio
contrario	misterio		
criterio			

TERMINACIONES: -ismo

activismo	anglicismo	cretinismo	favoritismo
albinismo	ascetismo	dramatismo	feudalismo
alcoholismo	astigmatismo	egoismo	humanismo
altruismo	bautismo	embolismo	humorismo
anacronismo	botulismo	estrabismo	ilusionismo
aneurismo	convencionalismo	fatalismo	intelectualismo

mechanism	occultism	professionalism	symbolism
metabolism	optimism	rickets	sinapism
mysticism	patriotism	regionalism	somnambulism
mongolism	pessimism	rheumatism	vandalism

ENDINGS: -ous

ambitious	envious	industrious	nervous
anxious	spacious	ingenious	prodigious
harmonious	studious	intravenous	religious
cancerous	famous	marvelous	suspicious
contagious	fibrous	melodious	talented
copious	furious	meticulous	verbose
curious	generous	mysterious	vigorous
defective	glorious	monstrous	
delicious	gracious	morbid	
desirous	impetuous	mucous	

ENDINGS: -ant, -ent

abundant	demented	important	president
agent	disinfectant	incoherent	Protestant
ambulant	deodorant	incompetent	recent
arrogant	different	independent	referring
assistant	diligent	infant	regent
brilliant	distant	imminent	repugnant
sedative	efficient	instant	resident
competent	stimulant	interesting	servant
complaisant	student	intermittent	solvent
conscious	excellent	latent	sufficient
constant	frequent	patient	tolerant
convalescent	gallant	permanent	turgid
correspondent	ignorant	pertinent	urgent
current	impatient	potent	vacant
decent	impertinent	present	vehement
deficient			

mecanismo	ocultismo	profesionalismo	simbolismo
metabolismo	optimismo	raquitismo	sinapismo
misticismo	patriotismo	regionalismo	sonambulismo
mongolismo	pesimismo	reumatismo	vandalismo

TERMINACIONES: -oso

ambicioso	envidioso	industrioso	nervioso
ansioso	espacioso	ingenioso	prodigioso
armonioso	estudioso	intravenoso	religioso
canceroso	famoso	maravilloso	sospechoso
contagioso	fibroso	melodioso	talentoso
copioso	furioso	meticuloso	verboso
curioso	generoso	misterioso	vigoroso
defectuoso	glorioso	monstruoso	
delicioso	gracioso	morboso	
deseoso	impetuoso	mucoso	

TERMINACIONES: -ante, -ente

abundante	demente	importante	presidente
agente	desinfectante	incoherente	protestante
ambulante	desodorante	incompetente	reciente
arrogante	diferente	independiente	referente
asistente	diligente	infante	regente
brillante	distante	inminente	repugnante
calmante	eficiente	instante	residente
competente	estimilante	interesante	sirviente
complaciente	estudiante	intermitente	solvente
consciente	excelente	latente	suficiente
constante	frecuente	paciente	tolerante
convaleciente	galante	permanente	turgente
correspondiente	ignorante	pertinente	urgente
corriente	impaciente	potente	vacante
decente	impertinente	presente	vehemente
deficiente			

ENDINGS: -ent

accompaniment	establishment	ligament	requirement
apartment	excrement	liniment	resentment
compartment	firmament	medication	rudiment
condiment	fomentation	moment	section
consent	fragment	monument	sentiment
corpulent	function	movement	somnolent
department	impediment	procedure	talent
discovery	implement	recognition	temperament
deterioration	instrument	refinement	torment
document	lament	regiment	treatment

ENDINGS: -ble

acceptable	fallible	insensible	probable
agreeable	flexible	inseparable	reasonable
amiable	impassive	unserviceable	removable
applicable	impossible	unsupportable	resistible
comparable	improbable	unreasonable	responsible
communicable	incomparable	irresistible	sensible
conservable	incommunicable	irritable	serviceable
considerable	uncontrollable	laudable	sociable
countable	incorrigible	maintainable	soluble
controllable	incredible	movable	supportable
credible	incurable	notable	sufferable
disagreeable	indicatable	observable	terrible
digestible	indigestible	obtainable	tractable
disposable	uneducable	operable	usable
durable	unstable	passable	variable
educable	immobile	possible	visible
emotional	unobservable	potable	vulnerable
stable	inoperable	presentable	

ENDINGS: -ty

amiability	atrocity	cavity	quality
amenity	calamity	clarity	debility
animosity	capacity	community	deformity
abnormality	charity	continuity	density

TERMINACIONES: -ento

acompañamiento	establecimiento	ligamento	requerimiento
apartamento	excremento	linimento	resentimiento
compartimiento	firmamento	medicamento	rudimento
condimento	fomento	momento	seccionamiento
consentimiento	fragmento	monumento	sentimiento
corpulento	funcionamiento	movimiento	soñoliento
departamento	impedimento	procedimiento	talento
descubrimiento	implemento	reconocimiento	temperamento
deterioramiento	instrumento	refinamiento	tormento
documento	lamento	regimiento	tratamiento

TERMINACIONES: -ble

aceptable	falible	insensible	probable
agradable	flexible	inseparable	razonable
amable	impasible	inservible	removible
aplicable	imposible	insoportable	resistible
comparable	improbable	irrazonable	responsable
comunicable	incomparable	irresistible	sensible
conservable	incomunicable	irritable	servible
considerable	incontrolable	laudable	sociable
contable	incorregible	mantenible	soluble
controlable	increíble	movible	soportable
creíble	incurable	notable	sufrible
desagradable	indicable	observable	terrible
digestible	indigestible	obtenible	tratable
disponible	ineducable	operable	usable
durable	inestable	pasable	variable
educable	inmovible	posible	visible
emocionable	inobservable	potable	vulnerable
estable	inoperable	presentable	

TERMINACIONES: -dad

amabilidad	atrocidad	cavidad	cualidad
amenidad	calamidad	claridad	debilidad
animosidad	capacidad	comunidad	deformidad
anormalidad	caridad	continuidad	densidad

difficulty	gravity	liberty	probability
durability	ability	maternity	regularity
infirmity	hospitality	morality	responsibility
stability	humanity	mobility	sanity
sterility	impossibility	nationality	security
eternity	improbability	naturalness	sensibility
facility	incapacity	necessity	similarity
faculty	identity	nervousness	solemnity
familiarity	instability	neutrality	solidarity
femininity	immobility	obesity	university
flexibility	immunity	opportunity	vanity
formality	insensibility	partiality	versatility
fragility	intensity	popularity	viscosity
generality	invisibility	possibility	visibility
generosity	irritability	priority	vitality
gentility	legality		

ENDINGS: -sis, -lis

acidosis	chlorosis	lordosis	psoriasis
alkalosis	diagnosis	mononucleosis	syphilis
amebiasis	dose	necrosis	synthesis
analysis	elephantiasis	paralysis	thesis
anuresis	sclerosis	paresis	phthisis
arteriosclerosis	halitosis	prognosis	torticollis
avitaminosis	hypnosis	prosthesis	trichinosis
brucellosis	hypochondriasis	psychoanalysis	thrombosis
cyanosis	hypothesis	psychosis	tuberculosis
cirrhosis			

ENDINGS: -itis

appendicitis	dermatitis	sclerotitis	mastoiditis
arthritis	diverticulitis	phlebitis	meningitis
bronchitis	encephalitis	gastritis	metritis
bursitis	encephalomyelitis	gingivitis	myocarditis
cystitis	endocarditis	hepatitis	osteomyelitis
colitis	enteritis	iritis	otitis
conjunctivitis	scleritis	laryngitis	pancreatitis

dificultad	gravedad	libertad	probabilidad
durabilidad	habilidad	maternidad	regularidad
enfermedad	hospitalidad	moralidad	responsabilidad
estabilidad	humanidad	movilidad	sanidad
esterilidad	imposibilidad	nacionalidad	seguridad
eternidad	improbabilidad	naturalidad	sensibilidad
facilidad	incapacidad	necesidad	similaridad
facultad	identidad	nerviosidad	solemnidad
familiaridad	inestabilidad	neutralidad	solidaridad
feminidad	inmovilidad	obesidad	universidad
flexibilidad	inmunidad	oportunidad	vanidad
formalidad	insensibilidad	parcialidad	versatilidad
fragilidad	intensidad	popularidad	viscosidad
generalidad	invisibilidad	posibilidad	visibilidad
generosidad	irritabilidad	prioridad	vitalidad
gentilidad	legalidad		

TERMINACIONES: -sis, -lis

acidosis	clorosis	lordosis	psoriasis
alcalosis	diagnosis	mononucleosis	sífilis
amebiasis	dosis	necrosis	síntesis
análisis	elefantiasis	parálisis	tesis
anuresis	esclerosis	paresis	tisis
arterioesclerosis	halitosis	prognosis	tortícolis
avitaminosis	hipnosis	prótesis	triquinosis
brucelosis	hipocondriasis	psicoanálisis	trombosis
cianosis	hipótesis	psicosis	tuberculosis
cirrosis			

TERMINACIONES: -itis

apendicitis	dermatitis	esclerotitis	mastoiditis
artritis	diverticulitis	flebitis	meningitis
bronquitis	encefalitis	gastritis	metritis
bursitis	encefalomielitis	gingivitis	miocarditis
cistitis	endocarditis	hepatitis	osteomielitis
colitis	enteritis	iritis	otitis
conjuntivitis	escleritis	laringitis	pancreatitis

parotitis	peritonitis	prostatitis	sinusitis
	pyelitis	retinitis	tonsillitis
pericarditis	poliomyelitis	rhinitis	vaginitis

parotiditis, parotitis	peritonitis	prostatitis	sinusitis
	pielitis	retinitis	tonsilitis
pericarditis	poliomielitis	rinitis	vaginitis

Numbers and Miscellaneous

Numbers	Numerals	Números
one	1	uno
two	2	dos
three	3	tres
four	4	cuatro
five	5	cinco
six	6	seis
seven	7	siete
eight	8	ocho
nine	9	nueve
ten	10	diez
eleven	11	once
twelve	12	doce
thirteen	13	trece
fourteen	14	catorce
fifteen	15	quince
sixteen	16	dieciséis, diez y seis
seventeen	17	diecisiete, diez y siete
eighteen	18	dieciocho, diez y ocho
nineteen	19	diecinueve, diez y nueve
twenty	20	veinte
twenty-one	21	veintiuno, veinte y uno
twenty-two	22	veintidós, veinte y dos
twenty-three	23	veintitrés, veinte y tres
twenty-four	24	veinticuatro, veinte y cuatro
twenty-five	25	veinticinco, veinte y cinco
twenty-six	26	veintiséis, veinte y seis
twenty-seven	27	veintisiete, veinte y siete
twenty-eight	28	veintiocho, veinte y ocho
twenty-nine	29	veintinueve, veinte y nueve

Numbers	Numerals		Números
thirty		30	treinta
forty		40	cuarenta
fifty		50	cincuenta
sixty		60	sesenta
seventy		70	setenta
eighty		80	ochenta
ninety		90	noventa
one hundred		100	cien, ciento
two hundred		200	doscientos, -as
three hundred		300	trescientos, -as
four hundred		400	cuatrocientos, -as
five hundred		500	quinientos, -as
six hundred		600	seiscientos, -as
seven hundred		700	setecientos, -as
eight hundred		800	ochocientos, -as
nine hundred		900	novecientos, -as
one thousand	1,000	1.000	mil
one million	1,000,000	1.000.000	un millón

Ordinal Numbers		Números ordinales	
first	1st	primer, primero, primera	1°, 1^a
second	2nd	segundo, -a	2°, 2^a
third	3rd	tercer, tercero, tercera	3°, 3^a
fourth	4th	cuarto, -a	4°, 4^a
fifth	5th	quinto, -a	5°, 5^a
sixth	6th	sexto, -a	6°, 6^a
seventh	7th	séptimo, -a	7°, 7^a
eighth	8th	octavo, -a	8°, 8^a
ninth	9th	noveno, -a	9°, 9^a
tenth	10th	décimo, -a	10°, 10^a

Months	Meses
January	enero
February	febrero
March	marzo
April	abril
May	mayo
June	junio
July	julio
August	agosto
September	septiembre
October	octubre
November	noviembre
December	diciembre

Days of the Week	Días de la semana
Sunday	domingo
Monday	lunes
Tuesday	martes
Wednesday	miércoles
Thursday	jueves
Friday	viernes
Saturday	sábado

Seasons of the Year	Estaciones del año
spring	primavera
summer	verano
fall, autumn	otoño
winter	invierno

Cardinal Points	Puntos cardinales
north, northern	norte, septentrional
south, southern	sur, meridional
east, eastern	este, oriental
west, western	oeste, occidental

Spanish-English Vocabulary

A

<u>a</u> at, to, per

<u>abajo</u> underneath

<u>abandonado</u>, <u>-a</u> left, abandoned

<u>abogado</u> lawyer

<u>aborto</u> abortion, miscarriage

<u>abrazar</u> to hug

<u>abrazo</u> hug

<u>abrigarse</u> to cover up, to wrap up

<u>abrigo</u> coat

<u>abrir</u> to open

<u>abrochar</u> to fasten

<u>absceso</u> abscess

<u>abstenerse</u> to abstain

<u>abuela</u> grandmother

<u>abuelo</u> grandfather

<u>aceite</u> (m.) oil

<u>acerca</u> about

<u>acidez</u> (f.) acidity

<u>acostarse</u> to go to bed; <u>la hora de acostarse</u>, bedtime

<u>acostumbrarse</u> to become accustomed to

<u>acupuntura</u> acupuncture

<u>adelante</u> come in

<u>adicto</u>, <u>-a</u> addicted, addict

<u>adiós</u> good-bye

<u>adormecer</u> to deaden, to put to sleep

<u>adquirir</u> to get, to acquire

<u>afectado</u>, <u>-a</u> affected

<u>afeitar(se)</u> to shave

<u>afuera</u> outside

<u>agua</u> water; <u>agua potable</u>, drinking water

<u>aguacate</u> (m.) avocado

<u>aguja</u> needle

<u>ahí</u> there, right there

<u>ahora</u> now; <u>ahora mismo</u>, right now, right away

<u>aire</u> (m.) air

<u>aireacondicionado</u> air conditioning

<u>aislamiento</u> isolation

<u>aislar</u> to isolate

<u>ajo</u> garlic

<u>ajustador</u> (m.) bra, brassiere

<u>al</u> + infinitive when + verb

<u>albaricoque</u> (m.) apricot

<u>alcanzar</u> to reach

<u>alegrarse</u> to be glad

<u>aletargamiento</u> lethargy, stupor

<u>alfiler</u> (m.) pin

<u>algo</u> something

<u>algodón</u> (m.) cotton

<u>alguno</u>, <u>-a</u> some, someone

<u>alimentar</u> to feed

<u>alimento</u> food

<u>almeja</u> clam

<u>almíbar</u> (m.) syrup

<u>almohada</u> pillow

<u>almorranas</u> piles, hemorrhoids

<u>almuerzo</u> lunch

<u>alto</u>, <u>-a</u> high; <u>alta presión</u>, high blood pressure

<u>allí</u> there

ama de casa housewife

amable kind

amamantar to breastfeed, to nurse

amar to love

amarillo, -a yellow

amígdalas tonsils

amigdalitis tonsilitis

amigo, -a friend

amoníaco ammonia

amor (m.) love

amplio, -a loose

ampolla blister

analizador (m.) analyzer; analizador del oxígeno de la sangre, blood oxygen analyzer

anchoa anchovy

andador (m.) walker

anestesiólogo anesthesiologist

anillo ring; IUD ring

ano anus

anteojos eyeglasses

antes, antes de before

anticoncepción (f.) birth control

anticuerpo antibody

antídoto antidote

antipático, -a disagreeable, unpleasant

ántrax (m.) anthrax

añadir to add

año year

apagar to turn off

aparato equipment; device; system

apartado postal post office box

apéndice (m.) appendix

apio celery

apósito dressing

apretado, -a tight

apretar to tighten

aprisa fast, quick; de prisa, in a hurry

aquí here

arañar to scratch

arañazo scratch

ardor (m.) burning

arete (m.) earring

armario closet, wardrobe

arreglar to fix

arriba on top, above; upstairs

arroz (m.) rice; arroz con leche, rice pudding; arroz con pollo, chicken and rice

articulación (f.) joint

asado, -a roasted

asar to roast

aseo cleanliness

así thus, like this; así, así, so-so

asiento seat; baño de asiento, sitz bath

asilo asylum

asma asthma

asoleado, -a sunburned

astilla splinter

atacar to attack, to rape

ataque (m.) attack, fit; ataque al cerebro, stroke; ataque al corazón, heart attack

atar to tie

atento, -a attentive

atraso setback

atún (m.) tuna

aumentar to gain; aumentar de peso, to gain weight

ausente absent

automóvil (m.) auto, automobile, car

avena oatmeal

axila armpit

ayer yesterday

ayuda aid, help; enema

ayudar to help

ayunar to fast

ayuno fast (abstention)

azúcar (m.) sugar

azul blue

azuloso, -a bluish

B

bacín (m.) basin, bowl; bedpan

bajar to lower; to come down; to get out

bajo, -a short, low

bala bullet; herida de bala, bullet wound

balanceado, -a balanced

bandeja tray, basin

bañadera bathtub

bañarse to take a bath

baño bath, bathroom; baño de inmersión, baño de tina, tub bath; cuarto de baño, restroom, bathroom; papel de baño, toilet tissue

barba chin, beard

barbacoa barbecue; costillas en barbacoa, barbecued ribs

barbilla chin

barbiturato barbiturate

bastante enough, sufficient

bastón (m.) cane (walking)

basura trash, garbage

bata robe

bazo spleen

bebé (m. or f.) baby

beber to drink

bebida drink; bebida caliente, hot drink; bebida fría, cold drink

benigno, -a benign; tumor benigno, benign tumor

berenjena eggplant

beso kiss

betabel (m.) beet

biberón (m.) baby bottle

bicarbonato bicarbonate

bidet (m.) bedpan

bien well

biftec (m.) steak

billetera billfold

bizcocho cookie, wafer

blanco, -a white

blanquillos eggs

boca mouth; resucitación boca a boca, mouth-to-mouth resuscitation

bolsa bag, handbag, purse; bolsa de agua caliente, hot water bottle; bolsa de hielo, icepack

bonito, -a pretty

borracho, -a drunk

bostezar to yawn

botella bottle

botiquín (m.) medicine chest, cabinet, kit

botón (m.) button

brazo arm

brécol, bróculi (m.) broccoli

bronquios bronchial tubes

buen, bueno, buena good; buenas noches, good evening, good night; buenas tardes, good afternoon; buenos días, good morning

bufanda scarf

busto breast, bust

C

cabecera head (of bed, table)

cabello hair

cabeza head

cabrito kid (goat)

cacahuate, cacahuete (m.) peanut

cacerola casserole (food container)

cada each, every

cadera hip

caer(se) to fall (down)

café coffee; brown color; café con crema, coffee with cream; café con leche, coffee with milk; café solo, café oscuro, café puro, black coffee

caída fall

caja box, cashier (window, office); caja de seguridad, safe

cajera cashier

calabaza squash, pumpkin

calambre (m.) cramp

calcetines (m.) socks

calcificado, -a calcified

cálculos stones; cálculos biliares, gallstones; cálculos renales, kidney stones

caldo broth

calefacción (f.) heat, heating system

caliente hot (temperature)

calma calm; tener calma, to be calm

calmante (m.) sedative

calmarse to be calm

calor (m.) heat; tener calor, to be hot

calzoncillos men's undershorts

calzones (m.) panties

callarse to be quiet

callo callus, corn

calloso, -a callous

cama bed

camarón (m.) shrimp

cambiar to change

cambio change

camilla stretcher, litter; camilla de cuidado crítico, critical care cot

caminar to walk

camisa shirt; camisa de noche, nightgown

camiseta undershirt

cáncer (m.) cancer

cangrejo crab

canica marble

cansado, -a tired

cansancio tiredness

capacidad (f.) vital vital capacity

capellán (m.) chaplain

cápsula capsule

cara face

carbohidrato carbohydrate

cárcel (f.) jail

cardiopulmonar cardiopulmonary; resucitador cardiopulmonar, cardiopulmonary resuscitator

cardioscopio cardioscope

cargar to carry

carie (f.) tooth decay, cavity (tooth)

cariño caress

carne (f.) meat; carne asada, roast beef; carne de puerco, pork

caro, -a expensive

carpintero carpenter

carro car

cartera billfold; handbag

casa house, home; a casa, (to) home; en casa, at home

casado, -a married

cáscara peel, rind, hull, shell

caso case

casualidad (f.) chance; por casualidad, by chance

cataplasma poultice

catarata cataract

catarro cold (disease)

catéter (m.) catheter

caudal (m.) abundance, capital

cebolla onion

ceja eyebrow

cena supper

centeno rye

centígrado centigrade

centímetro centimeter; centímetro cúbico, cubic centimeter (cc.)

centro center

cepillo brush; cepillo de cabeza, hairbrush; cepillo de dientes, tooth-brush

cerca near, close

cerdo pork

cerebro brain

cereza cherry

cerradura lock

cerrado, -a closed

cerrar to lock

cerveza beer

cicatriz (f.) scar

ciego, -a blind

ciento one hundred; por ciento, percent

cierto certain

cinta ribbon, tape

cintura waist

cinturón (m.) belt

ciruela plum; ciruela pasa, prune

cirugía surgery

cirujano surgeon

ciudad (f.) city

clara egg white

claro, -a clear; claro, certainly, of course

clase (f.) kind, type, class

clave (f.) code, key

clínica de reposo nursing home

cloro bleach

cobalto cobalt

coca cola drink

cocido, -a cooked, stewed

coctel (m.) coctail; coctel de fruta, fruit cocktail

coche (m.) car

codo elbow

coito intercourse, coitus; interrupción de coito, coitus interruptus

cojo, -a lame

col (f.) cabbage; col de Bruselas, Brussels sprout

colapso nervioso nervous breakdown

cólera cholera

colesterina (f.), colesterol (m.) cho-lesterol; nivel de colesterol, choles-terol count

colgar to dangle, to hang

coliflor (f.) cauliflower

colmillo eyetooth

colon (m.) colon

columna vertebral spinal column

coma coma

comer to eat

comida food, meal, dinner

como as, like, how; cómo, how? what? how . . .!; ¿cómo no? or ¡cómo no! of course

cómodo, -a comfortable

complaciente pleasing

componer to set (a fracture)

comprar to buy

comprender to understand

compresa compress

compuesto, -a compound; fixed (repaired)

con with; con frecuencia, frequently, often; con mucho gusto,
gladly; con permiso, with your
permission; con regularidad,
regularly

concentrado, -a concentrated

condado county

condón (m.) condom

conejo rabbit; examen de conejo,
rabbit test

confuso, -a confused

congelado, -a congealed, frozen, frostbitten

congénito, -a congenital

conseguir to get, to obtain

conservar to keep

constipación head cold, stuffy nose;
constipación de vientre, constipation

constipado, -a constipated

consulta consultation

contado: al contado cash

contagiar to infect

contaminado, -a contaminated

contaminar to contaminate, to infect

contento, -a happy

conteo count, blood count

contra against

contracepción (f.) birth control,
contraception

corazón (m.) heart

corbata necktie

corcho cork

cordal (m.) wisdom tooth

cordero lamb

córnea cornea

corona crown

corpiño bra, brassiere

corral (m.) playpen

correa strap

correos post office

corriente (f.) de aire draft

corrompido, -a putrid, rotten

cortar to cut

cortado, -a cut

cortés courteous

cortinas blinds, drapes

cosa thing

costilla rib; costillas asadas, pork
ribs

coyuntura joint

cráneo cranium

creer to believe

crema cream, ointment

cruzar to cross; cruzar pruebas, to
cross-match

cuajado, -a set, curdled; leche
cuajada, junket

cuál, cuáles what?, which?

cualquier any

cuándo when?; cuando usted quiera, whenever you want; desde cuándo?, how
long?

cuánto, -a how much?

cuántos, -as how many?

cuarto quarter; quart; room; cuarto de
niños, nursery

cubrir cover

cuchara spoon

cucharada tablespoonful

cucharadita teaspoonful

cucharilla, cucharita teaspoon

cuchilla de afeitar razor blade

cuchillo knife

cuello neck; cuello uterino, cuello de la matriz, cervix

cuenta bill

cuerda string

cuerpo body; cuerpo extraño, foreign body

cuesta it costs, does it cost

cuidado care; cuidado intenso, intensivo, intensive care

cuidarse to take care of oneself

cuna cradle, crib

cuña bedpan

cuñada sister-in-law

cuñado brother-in-law

cura (m.) priest

cura (f.) cure

curar to cure

curita Band-Aid

cutis (m.) complexion, skin

Ch

chaleco vest

champiñón (m.) mushroom

chancro chancre

chaqueta jacket

chata bedpan

cheque (m.) check

chícharo pea

chile (m.) hot pepper; chile relleno, stuffed pepper

choque (m.) shock; choque anafiláctico, anaphylactic shock

chorizo sausage

chuleta chop; chuleta de puerco, pork chop

chupar to suck

D

dama lady

dar to give; dar de alta, to discharge, dismiss; dar de comer, to feed; dar de mamar, to nurse; dar el pecho, to breastfeed

de from, of

debajo, debajo de under

deber ought, should; to owe

débil weak

debilidad (f.) weakness

decir to say, tell

dedo finger; dedo del pie, toe

defecar to defecate, to have a bowel movement

defecto defect

defribrilador (m.) defibrillator

deglutir to swallow

dejar to leave (behind)

delantal (m.) apron

delante, delante de in front, in front of

delgado, -a thin, slender

delirando delirious

demasiado too much

demora delay

dentadura denture, set of teeth; dentadura parcial, partial plate

dentista (m. or f.) dentist

depósito deposit

derecho, -a right; a la derecha, to the right

desagradable unpleasant

desangrarse to bleed profusely

desastre (m.) disaster

desayunar(se) to eat breakfast

desayuno breakfast

descansar to rest

descanso rest

descremar to skim; leche descremada, skimmed milk

desde since

desecho discharge; desecho de sangre, discharge of blood

deshidratado, -a dehydrated

desmayar to faint

desmayo fainting spell

despacio slowly; más despacio, more slowly

despertarse to wake up; despiértese, wake up (imperative)

después later; después de, after

destemplanza malaise, indisposition

desventaja disadvantage

detrás, detrás de behind

día (m.) day

diabetes (f.) diabetes

diafragma (m.) diaphragm

diario newspaper; daily

diarrea diarrhea

dice you say; he, she says

diente (m.) tooth; dientes postizos, bridgework, dentures

dieta diet

dietista (m. or f.) dietitian

difunto, -a dead person

diga, dígame tell me

diligente hard-working

dinero money

dirección (f.) address

disco disc; disco calcificado, calcified disc; disco desplazado, slipped disc

dispositivo device; dispositivo intrauterino, intrauterine device, IUD

distrofía muscular muscular dystrophy

divorciado, -a divorced, divorcée

doblar to bend, to fold

doble double

docena dozen

dólar dollar

doler to ache, to be sore, to have pain;

dolor (m.) pain; dolor expulsivo, expulsive pain; dolor fantasma, ghost pain; dolor de parto, labor pain; tener dolor, to be in pain

dónde where?; a dónde, (to) where?; de dónde, (from) where?

dormir sleep

dracma (m.) dram

droga drug

ducha shower, douche

duele it aches; me duele, my . . . aches; le duele, your, his her . . . aches

dulces candy, sweets

durante during

durar to last

durazno (m.) peach

E

efectivo, -a effective; en efectivo, cash

eficaz effective

ejercicio exercise

ejote (m.) green bean

el (m.) the

electrocardiograma (m.) electrocardiogram

eliminar to eliminate, to have a bowel movement, to urinate

elote (m.) corn on the cob

embarazada pregnant

embarazo pregnancy; embarazo tubárico, tubal pregnancy, ectopic pregnancy

embolia embolism, embolus

embriagado, -a intoxicated

embrujado, -a bewitched

emergencia emergency; sala de emergencia, emergency room

empaste (m.) filling (of a tooth)

empezar to begin; empieza, you begin; he, she begins

emplasto poultice

en in, on, at, around; en frente, in front

enagua slip (lingerie)

encantar to like very much, to love; me encanta(n), I love it (them); le encanta(n), you love it, them; he, she loves it (them)

encías gums

encinta pregnant

encubrir to cover over, to cover up

enderezar to straighten

enema enema

enfermedad (f.) disease, illness

enfermería nursing

enfermero, -a nurse; enfermera especial, special nurse

enfermo, -a sick

enfisema emphysema

enfriar(se) to chill, to cool, to get cold

enjuagar(se) to rinse

enlatado, -a canned

enojado, -a angry

enredado, -a tangled

ensalada salad

ensuciar to dirty; to have a bowel movement, to defecate

enterrado, -a ingrown

entierro burial

entonces then

entrada entrance, admission, admittance

entrar to enter

entrepierna crotch

enyesar to put in a plaster cast

eructar to belch

eructo belch

erupción (f.) rash

es you are; he, she is; es cierto, it is true; es seguro, it is certain

escalofrío chill

escarlatina scarlet fever

escaso, -a scarce, sparse

escoger to choose, to select

escribir to write

escudo shield, IUD shield

escupir to spit

esófago esophagus

espalda back

espárrago asparagus

espasmo spasm

especializado, -a specialized, specialist

espejo mirror

espejuelos eyeglasses

esperanza hope

esperar to wait, to hope

espermatozoide (m.) spermatozoid

espermicida spermicide

espeso, -a thick

espinaca spinach

espiral (f.) spiral (IUD)

esplín (m.) spleen

esponja sponge

esposa wife

esposo husband

esputo sputum, saliva

esquite (m.) popcorn

esta (f.), este (m.), esto (n.) this

está you are; he, she is; ¿cómo está? how are you?, how is he, she?

estado state, stage; en estado, en estado de gestación, pregnant; estado secundario, secondary stage

Estados Unidos United States

estampilla stamp

están you (pl.) are; they are

estar to be, to stay

estas, estos those

esterilizador (m.) sterilizer

estómago stomach

estornudar to sneeze

estreñido, -a constipated

estricto, -a strict

estuche (m.) case; estuche de drogas de emergencia, emergency drug kit

estupor (m.) stupor

etiqueta label

evacuación (f.) bowel movement, BM, stool

evitar to avoid

examen (m.) examination

exánime lifeless, limp

excusado toilet

explosión (f.) boom, explosion

exponer to expose

expulsivo, -a expulsive

extraer to extract

F

factor factor; factor Rhesus, Rh factor

faja girdle, belt

falda skirt

Falopio Fallopian; trompa de Falopio, Fallopian tube

falta lack; falta de aire, shortness of breath

fallar to fail

fallo cardíaco cardiac arrest

fatiga fatigue

favor de + infinitive please + verb; por favor, please

fecha date; fecha de nacimiento, date of birth

feliz happy

feo, -a ugly

fibroma fibroma, cyst, fibrous tumor

fibrosis (f.) quística cystic fibrosis

fideo noodle, spaghetti

fiebre (f.) fever; fiebre amarilla, yellow fever; fiebre reumática, rheumatic fever; fiebre tifoidea, typhoid fever

firma signature

firmar to sign

fisioterapia physiotherapy

flaco, -a skinny

flan (m.) custard, pudding

flema phlegm

flojo, -a loose

flor (f.) flower

florero vase

flujo flow; flujo purulento, pus

fondo bottom; slip (lingerie)

fosa nasal nostril

fractura fracture

fracturado, -a fractured

fracturar to fracture

frambuesa raspberry

frasco bottle, flask, vial

frazada blanket

frecuentemente frequently

freír to fry

frente (m.) front

frente (f.) forehead

fresa strawberry

fresco, -a fresh, impudent

frijol (m.) bean; frijol blanco, navy bean

frío, -a cold (temperature)

frito, -a fried

frotis (m.) smear; frotis de Papanicolaou, Pap smear

fruta fruit

fuente (f.) bag of waters; fountain, drinking fountain

fuerte strong, intense

fuerza strength

fumar to smoke

funda pillowcase

funeral (m.) funeral

funeraria funeral home

G

gabinete (m.) cabinet, closet; gabinete para la ropa, clothes closet

galón (m.) gallon

galleta cookie, cracker; galleta blanca, soda cracker

ganar to gain, to win, to earn

ganas: tener ganas de + infinitive to feel like + -ing

gangrena gangrene

garganta throat

garrapata tick (insect)

gas (m.) gas, flatulence

gasa (m.) gauze

gelatina gelatin; gelatin dessert; vaginal jelly; gelatina de fruta, fruit gelatin

gemelos twins

genitales (m., pl.) genitals

gente (f.) people

germen (m.) germ

germicida (m.) germicide

globo globe; globo del ojo, eyeball

glóbulo corpuscle; glóbulo blanco, white corpuscle; glóbulo rojo, red corpuscle

glucosa glucose

golpe (m.) blow, contusion

goma rubber, condom; glue

gonorrea gonorrhea

gordo, -a fat, thick

gorro cervical cervical cap

gota gout

gracias thanks; muchas gracias, many thanks, thanks a lot

gracioso, -a funny

grado degree

gramo gram

grande large

grano sore, pimple; grain

grasa fat, grease

grasoso, -a greasy, fatty

grave serious, seriously ill

gripe (f.) flu, influenza

gris gray

gritar to yell, to scream

grito yell, scream

grueso heavy, thick

guajalote, guajolote (m.) turkey

guapo, -a handsome

guardar to keep, to put away

guisante (m.) pea

gustar to like; me gusta(n), I like; le gusta(n), you like; he, she likes

gusto taste, pleasure; con mucho gusto, gladly; mucho gusto, pleased to meet you

H

ha (auxiliary verb) you have; he, she has; ha sentido, you have felt; he, she has felt; ha tenido, you have had; he, she has had

haba lima bean, large bean

habichuela green bean

hablar to speak

hacer to do, to make; hago, I make, do; hace, you make, do; he, she makes, does; hace calor, it is hot; hace frío, it is cold; hace + time, for + duration of time

hambre (f.) hunger; tener hambre, to be hungry

hamburguesa hamburger

harina flour

hasta until

hay there is, there are; hay que +
  infinitive, one should, one must

heces feces

helado ice cream

hemorragia bleeding, hemorrhaging;
  hemorragia nasal, nosebleed

hemorroides (f.) hemorrhoids

herida incision, wound; herida de bala,
  gunshot wound

herido, -a injured

hermana sister

hermano brother

hermoso, -a beautiful

hervido, -a boiled

hervir to boil

hervor (m.) heartburn

hiedra venenosa poison ivy

hielo ice; sherbet

hierro iron

hígado liver

hija daughter

hijo son

hijos children

hinchado, -a swollen

hinchar to swell

hinchazón (m.) swelling

hipo hiccough

hombre (m.) man; hombre de negocios,
  businessman

hombro shoulder

hongo mushroom

hora time, hour

hormigueo tingling

horno oven; al horno, baked

hospicio orphanage

hoy today

hueso bone

huevo egg; huevo duro, hard-boiled
  egg; huevo frito, fried egg; huevo
  hervido en agua, poached egg; huevos
  con jamón, ham and eggs; huevo pasado
  por agua, soft-boiled egg; huevos
  revueltos, scrambled eggs; huevos con
  tocino, bacon and eggs

humano, -a human

humilde humble

I

ictericia jaundice

impactado, -a impacted

impétigo impetigo

incapacidad (f.) disability

incubación (f.) incubation

incubadora incubator

infancia childhood, infancy

infarto infarct

infectado, -a infected

inferior lower, inferior

inflamado, -a inflamed

influenza flu, influenza

ingle (f.) groin

inglés English

ingresar to be admitted

injerto graft

inmunizar to immunize

inodoro toilet

insecticida insecticide

insolación (f.) sunstroke

insomnio insomnia

intensivo, -a intensive

intenso, -a intensive

interior inner

intestino intestine

intrauterino, -a intrauterine; dispositivo intrauterino, intrauterine device,
  IUD

inyección (f.) injection, shot;
  inyección secundaria, booster shot

ir to go

izquierdo, -a left; a la izquierda, to
  the left

J

jabón (m.) soap; jabón germicida, germicidal soap

jalea jelly

jamón ham

jaqueca headache, migraine headache

jarabe (m.) syrup; jarabe para la tos,
  cough syrup

jarra pitcher

jefe (m.) head, chief, boss; jefe de la
  casa, head of household

jeringuilla syringe

jorobado, -a hunchback, hunchbacked

judío, -a Jewish

jugar to play

jugo juice; jugo gástrico, gastric
  juice; jugo de naranja, orange juice;
  jugo de tomate, tomato juice

juguete (m.) toy

justillo bra, brassiere

K

kilogramo kilogram

kleenex (m.) face tissue

L

la, las the, her, them (direct object
  pronoun)

labio lip

labor (f.) labor

laboratorio laboratory

ladillas crab lice

lado side; al lado, beside, next to;
  ponerse de lado, to turn on one's
  side

lámpara lamp

laparoscopía laparoscopy

lápiz (m.) pencil; lápiz de cejas, eyebrow pencil; lápiz de labios, lipstick

laringe (f.) larynx

laringitis (f.) laryngitis

lástima shame, pity; ¡qué lástima!,
  what a pity!

lastimado, -a injured, hurt

lastimar to hurt, to injure

lata can (container)

latido heartbeat, throb

latir to beat, to throb

lavado enema

lavamanos (m., sing.) lavatory,
  washbowl

lavar(se) to wash (oneself); lavarse
  los dientes, to brush one's teeth

lavativa enema

laxante (m.) laxative

lazo loop (IUD)

lección (f.) lesson

leche (f.) milk; leche con chocolate,
  chocolate milk; leche condensada, con-
  densed milk; leche descremada, skimmed
  milk; leche evaporada, evaporated
  milk; leche de magnesia, milk of magnesia; leche en polvo, powdered milk

lechuga lettuce

legumbre (f.) vegetable, legume

lejía lye

lejos far away, far

lengua tongue

lentes (m.) lenses, glasses; lentes
  de contacto, contact lenses

lesión (f.) sore, injury

letargo lethargy

levantar to raise; levantarse, to get
  up, to stand up; levantarse la manga,
  to roll up one's sleeve

leve minor, light

libra pound

libro book; libro de cheques, checkbook

liendre (f.) nit

ligadura tie, bond, ligature

ligar to tie

lima lime

limón (m.) lemon

limpiar to clean

limpieza cleaning, cleanliness; agente
de limpieza, cleaning fluid

limpio, -a clean

líquido liquid

lisiado, -a crippled, maimed

lisiar to cripple

listo, -a ready

litro liter

lívido, -a livid

lo him, you, it

local local

loco, -a crazy, insane

locura insanity

lombriz (f.) worm

los (m., pl.) the

lucidez (f.) sanity

lucha fight

luego later, then

lumbre (f.) fire

lunar (m.) mole, blemish

luz (f.) light; encender la luz,
turn on the light

Ll

llamar(se) to call, to be named; me
llamo, my name is; se llama, your,
his, her name is

llanto cry

llave key

llevar to wear, to take with one,
to carry

llorar to cry

M

madrastra stepmother

madre (f.) mother

maíz (m.) corn; maíz tierno, sweet corn

mal bad, badly

maleta suitcase

maletín (m.) kit; maletín de drogas de
emergencia, emergency drug kit

malo, -a bad; ill, sick

mamar to suck, to suckle; dar de mamar,
to breastfeed

manco, -a maimed or crippled in the
hand

mancha spot, stain

manchado, -a stained, spotted

mandíbula jaw

manejar to drive, to handle

manga sleeve

mango mango (fruit); a handle

manicomio mental institution, insane
asylum

mantequilla butter

manzana apple

mañana tomorrow; morning; de la
mañana, A.M.; por la mañana, en la
mañana, in the morning

maquillaje (m.) makeup

maquillarse to put on makeup

máquina de afeitar razor

marca mark

marcar to mark

mareo dizziness

marido husband

marisco shellfish

mármol (m.) marble

más more, most; más despacio, more slowly; más rapido, more quickly

masaje (m.) massage

mascar to chew

mascarilla mask

mastectomía mastectomy

masticar to chew

matriz (f.) uterus

mayonesa mayonnaise

mayor older, oldest; major

me me, to me

mear to urinate

mecánico mechanic

medianoche (f.) midnight

medias hose, stockings; medias pantalón, panty hose

médico doctor

medida measure

medio, -a half

mediodía (m.) noon

medir to measure

mejilla cheek

mejor better; mejorarse, to get better; que se mejore, I hope you get better

melocotón (m.) peach

melón melon; melón de agua, watermelon

membrana membrane

menor younger, youngest; menor de edad, (a) minor

menos less, least, minus

mente (f.) mind

merienda snack

mermelada jam

mertiolato Merthiolate

mes (m.) month; al mes, per month; por meses, by the month

mesa table

metadona methadone

método method

metro meter

mi, mis my

microbio germ, microbe

microscopio microscope

miedo fear; tener miedo, to be afraid

miel (f.) honey

miembro limb, member; miembro artificial, artificial limb

miligramo milligram

mililitro milliliter

ministro minister, pastor

mirar to look at

mitad (f.) a half

moderado, -a moderate

mojado, -a wet

mojar to wet; mojarse, to get wet

molestar to bother, to annoy

molestia discomfort

momentáneo, -a of short duration

moneda coin

monja nun

mono, -a cute

morder to bite, to chew

mordida bite; mordida de serpiente, snakebite

morir to die

mortificado, -a worried, upset

mover to move

mucosidad (f.) mucus

mucoso, -a mucous

muchacha girl

muchacho boy

mucho, -a much, a lot

muchos, -as many

muela molar, tooth; muela del juicio, wisdom toot

muerte (f.) death

muerto, -a dead

muestra sample, specimen

mujer (f.) woman, wife

muleta crutch

muñeca wrist; doll

murmullo murmur

músculo muscle

muslo thigh

muy very

N

nacer to be born

nacimiento birth

nació you were born; he, she was born

nada nothing; de nada, you are welcome, don't mention it

nalga buttock

naranja orange; color de naranja, orange color

nariz (f.) nose; nariz tapada, tupida, stuffy nose

nasal nasal; congestión nasal, nasal congestion; fosa nasal, nostril

náusea(s) nausea

necesario, -a necessary

necesidad (f.) need, necessity

necesitar to need

negativo, -a negative

negocios business

negro, -a black, dark

nervio nerve

nerviosidad (f.) nervousness

nervioso, -a nervous

nieta granddaughter

nieto grandson

nieve (f.) snow; sherbet, ice cream

ninguno no one, none

niña girl, baby girl

niño boy, baby boy, child

niños children

no no, not

noche (f.) night; de noche, at night; de la noche, P.M.; por la noche, in the evening, during the night

nombre (m.) name

notificar to notify

novia fiancee, steady girlfriend, sweetheart

novio fiance, steady boyfriend, sweetheart

nudo knot, bow (IUD)

nuera daughter-in-law

nuevo, -a new

número number

nunca never

O

obeso, -a obese

obscuro, -a dark

obstruir to block, to obstruct

oficina office

oído inner ear; hearing

ojalá I hope so

ojo eye

olor (m.) odor, smell

ombligo umbilical cord; navel

onza ounce

orden (m.) order, series

orden (f.) order, authorization; orden escrita, written order

oreja outer ear; ear lobe

orgullo pride

orgulloso, -a proud

orinal (m.) urinal

ortopédico dental orthodontist

ortopedista (m. or f.) orthopedist

orzuelo sty

ostra oyster

otro, -a other, another

oxígeno oxygen

P

paciente (m. or f.) patient

padezco I suffer

padrastro stepfather

padre (m.) father

padres (m.) fathers, parents

pagar to pay

pago payment, fee; I pay

paja speck, straw

pajamas, pijamas pajamas

palangana washbowl

paleta bedpan; shoulderblade

palidez (f.) paleness

pálido, -a pale

palma de la mano palm of the hand

palta avocado

paludismo malaria

pan (m.) bread; pan blanco, white bread; pan dulce, sweet roll; pan duro, stale bread; pan moreno, dark bread; pan tostado, toast

páncreas (m.) pancreas

pantaletas panties

pantalón (m.) pants, panties

pantalones (m.) pants, slacks, trousers

pantuflas slippers (bedroom)

pañal (m.) diaper

papa potato; papa asada, baked potato; papas fritas, French fries; puré de papas, mashed potatoes

papá daddy, papa

papel (m.) paper; papel de baño, toilet tissue; papel de escribir, stationery

paperas mumps

para for, in order to, to

parálisis (f.) infantil infantile paralysis

paralizado, -a paralyzed

parásito parasite

parche (m.) dressing, patch

parejo, -a even, smooth

parentesco relationship

pariente (m. or f.) relative

paro cardíaco cardiac arrest

parótidas parotid glands

parotiditis (f.) mumps

párpado eyelid

parrilla grill, broiler; a la parrilla, grilled, broiled, barbecued

parte (f.) part

parto childbirth, birth, delivery; parto cesáreo, Cesarean birth; parto natural, natural childbirth

pasa raisin

pasa: ¿qué pasa?, what is the matter?; ¿qué le pasa?, what is the matter with with you?

pasar to pass; to happen, to occur; to enter

pase come in (imperative)

pasillo hall

paso step

pastel (m.) pie, pastry; pastel de cereza, cherry pie; pastel de limón, lemon pie; pastel de manzana, apple pie

pastilla tablet, lozenge, pill

patata potato

pato duck; bedpan (male)

pavo turkey

peca freckle

pecho chest; dar el pecho, to breast-feed

pedazo piece

pedir to ask for; pedir prestado, to borrow

peinar(se) to comb (one's hair)

peine (m.) comb

pelar to peel; to cut (hair)

peligro danger

pelo hair

peluca wig

pelvis (f.) pelvis

pena pity; ¡qué pena!, what a pity!

pene (m.) penis

pensar to think, to believe

pentotal (m.) de sodio sodium pentothal

peor worse

pepinillo pickle

pepino cucumber

pequeño, -a little, small (size)

pera pear

perder to lose

pérdida loss

perdido, -a lost

perejil (m.) parsley

perineo perineum

periódico newspaper, periodical

período menstrual period

permiso permission; con permiso, excuse me

persona person

pesar(se) to weigh; to get weighed

pescado fish

peso weight

pestaña eyelash

peste bubónica plague

peticote (m.) slip (lingerie)

pezón (m.) nipple (of female breast)

picada, picadura insect bite

picante spicy (hot)

picar to itch; me pica, it itches; ¿le pica?, does it itch?

picazón (f.) itching

pie foot; pie de la cama, foot of the bed

piedra stone

piel (f.) skin, fur

pierna leg

pijamas pajamas

píldora pill; píldoras para dormir, sleeping pills

pimienta pepper (table)

pimiento bell pepper

pinchar to prick, to puncture

pinta pint

pintura de labios lipstick

pinza pliers, forceps, tweezers

piña pineapple

piojos lice

piorrea pyorrhea

pisada step

pisar to step on

piso floor (of a building)

placa plate; placa de metal, metal plate; placa de rayos X, x-ray picture

plástica: cirugía plástica plastic surgery

plátano banana

platillo saucer

plato dish, plate

plazo: a plazos on terms, on credit

pluma pen, feather

población (f.) population

pobre poor

poco, -a little (amount)

poder to be able, can; power

poliomielitis (f.) polio, poliomyelitis

póliza policy

polvo powder, dust

pollo chicken; pollo asado, baked chicken; pollo frito, fried chicken; caldo de pollo, chicken broth; sopa de pollo, chicken soup

pomada salve

poner to put, to turn on, to give;
  ponerse, to put on; ponerse de lado,
  to turn on one's side; póngase, put
  on (imperative)

por for, per; por favor, please;
  ¿por qué?, why?; porque, because

por ciento percent

positivo, -a positive

postilla scab

postizo, -a false; dentadura postiza,
  false teeth

postoperativo, -a postoperative

postración (f.) del calor heat prostration

postre (m.) dessert

potable: agua potable drinking water

precioso, -a darling, precious

pregunta question

preguntar to ask (a question)

prenatal prenatal, predelivery

prender to turn on; to fasten

preocupado, -a worried

presentar to introduce; presentarle,
  to introduce to you, him, her

presilla clip, fastener, loop

presión (f.) pressure; presión alta,
  high blood pressure; presión baja,
  low blood pressure; presión de la
  sangre, blood pressure

prestado, -a lent

prestar to lend

preventivo, -a preventive

primero, -a first; primeros auxilios,
  first aid

primo, -a cousin

principal main, principal

privado, -a private

privar to deprive

probar to taste; to test

problema (m.) problem

profundo, -a deep(ly); profundamente,
  deeply

prolongado, -a prolonged

promesa promise

prometer to promise

pronto soon

próstata prostate

proteger(se) to protect (oneself)

prueba test; pruebas cruzadas, cross-
  match

puede you, he, she can; se puede, one
  can

puedo I can

puerco pork; chuleta de puerco, pork
  chop

pujar to push

pujo expulsive contraction, a pushing
  sensation

pulga flea

pulgada inch

pulgar (m.) thumb

pulmón (m.) lung; pulmón de acero,
  pulmotor, iron lung, pulmotor

pulmonía bronquial bronchopneumonia

pulsación (f.) beat, throb, pulse

pulsera bracelet

pulso pulse

puntada stitch

punto stitch; period; puntos negros,
  black spots

puño fist; cerrar el puño, to make a
  fist

pupila pupil

purgante (m.) laxative, purgative

pus (m.) pus

pústula pustule, pimple

Q

que which, that; lo que, that which

qué? what? which?; ¿qué tal? how are
  things?

quebrado, -a broken

quebrar to break

quedar(se) to stay, to remain

quemado, -a burned, sunburned

quemar(se) to burn; to get burned

queque (m.) cake

querer to want, to wish; to love

querido, -a dear, darling

queso cheese; queso amarillo, yellow
cheese; queso blanco, white cheese;
queso crema, cream cheese; queso
requesón, cottage cheese

quien who, whom; quienes, who (pl.);
a quien(es), whom

quién who?; quiénes?, who (pl.)?

quiere you want; he, she wants

quiero I want

quitar to take (from someone); quitarse,
to take off; quítese, take off
(imperative)

R

rábano radish

rabia rabies

radio radio; radius; radium

radiografía x-ray

radioterapia x-ray therapy; radium
therapy

raíz (f.) root; canal (m.) de la raíz,
root canal

rápido, -a quick, fast, rapid(ly);
rápidamente, rapidly

raquídea spinal anesthesia

rascar(se) to scratch (oneself)

rasgar to tear, to rip

rasurar to shave

rebanada slice

receta prescription; recipe

recibir to receive

recibo receipt

reconocimiento examination; reconocimiento completo, complete examination; reconocimiento médico, physical examination

recto rectum

recuento blood count

regadera shower; baño de regadera,
shower

regla menstrual period; rule

reglamento regulation

reír(se) to laugh; se ríe, you laugh,
he, she laughs, smiles

relaciones (f.) sexuales intercourse,
sexual relations

relajar to relax

reloj (m.) watch, clock

relleno dressing, stuffing; stuffed

remolacha beet

repente: de repente suddenly

repollo cabbage

resfriado, resfrío cold (disease)

resfriarse to catch a cold

residuo residue; residuo bajo, low
residue

respiración (f.) breath, breathing;
respiración artificial, artificial
respiration; respiración boca a boca,
mouth-to-mouth resuscitation; respiración corta, shortness of breath;
respiración profunda, deep breath

respirar to breathe

responsable responsible party

resto remainder, residue; el resto,
the rest

resucitador (m.) resuscitator;
resucitador cardiopulmonar, cardiopulmonary resuscitator

resultado result

retirada withdrawal

revés (m.) setback

revista magazine

revuelto, -a upset, stirred up

rico, -a rich; delicious

riñón (m.) kidney

ritmo rhythm

rodilla knee

rojo, -a red

rollo roller, curler

romper to break, to tear

ronquera hoarseness

ropa clothes, clothing; ropa de cama, bed linens; ropa de dormir, night-clothes

ropero closet

rosa rose; color de rosa, pink

rosbif (m.) beef, roast beef

roto, -a broken

rubéola German measles

ruído noise

S

sábana sheet

saber to find out, to know

sabio, -a wise

sabor (m.) taste, flavor

sabroso, -a delicious

sacar to take out

sal (f.) salt

sala room; sala de emergencia, sala de urgencia, emergency room; sala de partos, delivery room; sala prenatal, predelivery room

salchicha sausage

salida exit

salir to leave (a place)

saliva saliva, spit

salpullido rash

salsa sauce; salsa de ensalada, salad dressing; salsa de tomate, catsup, tomato sauce

salubridad (f.) public health

salud (f.) health

saludar to greet

saludo greeting; saludo de mano, hand-shake

salvavidas (m. or f.) lifeguard, life preserver

sanar to heal

sandía watermelon

sangrando bleeding

sangrar to bleed

sangre (f.) blood

sarampión (m.) measles

se + verb one + verb

sé (saber) I know

sebáceo, -a sebaceous

sebo fat

secar to dry

seco, -a dried, dry

sed (f.) thirst; tener sed, to be thirsty

seguida succession, continuation; en seguida, right away

seguir to follow

según according to

seguro insurance; es seguro, it's certain; seguro social, social security

seleccionar to choose, to select

sello stamp, seal

semana week; a la semana, per week

semilla seed, sperm

sencillo, -a simple, plain

sensible sensitive, feeling; reasonable

sensitivo, -a sensitive, touchy

sentimiento feeling

separado, -a separated

separar to put away from, to spread apart, to separate

sequedad (f.) dryness

ser to be

serio, -a serious

servilleta napkin; servilleta sanitaria, sanitary napkin

servir to serve

si if

sí yes, indeed

siente (sentir): se siente you feel;
  he, she feels

siéntese (sentarse) sit down (imperative)

siento: lo siento I'm sorry; me siento,
  I feel

signos vitales vital signs

silla chair; silla de ruedas, wheelchair

silleta bedpan

simpático, -a pleasing, nice

sin without

síncope (m.) syncope; fainting spell

síntoma (m.) symptom

sirve you serve; he, she serves; se
  sirve it is served

sobaco armpit

sobre (m.) envelope

sobre over, above

sobrecama bedspread

sobrina niece

sobrino nephew

socorro help

soda soda pop, carbonated beverage

solo, -a alone

sólo, solamente only

soltero, -a single (not married)

son you (pl.) are; they are

sonar to ring, to sound; sonarse la
  nariz, to blow one's nose

sonda catheter

sondear to catheterize

sopa soup

sopero soup bowl

soplar to blow; soplarse la nariz, to
  blow one's nose

soplo murmur (heart)

soporte (m.) brace, support, base

sorbete (m.) sherbet

sordo, -a deaf

sortija jeweled ring

sospechar to suspect

sostén (m.) bra, brassiere

sostener to support, to hold

su, sus his, her, your, their

sucio, -a dirty, soiled

sudar to perspire, to sweat

sudor (m.) sweat, perspiration

suegra mother-in-law

suegro father-in-law

suelo ground, floor

suero serum; suero intravenoso, intravenous serum, IV fluid

suéter (m.) sweater

suficiente sufficient, enough

sufrir to suffer

suicidarse to commit suicide

suicidio suicide

sujetar to hold

sulfa sulfa

superior upper

supermercado supermarket

supurar to suppurate, to discharge

susto scare, frightening experience;
  ¡qué susto!, how frightening!

T

tableta tablet

tacto touch; tacto rectal, rectal
  examination

tachar to scratch out

tajada slice

talco talcum powder

talón (m.) heel

tallarines (m., pl.) noodles

tamaño size

tampón (m.) tampon

tanto, -a so much, as much

tantos, -as many, as many, so many

tapa cover

tapioca pudding

tapón (m.) plug, cap, cork, tampon

tarde (f.) afternoon; de la tarde, P.M.; por la tarde, en la tarde, in the afternoon

tarde late

tartamudo, -a stutterer

taza cup; bedpan; dentist's bowl; taza de medir, measuring cup; taza de orinar, bedpan; taza de vomitar, emesis basin

tazón (m.) basin, bowl

té (m.) tea; té helado, iced tea

tejido tissue (body); fabric

tela adhesiva adhesive tape

televisor (m.), televisión (f.) television

temblor (m.) tremor

temperatura temperature

temprano, -a early

tenazas forceps

tenedor (m.) fork

tener to have; tener calor, to be hot; tener frío, to be cold; tener hambre, to be hungry; tener miedo, to be afraid; tener razón, to be right; tener sed, to be thirsty; tener sueño, to be sleepy; tener que + infinitive, to have to + verb

tengo I have

termómetro thermometer

termoterapia heat therapy

ternera veal

testículo testicle

testigo witness

teta nipple, teat

tétano tetanus

tetera, teto nipple (of nursing bottle)

tetracloruro de carbón carbon tetrachloride

tía aunt

tibio, -a warm

tiene you have; he, she has; ¿qué tiene?, what's the matter?

tifo typhus

tifoidea typhoid

tijeras scissors

timbre (m.) bell

tina tub

tío uncle

tipo type; tipo y cruzar pruebas, type and cross-match

tira strap

tiro shot (gun); tiro de bala, gunshot

tiroides (f.) thyroid

toalla towel

toallita washcloth

tobillo ankle

tocar to ring (bell); to touch

tocino bacon; huevos con tocino, bacon and eggs

todavía yet; todavía no, not yet

todo, -a all, everything, every; todos, -as, everybody; todas las noches, every night; todos los días, every day

tomar to drink, to take; tome, drink, take (imperative)

tomate (m.) tomato

torcido, -a twisted

torniquete (m.) tourniquet

toronja grapefruit

tortícolis (m.) wry neck, torticollis

tos (f.) cough; tos ferina, whooping cough

toser to cough

total complete, total

trabajar to work

trabajo work, job

trabilla small strap, clasp

traer to bring

tragar to swallow

traigo I bring

traje (m.) suit; traje pantalón, pants suit

tranquilizante (m.) tranquilizer

tranquilo, -a calm; estar tranquilo, to be calm, to be resting

transmisible communicable

tráquea trachea

tratar to try, to deal; tratar de + infinitive, to try to + verb

trauma (m.) trauma

trementina turpentine

tripa intestine; tripe

triste· sad

trompa tube; horn; trompa de Eustaquio, Eustachian tube; trompa de Falopio, Fallopian tube

tronco trunk

tu, tus your (familiar)

tú you (familiar)

tubárico tubal; embarazo tubárico, tubal pregnancy

tubo tube

tullido, -a crippled (any limb)

turno turn, appointment; de turno, on duty; es su turno, it's your turn; turno de día, day shift; turno de noche, night shift

U

úlcera ulcer

último, -a last

un, uno, una a, an, one

ungüento ointment

unos, -as some

unto smear; unto de Papanicolaou, Pap smear

uña nail; uña enterrada, ingrown nail

uréter (m.) ureter

uretra urethra

urgencia emergency; llamado de urgencia, emergency call

urticaria hives

usar to use

usted you (formal) (abbrev. Ud., Vd., V.)

utensilio utensil, silverware

útero uterus

uva grape

V

va you go; he, she goes

vacante empty

vacío vacuum

vacío, -a empty

vacuna vaccination, vaccine

vamos we go, let's go

van you (pl.) go; they go

vapor (m.) steam

vaporizador (m.) vaporizer

varicela chickenpox

várices (f., pl.) varicose veins

varicoso, -a varicose

varilla rod; varilla de metal, metal rod

varios, -as some, various

vasija basin, bowl, container

vaso glass

vecino, -a neighbor

vegetal (m.) vegetable

vejiga bladder

vello body hair, fuzz

vena vein; venas varicosas, varicose veins

venda bandage

vendaje (m.) bandage

vender to sell

veneno poison

venéreo, -a venereal

venir to come; vengo, I come

ventaja advantage

ver to see; veo, I see

verdad (f.) truth; es verdad, it's true

verde green

verdura green vegetables, greenery, foliage

verruga wart

vesícula gallbladder

vestido dress

vez (f.) time; veces, times; a veces, at times, sometimes; muchas veces, many times; pocas veces, few times, seldom; la primera vez, the first time; una vez, one time

viajar to travel

viejo, -a old

vientre (m.) stomach, abdomen

vigilante (m.) watchman

vigilar to watch

vinagre (m.) vinegar

vino wine

violar to rape

viruela smallpox

viruelas locas chickenpox

visión (f.) sight

visita visitor, visit

viuda widow

viudo widower

vivir to live, to reside

vivo, -a alive

volar to fly

voltearse to turn (oneself) over

volver to return

vómito vomit; vómitos de sangre, vomiting blood; vómitos de embarazo, morning sickness

voy I go, I am going

Y

y and

ya already

yarda yard (unit of measure)

yema yolk, heart, center; yema del dedo, fingertip; yema del huevo, egg yolk

yerno son-in-law

yeso plaster cast

yo I

yodo iodine

Z

zanahoria carrot

zapatilla slipper

zapato shoe

zona zone; zona postal, zip code, postal zone

English-Spanish Vocabulary

A

a, an un, una

abdomen abdomen (m.), vientre (m.)

able cápaz, hábil; to be able, poder

abortion aborto

about, concerning acerca de

about, nearly casi

above arriba, encima, sobre

abscess absceso

to abstain abstenerse

according to según

accustomed acostumbrado, -a; to become accustomed, acostumbrarse

ache dolor (m.)

to ache doler; my . . . aches, me duele; your, his, her . . . aches, le duele; they ache, duelen

acidity acidez (f.)

acupuncture acupuntura

to add añadir

added añadido, -a

addict, addicted adicto, -a

address dirección (f.)

adhesive adhesivo, -a; adhesive tape, tela adhesiva

admission, admittance admisión (f.), entrada; admission desk, admission office, oficina de admisión

to admit admitir

advantage ventaja

affected afectado, -a

afraid: to be afraid, tener miedo

after después de

again otra vez

against contra

air aire (m.)

air conditioning, air-conditioned aire-acondicionado

alive vivo, -a

all todo, -a

alone solo, -a

already ya

A.M. de la mañana

ammonia amoníaco

amputee, amputated amputado, -a

to analyze analizar

analyzer analizador (m.); blood oxygen analyzer, analizador del oxígeno de la sangre

anchovy anchoa

and y

anesthesiologist anestesiólogo, -a

angry enojado, -a; to become angry, enojarse

ankle tobillo

anthrax ántrax (m.)

antibody anticuerpo

antidote antídoto

antispasmodic antiespasmódico

antitetanic antitetánico

anus ano

any algún, alguno, alguna; cualquier, cualquiera

appendix apéndice (m.)

appetite apetito

apple manzana; apple pie, pastel (m.) de manzana

appointment turno, cita

apricot albaricoque (m.)

apron delantal (m.)

are: you are (sing.), es, está; you (pl.), they are, son, están; we are, somos, estamos; there are, hay

arm brazo

armpit axila, sobaco

around en

arrest: cardiac arrest, paro cardíaco

artificial respiration respiración (f.) artificial

ask: to ask for, pedir; to ask a question, preguntar

asparagus espárrago

assistance ayuda

assistant ayudante, asistente

asthma asma

asylum asilo; insane asylum, manicomio

at a, en

to attach añadir, unir

attached añadido, -a

attack ataque (m.); heart attack, ataque al corazón

to attack atacar, violar

attentive atento, -a

aunt tía

avocado aguacate (m.), palta

to avoid evitar

away lejos; far away, muy lejos; go away, váyase (imperative)

awful antipático, -a; horrible, terrible

B

baby bebé (m. or f.); niño, -a

back espalda; backache, dolor (m.) de espalda

bacon tocino; bacon and eggs, huevos con tocino

bad mal, malo, mala; badly, mal

baffled confundido, -a; confuso, -a

bag bolsa, bolso, cartera; ice bag, bolsa de hielo; bag of waters, fuente (f.)

to bake asar

baked asado, -a

baking soda bicarbonato

balanced balanceado, -a

banana plátano

bandage venda, vendaje (m.)

to bandage vendar

Band-Aid curita

barbecue barbacoa

base base (f.), soporte (m.)

basin bacín (m.), tazón (m.), vasija, bandeja, palangana

bath baño; to take a bath, bañarse

bathroom baño, cuarto de baño; bathroom tissue, papel (m.) de baño

be: to be, ser, estar

bean frijol (m.); green bean, ejote (m.) habichuela; lima bean, large bean, haba; navy bean, frijol blanco

beard barba

beautiful hermoso, -a; lindo, -a

because porque

bed cama; bed linens, ropa de cama; bedspread, sobrecama; to go to bed, acostarse

bedpan bacín (m.), bidet (m.), cuña, chata, pato, paleta, silleta, taza

bedtime la hora de acostarse

beef carne (f.) de res; roast beef, carne asada, rosbif (m.)

beer cerveza

beet remolacha, betabel (m.)

before antes de

to begin empezar; you (sing.) begin, empieza

behind detrás de

belch eructo

to belch eructar

to believe creer

bell timbre (m.)

belt cinturón (m.), faja

to bend doblar

benign benigno, -a

beside al lado de

best mejor

better mejor; to get better, mejorarse; I hope you get better, que se mejore

bewitched embrujado, -a

bill cuenta

billfold billetera, cartera

birth nacimiento; birth certificate, certificado de nacimiento; birth control, anticoncepción, contracepción; date of birth, fecha de nacimiento

biscuit panecillo

bite mordida; snakebite, mordida de serpiente; insect bite, picadura, picada, piquete (m.)

to bite morder

black negro, -a

bladder vejiga; gallbladder, vesícula

blade cuchilla, hoja; razor blade, cuchilla de afeitar

bland blando, -a; suave

blanket frazada, manta

bleach cloro

to bleed sangrar; to bleed profusely, desangrarse

bleeding sangrando; profuse bleeding, hemorragia

blind ciego, -a

blinds cortinas

blister ampolla

block obstrucción (f.)

to block obstruir, adormecer

blood sangre (f.); blood count, conteo de sangre, recuento; blood pressure, presión; blood test, examen (m.) de sangre

blouse blusa

blow golpe (m.)

to blow soplar; to blow one's nose, soplarse la nariz, sonarse la nariz

blue azul

bluish azuloso, -a

body cuerpo

boil forúnculo, grano

to boil hervir

boiled hervido, -a

bone hueso

book libro

boom explosión (f.)

booster shot inyección secundaria

born: to be born, nacer; you were born, he, she was born, nació

to borrow pedir prestado, -a

to bother molestar

bottle botella; baby bottle, biberón

bottom fondo

bow (IUD) nudo

bowel intestino, tripa; bowel movement, BM, evacuación (f.), eliminación (f.); to have a bowel movement, defecar, eliminar, evacuar, ensuciar

bowl bacín (m.), taza; dentist's bowl, taza

box caja; post office box, apartado postal

boy niño, muchacho, hijo

bra, brassiere sostén (m.), ajustador (m.), justillo, corpiño

brace soporte (m.)

bracelet pulsera

brain cerebro, seso

bread pan (m.); white bread, pan blanco; dark bread, pan moreno

to break quebrar, romper, fracturar

breakfast desayuno; to eat breakfast, desayunarse

breast seno, pecho, busto; to breast-feed, dar el pecho, dar de mamar breath respiración; deep breath, respiración profunda; shortness of breath, falta de aire; to hold one's breath, sostener la respiración

to breathe respirar

bridgework dientes postizos

to bring traer; I bring, traigo

broccoli bróculi (m.), brécol (m.)

broken quebrado, -a; roto, -a; fracturado, -a

bronchial tubes bronquios

broth caldo

brother hermano

brother-in-law cuñado

brown café; moreno, -a; pardo, -a

brush cepillo; toothbrush, cepillo de dientes

to brush one's teeth cepillarse los dientes, lavarse los dientes

brussels sprout col (f.) de Bruselas

bubonic plague peste (f.) bubónica

burial entierro

burn quemadura

to burn quemar

burned quemado, -a

burning ardor (m.)

to burp eructar

businessman hombre (m.) de negocios

bust busto

butter mantequilla

buttock nalga

button botón (m.); buttonhole, ojal (m.)

to buy comprar

C

cabbage col (f.), repollo

cabinet gabinete (m.)

cake queque (m.), torta

calficied calcificado, -a

call llamada

to call llamar

callus callo

calm calma; to be calm, calmarse, estar tranquilo, -a; be calm (imperative), cálmese

can (container) lata; canned, en lata, enlatado, -a

can, to be able poder; I can, puedo; you, he, she can, puede

candy dulce (m.)

cane (walking) bastón (m.)

canker sore ulceración (f.)

cap gorro, -a; cervical cap, gorro cervical

capacity: vital capacity, capacidad (f.) vital

capsule cápsula

car carro, coche (m.), automóvil (m.)

carbohydrate carbohidrato

carbon tetrachloride tetracloruro de carbón

cardiac cardíaco, -a; cardiac arrest, fallo cardíaco

cardiopulmonary resuscitator resucitador (m. or f.) cardiopulmonar

cardioscope cardioscopio

care cuidado; intensive care, cuidado intensivo, cuidado intenso; to take care of oneself, cuidarse

caress caricia, cariño

carpenter carpintero

carrot zanahoria

to carry cargar, llevar

case caso, caja

cash efectivo; en efectivo, al contado

cashier cajera; cashier's office, cashier's window, caja

casserole cacerola

cast yeso; to put in a plaster cast, enyesar

cataract catarata

catheter catéter (m.), sonda

to catheterize sondear

catsup salsa de tomate

cauliflower coliflor (f.)

cavity cavidad (f.); (tooth) carie (f.)

cc. centímetro cúbico

celery apio

cell célula; blood cell, glóbulo

center centro

centigrade centígrado

centimeter centímetro

cereal cereal; cooked cereal, cereal cocido

cerebral palsy parálisis (f.) cerebral

certain cierto, -a; seguro, -a

certainly claro, ciertamente

cervix cuello uterino, cuello de la matriz

chair silla

chance casualidad (f.); by chance, por casualidad

chancre chancro

change cambio

to change cambiar

chaplain capellán (m.)

check cheque (m.); checkbook, libro de cheques

checkup reconocimiento médico

cheek mejilla

cheese queso; cottage cheese, queso requesón; cream cheese, queso crema; white cheese, queso blanco; yellow cheese, queso amarillo

cherry cereza

chest pecho

to chew masticar, mascar

chicken pollo; baked chicken, pollo asado; chicken broth, caldo de pollo; chicken soup, sopa de pollo; fried chicken, pollo frito

chickenpox varicela, viruelas locas

child niño, -a; hijo, -a

childbirth parto; natural childbirth, parto natural

childhood infancia

children hijos, niños

chill escalofrío

to chill enfriar

chin barba, mentón (m.)

chocolate chocolate (m.); chocolate milk, leche con chocolate; hot chocolate, chocolate caliente

cholera cólera

cholesterol colesterol (m.), colesterina; to lower the cholesterol count, bajar el nivel del colesterol

to choose escoger, seleccionar

chop chuleta; pork chop, chuleta de puerco

city ciudad (f.)

clam almeja

clasp presilla

class, kind clase

clean limpio, -a

to clean limpiar

cleaning, cleanliness limpieza, aseo

clear claro, -a; limpio, -a

clip presilla

clock reloj (m.)

to close cerrar

closed cerrado, -a

closet closet (m.), gabinete (m.) para la ropa, ropero

clothes, clothing ropa; night clothes, ropa de dormir

coat, overcoat abrigo, saco

cocktail coctel (m.)

code (key) clave; zip code, zona postal

coffee café (m.); black coffee, café obscuro, café puro, café solo; coffee with cream, café con crema; coffee with milk, café con leche

coin moneda

coitus coito; coitus interruptus, interrupción (f.) de coito

cola drink coca

cold (disease) resfriado, catarro, resfrío; to catch a cold, resfriarse

cold (temperature) frío, -a; cold drink, bebida fría; to be cold, tener frío

colon colon (m.)

comb peine (m.), peinete (m.), peineta; to comb one's hair, peinarse

to come venir; come in (imperative), adelante, entre, pase

comfortable cómodo, -a; amplio, -a

communicable transmisible

complete total; completo, -a

complexion cutis (f.), piel (f.)

compliment cumplido

compound compuesto, -a

to concentrate concentrar

concentrated concentrado, -a

condom condón (m.)

to confuse confundir

confused confundido, -a; confuso, -a

congenital congénito, -a

to constipate estreñir

constipated constipado, -a; estreñido, -a

consultation consulta

contact contacto; contact lenses, lentes (m.) de contacto

to contaminate contagiar, contaminar

contaminated contagiado, -a; contaminado, -a

to contract contraer

contraction contracción (f.), pujo

contusion golpe (m.)

cook cocinero, -a

to cook cocinar

cooked cocido, -a

cookie galleta; wafer, bizcocho

cool fresco, -a

to cool refrescar, enfriar

cork corcho, tapón de corcho

to cork tapar con corcho

corn (callus) callo

corn (vegetable) maíz, maíz tierno; corn on the cob, elote (m.), mazorca de maíz

cornea córnea

corpuscle glóbulo; red corpuscles, glóbulos rojos; white corpuscles, glóbulos blancos

cost costo

to cost costar; it costs, cuesta

cot catre (m.), camilla; critical care cot, camilla de cuidado crítico

cotton algodón (m.)

cough tos (f.); cough syrup, jarabe (m.) para la tos

to cough toser

count conteo, recuento; cholesterol count, nivel de colesterol

to count contar

county condado

courteous cortés

courtesy cortesía

cousin primo, -a

cover tapa, cubierta; (blanket) frazada, manta

to cover cubrir; to cover up (conceal), encubrir; to cover up, to wrap up, abrigarse

crab cangrejo

crab lice ladillas

cracker galleta; soda cracker, galleta blanca

cradle cuna

cramp calambre (m.)

cranium cráneo

crazy loco, -a

cream crema

credit: on credit, a plazos

crib cuna

to cripple incapacitar, lisiar, tullir

crippled lisiado, -a; tullido, -a; in the hand, manco, -a; in the foot, cojo, -a

crossmatch pruebas cruzadas

crotch entrepierna

crown corona

crutch muleta

cry llanto, grito

to cry llorar

cucumber pepino

cup taza

curdle cuajar

curdled cuajado, -a

cure cura

to cure curar

cured curado, -a

custard flan (m.)

cut cortada

to cut cortar

cute mono, -a

cyst quiste (m.)

cystic fibrosis fibrosis quística

D

dad, daddy papá

danger peligro

dangerous peligroso, -a

to dangle colgar

dark obscuro, -a

darling querido, -a; precioso, -a

date fecha, cita; date of birth, fecha de nacimiento

daughter hija

daughter-in-law nuera

day día (m.)

dead muerto, -a; dead person, difunto, -a

to deaden adormecer

deaf sordo, -a

dear querido, -a

death muerte (f.)

deep profundo, -a; deeply, profundamente

to defecate defecar, eliminar, ensuciar

defect defecto; birth defect, defecto de nacimiento

defibrillator defibrilador (m.)

degree grado

dehydrated deshidratado, -a

delay demora

delicious delicioso, -a; rico, -a; sabroso, -a

delirious delirando; delirante

delivery (birth) parto

dentist dentista (m. or f.)

denture dientes (m. pl.), postizos, dentadura

deposit depósito

to deposit depositar

to deprive privar

dessert postre (m.)

device aparato; intrauterine device, dispositivo uterino

diabetes diabetes (f.)

diaper pañal (m.), paño

diaphragm diafragma (m.)

diarrhea diarrea

to die morir; he, she died, murió; they died, murieron

diet dieta

dietitian dietista (m. or f.)

dinner comida

dirt lodo, polvo, tierra, mugre (m.)

dirty sucio, -a

disability incapacidad (f.)

disadvantage desventaja

disagreeable antipático, -a; desagradable

disaster desastre (m.)

disc disco; calcified disc, disco calcificado; slipped disc, disco desplazado

discharge (fluid) desecho, flujo, supuración

to discharge from the hospital dar de
alta

disease enfermedad (f.)

dish plato

dismiss (from the hospital) dar de alta

divorced, divorcé, divorcée divorciado, -a

dizziness mareo

dizzy mareado, -a; to become dizzy,
marearse

do hacer; I do, hago; you do, he, she
does, hace

doctor doctor, -a; médico

doll muñeca

dollar dólar (m.)

douche ducha

down bajo, abajo

dozen docena

draft (wind) corriente (f.) de aire

dram dracma (m.)

drapes cortinas

drawer gaveta, cajón (m.)

dress vestido

dresser tocador (m.)

dressing apósito, emplaste (m.),
parche (m.); (food stuffing) relleno

dried seco, -a

drink bebida

to drink beber, tomar

to drive manejar

drug droga

drunk borracho, -a; embriagado, -a

dry seco, -a

to dry secar

dryness sequedad (f.)

during durante

duty: on duty, de turno

E

each cada

ear (outer) oreja; (inner) oído; ear
lobe, lóbulo de la oreja

early temprano, -a

to earn ganar

earring arete (m.)

to eat comer; to eat breakfast,
desayunar(se); to eat lunch, almorzar;
to eat supper, cenar

effective eficaz; efectivo, -a

egg huevo, blanquillo; egg yolk, yema
de huevo; fried egg, huevo frito;
hard-boiled egg, huevo duro; poached
egg, huevo hervido en agua; scrambled
eggs, huevos revueltos; soft-boiled
egg, huevo pasado por agua; egg white,
clara de huevo

eggplant berenjena

elbow codo

electrocardiogram electrocardiograma (m.)

embolism embolia

emergency emergencia, urgencia; emergency drug kit, estuche (m.) de drogas
de emergencia; emergency room, sala
de urgencia

emesis vómito; emesis basin, taza de
vómito

emphysema enfisema

empty vacío, -a

enema ayuda, enema, lavado, lavativa

English inglés

enough bastante, suficiente

entrance entrada

envelope sobre (m.)

equipment aparato, equipo

esophagus esófago

even (equal) parejo, -a

evening tarde (f.), noche (f.)

every cada; every day, todos los días
every night, todas las noches

everybody, everyone todos, -as

everything todo, -a

examination examen (m.); physical examination, reconocimiento médico; rectal examination, tacto rectal

excuse me (permission) con permiso; (pardon) perdón, lo siento

exercise ejercicio

to exercise hacer ejercicio

expensive caro, -a

to expose exponer

expulsive expulsivo, -a; expulsive pain, dolor expulsivo, pujo

to extract extraer

eye ojo

eyeball globo del ojo

eyebrow ceja

eyeglasses anteojos, espejuelos, lentes

eyelash pestaña

eyelid párpado

eyetooth colmillo

F

factor factor (m.); Rh factor, factor Rhesus

to fail faltar

to faint desmayarse

fainting desmayos, síncope (m.)

fall caída

to fall down caerse

Fallopian Falopio; Fallopian tube, trompa de Falopio

far lejos

fast (abstinence) ayuno; (speed) rápido, -a; faster, más rápido

to fast ayunar

to fasten abrochar, asegurar

fat (obese) gordo, -a, grueso, -a; (grease) grasa; fatty, sebáceo, -a; grasoso, -a

father padre (m.)

father-in-law suegro

fatigue fatiga

fear temor (m.)

feces heces fecales

to feed dar de comer, alimentar

to feel sentir; I feel, me siento; you feel, he, she feels, se siente; to feel like + ing, tener ganas de + infinitive; to have no feeling, no sentir nada

feet pies (m., pl.)

fever fiebre (f.); rheumatic fever, fiebre reumática; typhoid fever, fiebre tifoidea; yellow fever, fiebre amarilla

fiancé, -ée novio, -a

fibroid fibroma, fibroide, fibroideo, -a

fibrous tumor tumor (m.) fibroso, fibroma

fight lucha

to fight luchar

filling (dental) empaste (m.); (food) relleno

to find out saber, averiguar, descubrir

finger dedo

fingertip yema del dedo, punta del dedo

fire lumbre (f.), quemazón (m.)

first aid primeros auxilios

fish pescado

fist puño; to make a fist, cerrar el puño

fit ataque (m.), convulsión (f.)

to fix arreglar

flask frasco

flea pulga

floor (of a building) piso; (flooring) suelo

flour harina

flow flujo, desecho

flower flor (f.)

flu gripe (f.), influenza

to fly volar

to fold doblar

to follow seguir

food comida, alimento

foot pie (m.); foot of the bed, pie de la cama

for para; for + duration of time, hace + time

forceps fórceps (m.), tenazas, pinzas

forehead frente (f.)

foreign body cuerpo extraño, paja

fork tenedor (m.)

fountain fuente (f.)

fracture fractura, quebradura

freckle peca

frequent frecuente; frequently, con frecuancia, frecuentemente

fresh fresco, -a

fried frito, -a

friend amigo, -a

to frighten asustar; to become frightened, asustarse; how frightening!, ¡qué susto!

from de

frostbite congelado

frostbitten congelado, -a

fruit fruta; fruit cocktail, coctel (m.) de fruta

to fry freír

full lleno, -a; completo, -a

funeral home funeraria

funny gracioso, -a

fuzz vello

fuzzy velloso, -a

G

to gain ganar, aumentar; to gain weight, aumentar de peso

gallbladder vesícula

gallon galón (m.)

gallstones cálculos biliares

gangrene gangrena

garbage basura

to gargle hacer gárgaras

garlic ajo

gauze gasa

gelatin gelatina; fruit gelatin, gelatina con fruta; medicinal gelatin, gelatina medicinal

genitals genitales (m., pl.)

germ germen (m.), microbio

German measles rubéola

germicidal, germicide germicida

to get conseguir, obtener; to get over, pasarse

to get up levantarse; to get up on the table, subir a la mesa

girdle faja

girl niña, muchacha

to give dar

glad: to be glad, alegrarse; I'm glad, me alegro; glad to know you, mucho gusto; gladly, con mucho gusto

gland glándula

glass vaso

glasses (eye) anteojos, lentes, espejuelos; contact lenses, lentes de contacto

glucose glucosa

glue goma

to glue pegar

gnat jején (m.), guasasa, mosquito

to go ir; I go, I am going, voy; you (sing.) go, he, she goes, va; you (pl.), they go, van; we go, vamos; to go down, bajar; to go up, subir; to go to bed, acostarse

gonorrhea gonorrea

good buen, bueno, buena; good afternoon, buenas tardes; good evening, good night, buenas noches; good morning, buenos días

good-bye adiós

gout gota

gown bata

graft injerto

grain grano

gram gramo

granddaughter nieta

grandfather abuelo

grandmother abuela

grandson nieto

grapefruit toronja

gray gris

grease grasa

greasy grasoso, -a

green verde; green beans, ejotes (m.), habichuelas

to greet saludar

greeting saludo

groceries comestibles (m.), víveres (m.)

groin ingle (f.)

to grow crecer

gums encías

gun pistola, carabina, rifle (m.)

gunshot tiro; gunshot wound, herida de bala

H

hair pelo, cabello, vello

hairbrush cepillo de cabeza

half medio, -a

hall pasillo

ham jamón (m.); ham and eggs, huevos con jamón

hamburger hamburguesa

hand mano (f.); palm of the hand, palma de la mano

handbag bolsa, bolso, cartera

handful puñado

handle mango, asa

to handle manejar

handsome guapo, -a

to hang colgar

hanger percha, perchero, gancho

happen pasar; what happened?, ¿Qué pasó?

happy contento, -a; feliz

hard (difficult) difícil; (consistency) duro, -a; hard-working, diligente

hat sombrero

has: he, she has, tiene; he, she has had, ha tenido; he, she has to + verb, tiene que + infinitive

have tener; you have, tiene; I have, tengo; you have had, ha tenido; I have had, he tenido; to have to + verb, tener que + infinitive

head cabeza; (of bed, table) cabecera; head of household, jefe de familia

headache jaqueca, dolor de cabeza

heal sanar

health salud (f.); healthy, saludable, sano, -a; public health, salubridad (f.) pública

to hear oír

hearing oído

heart corazón (m.); heart attack, ataque (m.) al corazón

heart beat latido

heartburn hervor (m.)

heat calor (m.); heat prostration, postración del calor

heat therapy termoterapia

heavy pesado, -a; grueso, -a

heel talón (m.)

help socorro, ayuda, asistencia

to help ayudar

hemorrhage, hemorrhaging hemorragia

hemorrhoids hemorroides (f.), almorranas

her (possessive) su, sus; (object pronoun) la, le

here aquí

hiccup, hiccough hipo

high alto, -a; mucho, -a; high blood pressure, presión alta; high up, arriba; muy alto, -a him lo, le

hip cadera

his su, sus

hives urticaria

hoarseness ronquera

to hold tener; (to keep) guardar; (to fasten) sujetar; to take hold of, coger; to hold away from, separar; to hold one's breath, sostener la respiración

hole agujero

home casa; (to) home, a casa; at home, en casa

honey miel (f.)

hook gancho, presilla

hope esperanza

to hope esperar

hose medias; panty hose, medias pantalón, pantimedias

hospitalization insurance seguro de hospitalización

hot (temperature) caliente; (spicy) picante; hot drink, bebida caliente; to be hot, tener calor

hour hora

house casa

housewife ama de casa

how cómo; how long, desde cuándo; how much, cuánto, -a; how many, cuántos, -as

hug abrazo

human humano, -a

humble humilde

hunchback jorobado, -a

hungry: to be hungry, tener hambre

hurt (injured) lastimado, -a; herido, -a; (a pain) dolor

to hurt tener dolor, doler

husband esposo, marido

hydrogen peroxide agua oxigenada

I

I yo

ice hielo

ice cream helado, nieve (f.), mantecado

ice pack bolsa de hielo

if si

ill enfermo, -a; seriously ill, grave, muy grave

illness enfermedad

immediate inmediato, -a; immediately, inmediatamente, en seguida

impacted impactado, -a

impetigo impétigo

impudent fresco, -a

in en

inch pulgada

incision herida, incisión

increase aumento

to increase aumentar

incubation period período de incubación

incubator incubadora

infantile paralysis parálisis infantil

infarct infarto

to infect contagiar, infectar

infected infectado, -a

inflamed inflamado, -a

influenza gripe (f.), influenza

ingrown enterrado, -a

injury lesión (f.), herida

inner interior

insanity locura

insect insecto; insect bite, picadura de insecto

inside dentro, adentro

insurance seguro

intensive intensivo, -a; intenso, -a; intensive care, cuidado intensivo intercourse relaciones sexuales, coito

intestine intestino, tripa

intoxicated borracho, -a; embriagado, -a

intrauterine device, IUD dispositivo intrauterino

to introduce presentar; (to introduce something into) introducir; I want to introduce you (him, her) to . . ., quiero presentarle a . . .

iodine yodo

iron hierro; iron lung, pulmón (m.) de acero, pulmotor (m.)

is: he, she, it is, es, está; there is, hay

to isolate aislar

isolation aislamiento

to itch picar; it itches, me pica; does it itch?, ¿le pica?

itching picazón (m.)

J

jacket chaqueta, saco

jail cárcel (f.)

jam mermelada

jaundice ictericia

jaw mandíbula, quijada

jelly jalea

jewelry joyas

Jewish judío, -a

to join añadir, unir, atar

joint articulación (f.), coyuntura

juice jugo

junket leche (f.) cuajada

K

to keep guardar, conservar

key (lock) llave (f.); (code) clave (f.); (typewriter) tecla

kid (goat) cabrito

kidney riñón; kidney stones, cálculos renales

to kill matar

kilogram kilogramo

kind (gentle) amable

kind (type) of clase (f.) de

kiss beso

to kiss besar

kit botiquín (m.); emergency kit, botiquín de emergencia; first aid kit, botiquín de primeros auxilios

knee rodilla

knife cuchillo

knob manilla, tirador (m.), perilla

knot nudo

to know (know facts, know how to) saber; (know people, places) conocer; I know, sé, conozco; you know, he, she knows, sabe, conoce

L

label etiqueta

labor labor (f.); labor pain, dolor (m.) de parto

lack falta

to lack faltar

lady dama, señora

lamb cordero

lame cojo, -a

lamp lámpara

large grande

larynx laringe (f.)

last último, -a

to last durar

late tarde; later, más tarde, luego, después

to laugh reírse

laughter risa

lavatory lavamanos (m., sing.)

lawyer abogado

laxative purgante (m.), laxante (m.)

least menos

to leave (a place) salir; (an object) dejar

left (abandoned) abandonado, -a

left (direction) izquierdo, -a; to the left, a la izquierda

leg pierna

lemon limón (m.); lemon pie, pastel (m.) de limón

less menos

lesson lección (f.)

lethargic aletargado, -a

lethargy aletargamiento, estupor (m.)

lettuce lechuga

lever palanca

lice piojos; crab lice, ladillas

lid tapa

life vida

lifeguard salvavidas (m. or f.)

lifeless exánime, sin vida

light luz (f.), lámpara; (weight, color) ligero, -a; claro, -a; (not serious) leve

to like (to enjoy) gustar; I like, me gusta(n); you like, he, she likes, le gusta(n)

like this así

limb miembro; artificial limb, miembro artificial

lime lima

limp cojera; (not stiff) flexible; flojo, -a; suelto, -a; blando, -a

to limp cojear

lip labio

lipstick pintura de labios

liquid líquido

liter litro

litter camilla

little (size) pequeño, -a; (amount) poco, -a

to live vivir

liver hígado

livid lívido, -a; pálido, -a

loan préstamo

to loan prestar

lock cerradura

to lock cerrar

to look (at) mirar; look (imperative), mire; what does . . . look like?, ¿cómo es . . . ?

loop lazo; IUD loop, lazo

loose flojo, -a; suelto, -a

to lose perder

loss pérdida

lot: a lot, mucho, -a

love amor (m.)

to love amar, querer; I love it, me encanta

low bajo, -a

lower inferior

to lower bajar

lozenge pastilla

lunch almuerzo, comida, lonche (m.)

lung pulmón (m.); iron lung, pulmón acero, pulmotor (m.)

lye lejía

M

made hecho

magazine revista

maid sirvienta, criada

maimed lisiado, -a; manco, -a

main principal

major mayor

to make hacer; I make, hago; you make, he, she makes, hace; to make a fist, cerrar el puño makeup maquillaje, cosméticos; to put on makeup, maquillarse

malaise destemplanza, malestar (m.)

malaria paludismo, malaria

man hombre (m.), señor (m.)

many muchos, -as; how many, cuántos, -as

marble canica, mármol (m.)

mark marca

to mark marcar

married casado, -a

mask mascarilla

massage masaje (m.)

to match emparejar; crossmatch, pruebas cruzadas

matter asunto, materia; what's the matter?, ¿qué tiene?, ¿qué (le) pasa?

mayonnaise mayonesa

me me

meal comida

measles sarampión (m.); German measles, rubéola

measure medida

to measure medir

measuring cup taza de medir

meat carne (f.)

medicine cabinet, chest botiquín (m.)

membrane membrana

menopause menopausia

menstrual period regla, menstruación, período

menu menú (m.)

Merthiolate mertiolato

meter metro

methadone metadona

method método

microscope microscopio

middle medio, -a; centro

midnight medianoche (f.)

migraine jaqueca, migraña

milk leche (f.); chocolate milk, leche con chocolate; milk of magnesia, leche de magnesia; skimmed milk, leche descremada; powdered milk, leche en polvo

milligram miligramo

milliliter mililitro

mind mente (f.)

minimum mínimo

minister ministro, pastor (m.)

minor menor, leve

minus menos

to mix mezclar

moderate moderado, -a

molar muela

mole lunar (m.)

money dinero

month mes; by the month, monthly, al mes, por meses

more más

most más

mother madre (f.)

mother-in-law suegra

mouth boca; mouth-to-mouth resuscitation, resucitación boca a boca

to move mover

movement movimiento; bowel movement, evacuación

much mucho, -a; too much, demasiado

mucous mucoso, -a

mucus mucosidad (f.)

multiple sclerosis esclerosis (f.) múltiple

mumps paperas, parótida, parotiditis (f.)

murmur murmullo; heart murmur, soplo

muscle músculo

muscular dystrophy distrofia muscular

mushroom champiñón (m.), hongo

my mi, mis

N

nail uña; ingrown nail, uña enterrada

name nombre (m.)

to name llamar; to be named, llamarse; what is your (his, her) name?, ¿cómo se llama?; my name is . . . , me llamo . . . ; his (her) name is . . . , se llama . . .

napkin servilleta; sanitary napkin, servilleta sanitaria

nausea náuseas

navel ombligo

navy marina; navy bean, frijol (m.) blanco

near cerca

neck cuello; stiff neck, tortícolis

need necesidad (f.)

to need necesitar

needle aguja

negative negativo, -a

neighbor vecino, -a

nephew sobrino

nerve nervio

nervous nervioso, -a; nervous breakdown, colapso nervioso; nervous system, sistema (m.) nervioso

nervousness nerviosidad (f.)

never nunca

new nuevo, -a

newborn recién nacido, -a

newspaper periódico, diario

next próximo, -a; next to, al lado de

nice simpático, -a

niece sobrina

night noche (f.); at night, de noche, por la noche; during the night, por la noche; nightclothes, ropa de dormir

nightgown camisa de noche, bata

nipple (of bottle) tetero, -a; teto; (of female) pezón (m.); (pacifier) chupete (m.), chupeta

nit liendre (f.)

no, not no

noise ruido

none ninguno, -a

noodle fideo

noon mediodía (m.)

nose nariz (f.)

nosebleed hemorragia nasal

nostril fosa nasal

nothing nada

to notify notificar

now ahora; right now, ahora mismo

numb entumecido, -a; to be numb, entumecer

number número

nun monja

nurse enfermera

to nurse (baby) dar de mamar, dar el pecho, amamantar

nursery cuarto de niños; newborn nursery, sala de los recién nacidos

nursing enfermería

nursing home clínica de reposo

O

oatmeal avena

obese obeso, -a

odor olor (m.)

of de; of course, claro, desde luego

off: to take off, quitar(se); to turn off, apagar

office oficina; office hours, horas de consulta

often con frecuencia, muchas veces

oil aceite (m.)

ointment ungüento, crema, pomada

old viejo, -a

on en

one un, uno, una

onion cebolla

only sólo, -a; solamente

to open abrir

orange naranja; orange color, color de naranja; orange juice, jugo de naranja

order (authorization) orden (f.); written order, orden escrita; (series) orden (m.)

organ órgano

orphan huérfano, -a

orphanage hospicio

orthodontist ortodontista (m. or f.); ortopédico dental

other otro, -a

ought deber

ounce onza

outside afuera, fuera

over sobre

overcoat abrigo

overdose dosis (f.) excesiva

to owe deber

oxygen oxígeno

oyster ostra

P

pacemaker marcador (m.) de ritmo, seno auricular

pacifier chupete (m.), chupeta

pack: ice pack, bolsa de hielo

pain dolor (m.); to be in pain, tener dolor, doler; ghost pain, dolor fantasma

pajamas pijamas, piyamas

pale pálido, -a

palm palma de la mano

pancreas páncreas (m.)

panties pantalón (m.), calzones (m., pl.), pantaleta; panty hose, medias pantalón, pantimedias

pants pantalones (m.); pants suit, traje pantalón (m.)

Pap smear frotis (f.) de Papanicolaou, unto de Papanicolaou

paper papel (m.)

parasite parásito

parents padres (m., pl.)

parotid parótida

parsley perejil (m.)

part parte (f.)

partial parcial; partial plate, dentadura parcial

to pass pasar

pastry pastel (m.)

to pay pagar

payment pago

pea chícharo, guisante (m.)

peach melocotón (m.), durazno

peanut cacahuate (m.), cacahuete (m.), maní (m.); peanut butter, crema de cacahuate, crema de maní, mantequilla de cacahuete

pear pera

peel, peeling cáscara

pelvis pelvis (f.)

pen pluma

penis pene (m.)

people gente (f., sing.)

pepper pimienta; bell pepper, pimiento; hot pepper, chile

per por; per month, al mes; per week, a la semana

percent por ciento

perineum perineo

period período; (menstrual) período, regla; (punctuation) punto

permission permiso

permit permiso, autorización (f.)

person persona

perspiration sudor (m.)

to perspire sudar

phlegm flema

physical físico, -a; physical examination, reconocimiento médico; physical therapy, fisioterapia

pickle pepinillo

pie pastel (m.); apple pie, pastel de
manzana; cherry pie, pastel de cereza;
lemon pie, pastel de limón

piece pedazo

piles almorranas

pill píldora, pastilla; sleeping pills,
píldoras para dormir

pillow almohada

pillow case funda

pimple grano

pin alfiler (m.)

pineapple piña

pink color de rosa

pint pinta

pitcher jarra

pity lástima, pena; what a pity!,
¡qué pena!

plague peste (f.) bubónica

plain (simple) sencillo, -a

plaster cast yeso

plastic plástico, -a; plastic surgery,
cirugía plástica

plate (dish) plato; (x-ray) placa;
denture, dentadura postiza; metal
plate, placa de metal; partial plate,
dentadura parcial

to play jugar

playpen corral (m.)

pleasant, pleasing agradable, complaciente, simpático, -a

please · por favor; favor de + infinitive

plenty (enough) suficiente, bastante

pliers pinzas

plum ciruela

P.M. de la tarde, de la noche

poison veneno; poison ivy, hiedra
venenosa

policy póliza

polio, poliomyelitis poliomielitis (f.)

poor pobre

popcorn esquite (m.), rositas de maíz

pork cerdo, carne de puerco; pork chop,
chuleta de puerco; pork ribs, costillas asadas

post office casa de correos, oficina de
correos; post office box, apartado
postal

postal zone zona postal

postoperative postoperativo, -a

to postpone aplazar, posponer

potato papa, patata; baked potato, papa
asada; fried potatoes, French fries,
papas fritas; mashed potatoes, puré
de papas

poultice emplaste (m.), cataplasma,
sinapismo

pound libra

powder polvo

power poder (m.)

predelivery prenatal

pregnancy embarazo; abdominal pregnancy,
embarazo extrauterino; ectopic pregnancy, embarazo ectópico; tubal pregnancy, embarazo tubárico

pregnant embarazada, en estado, en estado de gestación, encinta

prescription receta

pressure presión; blood pressure,
presión de sangre

pretty bonito, -a

to prevent prevenir, evitar

preventive preventivo, -a

to prick pinchar

priest cura (m.)

private privado, -a

to probe reconocer, sondear

problem problema (m.)

prolonged prolongado, -a

promise promesa

to promise prometer

prostate próstata

prosthesis prótesis, miembro artificial

to protect (oneself) proteger(se)

proud orgulloso, -a

prune ciruela pasa

pubic hair vello púbico

pudding flan (m.), pudín (m.); rice pudding, arroz (m.) con leche; tapioca pudding, tapioca

pulse pulso

pumpkin calabaza

pupil pupila

purse bolsa, bolso, cartera

pus flujo purulento, pus (m.)

pustule pústula

to put poner; to put away, guardar; to put away from (separate), separar; to put on, ponerse; put on (imperative), póngase

putrid podrido, -a

pyorrhea piorrea

Q

quart cuarto

quarter cuarto

question pregunta; to ask a question, preguntar

quick rápido, -a; quickly, rápidamente, en seguida

quiet tranquilo, -a; quieto, -a; to be quiet, estar tranquilo, callarse

R

rabbit: rabbit test, examen (m.) de conejo

rabies rabia

radish rábano

radium radio

radium therapy radioterapia

radius radio

to raise levantar

raisin pasa

to rape atacar, violar

rapid rápido, -a; rapidly, rápidamente

rash erupción (f.), salpullido

raspberry frambuesa

razor máquina de afeitar; razor blade, cuchilla de afeitar

to reach alcanzar

ready listo, -a

receipt recibo

to receive recibir

recipe receta

rectum recto

red rojo, -a; colorado, -a

regularly con regularidad (f.)

regulations reglamento

relationship parentesco

relatives parientes (m. or f.), familia

to relax relajar(se)

relaxation relajamiento

to repair reparar, componer

respirator respirador (m.)

rest descanso; the rest (remainder), el resto

to rest descansar

restroom baño, cuarto de baño, servicio

result resultado

resuscitation resucitación; mouth-to-mouth resuscitation, respiración boca a boca

to return volver

Rh factor factor Rhesus

rheumatic fever fiebre (f.) reumática

rheumatism reumatismo

rhythm ritmo

rib costilla

ribbon cinta

rice arroz (m.)

rich rico, -a

right (direction) derecho, -a; to the right, a la derecha; right away, en seguida, ahora mismo; to be right, tener razón

rind cáscara

ring anillo; IUD ring, anillo; jeweled ring, sortija

to ring tocar, sonar

to rinse enjuagarse

roast asado, -a; roast beef, carne asada, rosbif (m.)

to roast asar

robe bata

rod varilla; metal rod, varilla de metal

roll pan (m.); sweet roll, pan dulce

to roll up one's sleeve levantarse la manga

roller, curler rollo

room cuarto; delivery room, sala de partos; emergency room, sala de emergencia, sala de urgencia; labor room, sala prenatal

root raíz (f.); root canal, canal (m.) de la raíz

rotten podrido, -a

roughage material áspero inabsorbible; low roughage, residuo bajo

rubber goma, hule (m.)

rule regla

S

sad triste

safe caja de seguridad (f.); seguro, -a

salad ensalada; salad dressing, salsa de ensalada

saliva esputo, expectoración (f.), saliva

salt sal (f.)

salve pomada

sample muestra

sanitary napkin servilleta sanitaria, kotex

sanity lucidez (f.)

sauce salsa

saucer platillo

sausage chorizo, salchicha

to say decir; I say, digo; you say, he, she says, dice

scab postilla

scar cicatriz (f.)

scarce escaso, -a

to scare asustar

scarf bufanda

scarlet fever fiebre escarlatina

scissors tijeras

scratch arañazo, rasguño, raspón (m.); to scratch oneself, rascarse; to scratch out, tachar

scream grito

to scream gritar

seal sello

to seal sellar

seasoning condimento, especia (spice)

seat asiento

sebaceous sebáceo, -a

secondary stage estado secundario

sedative calmante (m.)

to see ver

seldom pocas veces

to select seleccionar

to sell vender

semen esperma, semen (m.)

sensitive sensitivo, -a; sensible

separated separado, -a

series serie (f.), orden (f.)

serious serio, -a; grave

serum suero

to serve servir; it is served, se sirve

to set (fracture) componer, reducir;
   (coagulate) coagular, cuajar

setback revés (m.), atraso

several varios, -as

sexual relations relaciones sexuales,
   coito

to shake sacudir; to shake hands, dar
   la mano

shame lástima; what a shame! ¡qué
   lástima!

to shave afeitar, rasurar; to shave
   oneself, afeitarse

sheet sábana

shellfish marisco

sherbet nieve (f.), sorbete (m.)

shield (IUD) escudo

shift turno; day shift, turno de día;
   night shift, turno de noche

to shift cambiar, mudar

shirt camisa

shock choque (m.), trauma (m.); anaphylactic shock, choque anafiláctico

shoe zapato

short bajo, -a

shortness of breath falta de aire,
   respiración corta

shorts (men's underwear) calzoncillos

shot inyección; gunshot, tiro

should deber; one should, hay que +
   infinitive, debe + infinitive

shoulder hombro; shoulderblade,
   paleta, paletilla, omóplato

shower ducha, baño de regadera

shrimp camarón (m.)

sick enfermo, -a

sickness enfermedad (f.)

side lado

sight visión (f.)

sign signo; vital signs, signos vitales

to sign firmar

signature firma

simple sencillo, -a

since desde

single (not married) soltero, -a

sinus trouble sinusitis (f.)

sister hermana

sister-in-law cuñada

to sit down sentarse; sit down (imperative) siéntese

sitz bath baño de asiento

to skim descremar; skimmed milk, leche
   descremada

skin piel (f.)

skinned (injured) arañado, -a; raspado,
   -a; abrasion, raspón (m.)

skinny flaco, -a

skirt falda

slacks pantalón (m.), pantalones

to sleep dormir; to be sleepy, tener
   sueño

sleeve manga

slice tajada, rebanada

to slice cortar en tajadas

slide (photographic) transparencia

to slide deslizarse

slip (lingerie) enagua, fondo, peticote (m.)

to slip resbalar(se)

slipper zapatilla, pantufla

slow lento, -a; slowly, despacio; more slowly, más despacio

small (size) pequeño, -a; (amount) poco, -a

smallpox viruela

to smash aplastar

smear unto, frotis (f.)

to smear untar

smell olor

to smell oler

smoke humo; smoke inhalation, inhalación de humo

to smoke fumar

snack merienda

to snack merendar

snake culebra, serpiente (f.), víbora

to sneeze estornudar

snow nieve (f.)

to snow nevar

so así; so-so, así, así

soap jabón (m.); germicidal soap, jabón germicida

Social Security seguro social

socks calcetines (m., pl.)

soda cracker galleta blanca

soda pop soda

sodium pentothal pentotal (m.) de sodio

soiled sucio, -a; manchado, -a

some unos, -as; varios, -as; algunos, -as

something algo

sometimes a veces

son hijo

son-in-law yerno

soon pronto

sore úlcera, lesión (f.), dolor (m.); to be sore, doler, tener dolor

sorry: to be sorry, sentir; I'm sorry, lo siento

soup sopa; soup bowl, sopero

spasm espasmo

to speak hablar

special especial; special delivery, entrega inmediata

specialist especialista (m. or f.)

specialized especializado, -a

specimen muestra

speck paja

spell desmayo, ataque (m.)

to spell deletrear

sperm esperma, semilla, espermato-zoide (m.)

spermicide espermicida

spice especia

spinach espinaca

spinal anesthesia raquídea

spinal column columna vertebral, espina dorsal

spiral (IUD) espiral

spit saliva

to spit escupir

spleen bazo, esplín (m.)

splinter astilla

spoiled corrompido, -a; podrido, -a

sponge esponja

spoon cuchara

spoonful cucharada

spot mancha; black spots, puntos negros

to spread apart, to spread out separar

squash calabaza

stab puñalada

to stab apuñalar, apuñalear

stage estado, etapa

stain mancha

to stain manchar

stained manchado, -a

stamp sello, estampilla

stand estante (m.), puesto

to stand estar de pie; to stand up, levantarse

state estado, condición

stationery papel para escribir

to stay quedarse, estar

steady firme, estable

steady (boyfriend, girlfriend) novio, -a

steak biftec (m.), bistec (m.), filete (m.)

steam vapor (m.); steam bath, baño de vapor

step paso, pisada

stepfather padrastro

stepmother madrastra

sterilizer esterilizador (m.)

stew guisado, cocido

stiff neck tortícolis (m.)

still quieto, -a; (yet) todavía

stillborn nació muerto, -a

to stir mezclar

stitch puntada, punto

stocking media

stomach estómago, vientre (m.)

stone piedra, cálculo; gallstones, cálculos biliares; kidney stones, cálculos renales

stool (bowel movement) excremento, eliminación (f.); (seat) banqueta, taburete

stopper tapón (m.)

storage depósito, almacenaje; in storage, guardado

store tienda

to store guardar

story (floor) piso; (tale) cuento

straight derecho, -a

to straighten enderezar

strap tira, correa

straw paja

strawberry fresa

strep throat infección (f.) de la garganta de estreptococo; estreptococia

stretcher camilla

strict estricto, -a

string cuerda

stroke ataque (m.) al cerebro

strong fuerte

student estudiante (m. or f.)

stuffed relleno, -a

stuffy nose nariz (f.) tapada, nariz tupida

stupor estupor (m.)

to stutter tartamudear

stutterer tartamudo, -a

sty orzuelo

success éxito

successive sucesivo, -a; seguido, -a

to suck chupar, mamar

sudden repentino, -a; suddenly, de repente

to suffer sufrir, padecer; I suffer, padezco

sufficient bastante, suficiente

to suffocate sofocar(se)

sugar azúcar (m. or f.)

suicide suicidio; to commit suicide, suicidarse

suit traje (m.)

suitcase maleta

sunburn quemadura de sol

sunburned quemado, -a del sol

sunstroke insolación (f.)

supermarket supermercado

supper cena

support soporte (m.), base (f.)

sure seguro, -a; I am sure, estoy
  seguro, -a

surgery cirugía

to suspect sospechar

to swallow tragar, deglutir

sweat sudor (m.)

to sweat sudar

sweater suéter (m.), chamarra

sweet dulce; a sweet, dulce (m.);
  sweets, dulces

to swell hinchar

swelling hinchazón (m.)

swollen hinchado, -a

symptom síntoma (m.)

syncope síncope (m.)

syringe jeringuilla

syrup jarabe (m.), almíbar (m.)

system (of the body) aparato

T

table mesa; to get up on the table,
  subir a la mesa

tablespoon cuchara

tablespoonful cucharada

tablet tableta

to take tomar; (with one) llevar;
  (from someone) quitar; to take out,
  sacar; to take off (clothing), quitarse; take off (imperative), quítese; to take (vaccine), prender;
  it took, prendió

talcum powder talco

tampon tapón (m.), tampón (m.)

to tangle enredar

tangled enredado, -a

tape (adhesive) tela adhesiva; (magne-
  tic) cinta, cinta magnética

taste sabor (m.), gusto

to taste probar

TB tuberculosis (f.)

tea té (m.); iced tea, té helado

tear (from crying) lágrima

to tear romper, rasgar

teaspoon cucharita, cucharilla

teaspoonful cucharadita

teeth dientes (m., pl.), dentadura

telephone teléfono

television televisor (m.)

to tell decir, avisar; tell me (imperative), dígame

temperature temperatura, fiebre (f.)

tepid tibio, -a

term plazo; on terms, a plazos

test examen (m.), análisis (m.)

to test probar, examinar

testicle testículo

tetanus tétano

thanks gracias, muchas gracias

the el (m., sing.), la (f., sing.), los
  (m., pl.), las (f., pl.)

their su, sus

then entonces, luego

there allí, ahí; there is, there are,
  hay

thermometer termómetro

these estos, -as

they ellos, -as

thick espeso, -a

thigh muslo

thin delgado, -a

thing cosa

to think creer, pensar

thirsty: to be thirsty, tener sed

this esto (n.), este (m.), esta (f.)

throat garganta

throb latido, pulso

to throb latir, pulsar

thumb dedo pulgar

thyroid   tiroides (m.)

tic   tic (m.) nervioso

tick   (insect) garrapata

tie   corbata

to tie   atar; to tie together, ligar

tight   apretado, -a

to tighten   apretar

time   (clock) hora; (number of times), vez (f.); the first time, la primera vez; one time, una vez; another time, otra vez

tingling   hormigueo

tip   punta fingertip, punta del dedo, yema del dedo

tired   cansado, -a

tiredness   cansancio, fatiga

tissue   tejido; facial tissue, papel (m.), kleenex (m.)

to   a, en

toast   pan (m.) tostado

today   hoy

toe   dedo del pie

toilet   excusado, inodoro; toilet tissue, papel (m.) de baño

tomato   tomate (m.); tomato juice, jugo de tomate

tomorrow   mañana

tongue   lengua

tonsillitis   amigdalitis (f.)

tonsils   amígdalas

too   también; too much, demasiado, -a

tooth   diente (m.), muela; eyetooth, colmillo; toothbrush, cepillo de dientes; toothpaste, pasta de dientes, pasta dentífrica

top   (lid) tapa; (direction) cima, arriba; on top, encima

touch   tacto

to touch   tocar

touchy   sensitivo, -a

tourniquet   torniquete (m.)

towel   toalla

toy   juguete (m.)

tranquilizer   tranquilizante (m.), apaciguador (m.)

trash   basura

trauma   trauma (m.)

to travel   viajar

tray   bandeja, charola

tremor   temblor (m.), convulsión (f.)

trip   viaje (m.); to take a trip, hacer un viaje

to trip   tropezar

trousers   pantalón (m.), pantalones

true   verdadero, -a

truth   verdad (f.)

trunk   tronco

to try: to try to, tratar de + infinitive

tub   bañadera, tina; tub bath, baño de tina, baño de inmersión

tubal pregnancy   embarazo tubárico

tube   tubo; Eustachian tube, trompa de Eustaquio; Fallopian tube, trompa de Falopio

tuna   atún (m.)

turkey   pavo, guajalote (m.), guajolote (m.)

turn   turno

to turn: to turn on, encender, poner, prender; to turn off, apagar; to turn on one's side, ponerse de lado; to turn over, voltearse

turpentine   trementina

tweezers   pinzas

twin   gemelo, -a; twins, gemelos, -as

twisted   torcido, -a

type   tipo

to type   escribir a máquina

to type blood   clasificar la sangre

typhoid   tifoidea

typhus   tifo

U

ugly feo, -a

ulcer úlcera

umbilical cord ombligo

uncle tío

underneath abajo

undershirt camiseta

to understand comprender

United States Estados Unidos

unpleasant desagradable; antipático, -a

until hasta

up arriba

upper superior

upset (emotional), mortificado, -a; upset stomach, estómago revuelto

to upset volcar

urethra uretra

urinal orinal (m.)

to urinate orinar, mear

urine orina

to use usar

used to acostumbrado, -a

useful útil

utensil utensilio

uterus útero, matriz (f.)

V

vacant vacante

vaccination vacunación (f.), inoculación (f.)

vaccine vacuna

vacuum vacío

varicose varicoso, -a; varicose veins, venas varicosas, várices (f.)

vase florero

veal ternera; veal cutlet, chuleta de ternera

vegetable vegetal (m.), verdura, legumbre (f.)

vein vena

venereal venéreo, -a; venereal disease, enfermedad (f.) venérea

very muy

vest chaleco

vial botella, frasco

victim víctima

vinegar vinagre (m.)

virus virus (m.)

visit, visitor visita

vital vital; vital signs, signos vitales; vital capacity, capacidad (f.) vital

vomit vómito; vomiting blood, vomitos de sangre

to vomit vomitar

W

waist cintura

to wait esperar

to wake up despertarse; wake up (imperative), despiértese

to walk caminar

walker andador (m.)

to want querer, desear; I want, quiero; you want, he, she wants, quiere

warm tibio, -a; warmer, más caliente

wart verruga

to wash lavarse

washbowl palangana, tina

washcloth toallita

watch (timepiece) reloj (m.)

to watch vigilar

watchman vigilante (m.), policía

water agua; drinking water, agua potable

watermelon sandía, melón de agua

weak débil

weakness debilidad (f.)

to wear llevar

weather tiempo, clima (m.)

week semana

to weigh pesar; to get weighed, pesarse

weight peso

well bien

what qué, cuál, cuáles

wheelchair silla de ruedas

when cuándo; al + infinitive

whenever you want cuando usted quiera

where dónde; (to where) a dónde; (from where) de dónde

whether si

which cuál, cuáles; that which, lo que

white blanco, -a

wish deseo

to wish desear

who quién, quiénes; whom, a quién, a quiénes

whooping cough tos ferina

why por qué

widow viuda

widower viudo

wife esposa, mujer

wig peluca

wine vino

wisdom tooth cordal (m.), muela del juicio

wise sabio, -a

with con

to withdraw sacar, retirar

withdrawal retirada

without sin

witness testigo

woman mujer (f.), señora

work trabajo

to work trabajar

worms lombrices (f., pl.)

worried preocupado, -a

worse peor

wound (injury) herida

to wrap: to wrap up, abrigarse

wrist muñeca

to write escribir

wrong: to be wrong, estar equivocado, -a; what's wrong?, ¿qué (le) pasa?

wryneck tortícolis (f.)

X

x-ray radiografía

x-ray therapy radioterapia

Y

yard yarda

to yawn bostezar

year año

yell grito

to yell gritar

yellow amarillo, -a

yes sí

yesterday ayer

yet todavía; not yet, todavía no

yolk (egg) yema (de huevo)

you (formal) usted; (familiar) tú

your (formal) su, sus; (familiar) tu, tus

you're welcome de nada, por nada

Z

zero cero

zip code zona postal

zone zona

Suggested Readings for Cultural Understanding

Berle, Beatrice Bishop. <u>Eighty Puerto Rican Families in New York City: Health and Disease Studied in Context</u>. New York: Columbia University Press, 1958.

A field survey which emphasizes the relationship of health and illness to the physical, emotional, and cultural aspects of a particular environment.

Clark, Margaret. <u>Health in the Mexican-American Culture: A Community Study</u>. Berkeley: University of California Press, 1959.

Discussion of overall aspects of social, economic, religious, and folkloric characteristics which affect problems of health and illness in a low-income Mexican-American community. The final chapter gives concrete recommendations as to how health care providers should deal with Mexican-American patients in terms of specific health problems.

Grabler, Leo, Joan W. Moore, and Ralph C. Guzmán. <u>The Mexican-American People</u>. New York: Free Press, 1970.

The most comprehensive data on Mexican-Americans in the United States; comparative charts and graphs that dispel some previously accepted stereotypes.

Kiev, Ari. <u>Curanderismo: Mexican-American Folk Psychiatry</u>. New York: Free Press, 1968.

A study in ethnopsychiatry exploring the influence of cultural factors as they relate to illness and treatment among Mexican-Americans.

Lewis, Oscar. <u>La Vida: A Puerto Rican Family in the Culture of Poverty -- San Juan and New York</u>. New York: Random House, 1966.

Case studies of the extended family in San Juan, Puerto Rico, and New York, with an introduction presenting contrasts between Puerto Ricans and Mexican-Americans in the culture of poverty.

Lewis, Oscar, with Douglas Butterworth. <u>A Study of Slum Culture: Backgrounds for La Vida</u>. New York: Random House, 1968.

Analyses of the subculture of poverty in San Juan, Puerto Rico, and New York.

Linehan, Edward. "Cuba's Exiles Bring New Life to Miami," <u>National Geographic</u> 144:(1), 68-95, 1973.

A portrait of Cuban culture in Miami.

Madsen, William. <u>The Mexican-Americans of South Texas</u>. New York: Holt, Rinehart and Winston, 1964.

A case study of classes and cultural attitudes, including four chapters dealing specifically with attitudes toward medicine, health, and healing.

Madsen, William. _Society and Health in the Lower Rio Grande Valley: A Guide for Medical and Welfare Workers among the Mexican-American_. Austin, Texas: Hogg Foundation for Mental Health, 1961.

> A study of cultural attitudes that influence health care, and specific recommendations for health care programs.

Menéndez Pidal, Ramón. _The Spaniards in Their History_. New York: W. W. Norton & Co., 1966.

> Discussion by a renowned Spanish scholar of characteristics of the Spaniard — traits evident to a greater or lesser extent in all Hispanic peoples.

Paz, Octavio. _The Labyrinth of Solitude: Life and Thought in Mexico_. New York: Grove Press, 1961.

> Descriptions by a contemporary Mexican poet and essayist of his views of the Mexican character as he sees it in the United States as well as in Mexico.

Ramos, Samuel. _Profile of Man and Culture in Mexico_. Austin: University of Texas Press, 1962.

> An in-depth study by a prominent Mexican philosopher and social anthropologist; the touchstone for many later studies of the Mexican character.

Rosaldo, Renato, Robert A. Calvert, and Gustav L. Seligman. _Chicano: The Evolution of a People_. Minneapolis: Winston Press, 1973.

> An anthology of the Mexican-American experience, through papers, articles, and book excerpts from various sources and regions.

Saunders, Lyle. _Cultural Differences and Medical Care: The Case of the Spanish-speaking People of the Southwest_. New York: Russell Sage Foundation, 1954.

> An exploration of cultural attitudes as they affect medical care; contrasts between Mexican-American and Anglo cultural values.

Grammar Index (by Lessons)

Numbers given are lesson numbers, not page numbers.

Minimum Spanish Communicator
for Medical Personnel

The minimum Spanish communicator is an outline of the essential communicating statements you have been practicing in the text. The communicator consists of lists of words that can be cut apart by section, mounted on cardboard or plastic, put in your pocket, and referred to for study or for use on the job.

The lists include basic expressions in English and Spanish and a range of infinitives, along with interrogatives to begin a question and completions to finish a sentence. Social amenities and useful phrases may be used by themselves. In order to make the lists initially more useful for reference, they are alphabetized by English.

Words and phrases are combined according to set formulas, as explained below. When you have learned how to combine the lists and how to restate ideas in terms of the words given, you have at your command a functional vocabulary for communicating idiomatically the majority of things you may need to say to a patient.

HOW TO USE THE COMMUNICATOR

Combine words according to the formulas given with the lists. There are two kinds of lists: those referred to by letter and those referred to by number. The lettered lists include social amenities and useful phrases, question words, basic expressions, and sentence completions. The numbered lists contain infinitives to be added to the basic expressions. The lists consist of the following:

S: "Social" -- Social amenities and useful phrases that can be used by themselves.

Q: "Question" -- Interrogative words that can precede basic expressions.

A: "Any, all" -- Basic expressions applicable to any person.

I: "I" -- Basic expressions that refer to things I say or do.

U: "You" -- Basic expressions that refer to things said or done to you.

1: General infinitives -- Verbs that can be added to any of the basic expressions (A, I, U).

2: Infinitives that refer to my body or actions that closely concern me -- Verbs for things that can happen without my will. Use with basic expressions I (but not A or U).

3: Infinitives that refer to my body or actions that closely concern me -- Verbs for things that either I do to myself or someone does to me. Can be added to all basic expressions (A, I, U).

4: Infinitives that refer to your body or actions that closely concern you -- Verbs for things that either happen to you or you do to yourself deliberately. Can be added to basic expressions A or U (but not I).

5: Infinitives that refer to your body or actions that closely concern you -- Verbs for things that someone does to you. Can be used with basic expressions <u>A</u> or <u>I</u> (but not <u>U</u>) and <u>must</u> be followed by a completion: a thing or a part of the body.

C: "Completions" -- Nouns, pronouns, and adverbs that can complete sentences; to be used wherever they make sense. If they make sense in English, they will make sense in Spanish; however, where English may use a possessive, Spanish needs only the word for <u>the</u> or <u>a</u>.

To give the opposite of any basic expression, use <u>no</u> with it. To make a question, simply show the question with your voice.

Many of the infinitives are repeated on the numbered lists to limit action according to the pronoun attached at the end. Examples of the various combinations are:

<u>A</u>		<u>List 1</u>		<u>C</u>
Es necesario	+	operar	+	mañana.
It's necessary to		operate		tomorrow.

<u>I</u>		<u>List 2</u>	
¿Voy a	+	mejorarme?	
Am I going to		get better?	

<u>A</u>		<u>List 3</u>	
Es necesario	+	operarme.	
It's necessary to		operate on me.	

<u>A</u>		<u>List 4</u>	
Es necesario	+	operarse.	
It's necessary to		operate on you.	

<u>A</u>		<u>List 5</u>		<u>C</u>
Es necesario	+	operarle	+	esto.
It's necessary to		operate on		this.

Some verbs that appear in lists 2, 3, 4, or 5 are not included in list 1. These are verbs that usually are not closely associated with one's body or one's immediate interests.

To practice the formulas given, make up statements of your own. (Other combinations will communicate, but not necessarily idiomatically.) Be flexible with words -- try to convey ideas rather than word-for-word translations. Think of how approximately the same thing may be said in another way that fits the words in the communicator. Try these substitutions:

<u>When you want to say:</u>		<u>Use:</u>
A command, ask someone to do something	Please	<u>Favor de</u> + inf.
Past tense	I have been able to You have been able to	<u>He podido</u> <u>Ha podido</u> + inf.
I like to You like to	I want to You want to	<u>Quiero</u> <u>Quiere</u> + inf.
I must You must	I have to You have to	<u>Tengo que</u> <u>Tiene que</u> + inf.
I need to You need to	It's necessary to	Es necesario + inf.

When you want to say:		Use:
I ought to You ought to	I should You should	$\underline{\text{Debo}}$ $\underline{\text{Debe}}$ + inf.
Perhaps	It's possible to	Es posible + inf.
I will You will	I'm going to You're going to	$\underline{\text{Voy a}}$ $\underline{\text{Va a}}$ + inf.
I won't You won't	I'm not going to You're not going to	$\underline{\text{No voy a}}$ $\underline{\text{No va a}}$ + inf.
Noun -- thing, part of body, article of clothing	this, that	esto, eso
Place, direction, or location	here, there	aquí, allá

He, she, it	same as you form	debe you should
		        he should
		        she should
		        it should

And if all else fails to communicate -- supplement with body language!

Q + A, I, or U   "Question"

Interrogative words--may be used alone or with basic expressions

How?	¿Cómo?
How much?	¿Cuánto?
What?	¿Qué?
When?	¿Cuándo?
Where?	¿Dónde?
Who?	¿Quién?
Why?	¿Por qué?

I + 1, 2, 3, or 5   "I"

Basic expressions referring to things I say or do

I can	(No)	Puedo
I have been able to	(No)	He podido
I have just	(No)	Acabo de
I have to	(No)	Tengo que
I'm going to	(No)	Voy a
I should	(No)	Debo
I want to	(No)	Quiero

A + 1, 3, 4, or 5 "Any, all"

Basic expressions applicable to any person

It's okay to	(No)	Está bien
It's necessary to	(No)	Es necesario
It's possible to	(No)	Es posible
Please		Favor de (no)

U + 1, 3, or 4   "You"

Basic expressions referring to things said or done to you

You can	(No)	Puede
You have been able to	(No)	Ha podido
You have just	(No)	Acaba de
You have to	(No)	Tiene que
You're going to	(No)	Va a
You should	(No)	Debe
You want to	(No)	Quiere

A, I, or U +   1

General infinitives--verbs of fundamental actions (not concerned with oneself)

be	estar
begin	empezar
bring	traer
buy	comprar
carry	llevar
clean	limpiar
close	cerrar
come	venir
cover	cubrir
die	morir
do	hacer
drink	tomar, beber
eat	comer
eliminate	eliminar
enter	entrar

feel	sentir
finish	terminar
follow	seguir
get (obtain)	obtener
give	dar
go	ir
have	tener
help	ayudar
keep	guardar
leave	salir
live	vivir
look at	mirar
lose	perder
lower	bajar
make	hacer
open	abrir
operate	operar
pay	pagar

A, I, or U +   1

General infinitives--verbs of fundamental actions (not concerned with oneself)

raise	levantar
rest	descansar
see	ver
sign	firmar
sleep	dormir
sterilize	esterilizar
take	tomar, llevar
use	usar
visit	visitar
walk	caminar
work	trabajar

I +   2

Infinitives whose object is me--body motion or state (I to myself)

fall	caerme
feel	sentirme
get better	mejorarme
go to sleep	dormirme
stay	quedarme
worry	preocuparme

Infinitives whose object is me--body motion or state (I to myself, you to me)

bend	doblarme
change	cambiarme
cut	cortarme
fix (up)	arreglarme
get up	levantarme
give	darme
go to bed, lie down	acostarme
lower	bajarme
move	moverme
operate	operarme
put on, in	ponerme
raise	levantarme
shave	afeitarme
sit down, up	sentarme
take a bath	bañarme
take care of myself, me	cuidarme
take off, away	quitarme
turn over	voltearme
wake up	despertarme
wash	lavarme

Infinitives whose object is you--body motion or state (you to yourself)

bend	doblarse
change	cambiarse
cut	cortarse
fall	caerse
feel	sentirse
fix	arreglarse
get better	mejorarse
get up	levantarse
give	darse
go to bed, lie down	acostarse
go to sleep	dormirse
lower	bajarse
move	moverse
put on, in	ponerse
raise	levantarse
shave	afeitarse
sit down, up	sentarse
stay	quedarse
take a bath	bañarse
take care of yourself	cuidarse
take off, away	quitarse
turn over	voltearse
wake up	despertarse
wash	lavarse
worry	preocuparse

A or I + 5 + C

Infinitives whose object is
you--body motion or state (I
to you + thing or part of
body)

bend	doblarle
change	cambiarle
cut	cortarle
fix	arreglarle
give	darle
lower	bajarle
move	moverle
operate	operarle
put in, on	ponerle
raise	levantarle
shave	afeitarle
take off, away	quitarle
wash	lavarle

S   "Social"

Social amenities, useful
phrases--may be used alone or
in combination with words from
other lists

Excuse me. (permission)	Con permiso.
Good morning.	Buenos días.
Good afternoon.	Buenas tardes.
Good evening, night.	Buenas noches.
How are you?	¿Cómo está usted?
How do you feel?	¿Cómo se siente?
I'm sorry.	Lo siento.
Pardon me.	Perdón.
Repeat, please.	Repita, por favor.
Slower, please.	Más despacio, por favor.
Thank you.	Gracias.
What's the matter?	¿Qué tiene?
You're welcome.	De nada.

Nouns, pronouns, and adverbs
to be used to complete sentences. (Where English uses
possessive, Spanish uses only
the word for <u>the</u> or <u>a</u>.)

anything	algo
bad, badly	mal
the bedpan the basin	el bacín
before	antes
better	mejor
earlier	más temprano
enough	bastante
every day	todos los días
fast	rápido
fever	fiebre
the food	la comida
here	aquí
home	a casa

an hour	una hora
an illness	una enfermedad
it (add only to words from List 1)	lo
it to you (add only to words from List 1)	selo
last night	anoche
late	tarde
later	después
a little	un poco
less	menos
a lot, much	mucho
more	más
never, ever	nunca
now	ahora
pain	dolor
quiet	quieto
a sample a specimen	una muestra
a shot, an injec- tion	una inyección
slow	despacio

Nouns, pronouns, and adverbs
to be used to complete sentences. (Where English uses
possessive, Spanish uses only
the word for <u>the</u> or <u>a</u>.)

soon	pronto
a test	un análisis
that	eso
there	allá
this	esto
this morning	esta mañana
this afternoon	esta tarde
today	hoy
tomorrow	mañana
tonight	esta noche
too much	demasiado
a treatment	un tratamiento
worse	peor
well	bien
yesterday	ayer